STEPS IN NURSING PROCESS

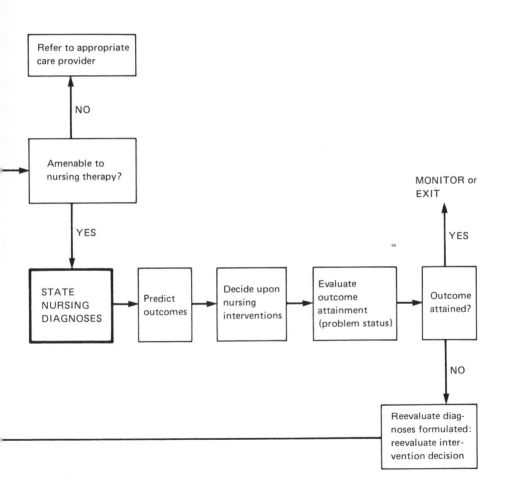

Refer to appropriate care provider

NO

Amenable to nursing therapy?

YES

STATE NURSING DIAGNOSES → Predict outcomes → Decide upon nursing interventions → Evaluate outcome attainment (problem status) → Outcome attained?

MONITOR or EXIT

YES

NO

Reevaluate diagnoses formulated: reevaluate intervention decision

NURSING DIAGNOSIS

PROCESS AND APPLICATION

NURSING DIAGNOSIS

PROCESS AND APPLICATION

Marjory Gordon, R.N., Ph.D., F.A.A.N.

Professor of Nursing
Boston College
and
Chairperson, Taskforce of the
National Group for Classification
of Nursing Diagnoses

McGRAW-HILL BOOK COMPANY
New York St. Louis San Francisco Auckland Bogota
Hamburg Johannesburg London Madrid Mexico Montreal New Delhi
Panama Paris São Paulo Singapore Sydney Tokyo Toronto

This book was set in Times Roman by Jay's Publishers Services, Inc.
The editors were David P. Carroll, Moira Lerner, and Stephen Wagley;
the production supervisor was Phil Galea.
The drawings were done by Jay's Publishers Services, Inc.
The cover was designed by Joe Cupani.
R. R. Donnelley & Sons Company was printer and binder.

NURSING DIAGNOSIS
Process and Application

34567890 DODO 898765432

ISBN 0-07-023815-4

Notice

As new medical and nursing research and clinical experience broaden our knowledge, changes in
treatment and drug therapy are required. The editors and the publisher of this work have made
every effort to ensure that the drug dosage schedules herein are accurate and in accord with the
standards accepted at the time of publication. Readers are advised, however, to check the product
information sheet included in the package of each drug they plan to administer to be certain that
changes have not been made in the recommended dose or in the contraindications for administration. This recommendation is of particular importance in regard to new or infrequently used drugs.

Library of Congress Cataloging in Publication Data

Gordon, Marjory.
    Nursing diagnosis.

    Bibliography: p.
    Includes indexes.
    1. Nursing. 2. Diagnosis. I. Title.
[DNLM: 1. Nursing process. WY 100 G664]
RT48.G67   610.73   81-17207
ISBN 0-07-023815-4   AACR2

Like hues and harmonies of evening—
Like clouds in starlight widely spread—
Like memory of music fled—
Like aught that for its grace may be
Dear, and yet dearer for its mystery.

Thy light alone—like mist o'er mountain driven,
or music by the night—wind sent
through strings of some still instrument,
or moonlight on a midnight stream,
Gives grace and truth to life's unquiet dream.

P. B. Shelley
Hymn to Intellectual Beauty

CONTENTS

PREFACE

In 1973 Kristine Gebbie and Mary Ann Lavin of St. Louis University called the First National Conference on Classification of Nursing Diagnoses. This began the national effort to identify, standardize, and classify health problems treated by nurses. The relevance of the work to practice, education, and research has sustained enthusiasm in the last decade. In addition, nursing diagnosis is a legally defined aspect of practice in a number of states. Actually, consumers in any state can expect nursing diagnosis to be included in their nursing care; national standards of practice specify this.

Diagnostic terminology is necessary, yet terminology without diagnostic skill leads to inaccurate clinical judgments. Similarly, diagnostic skill without terminology is akin to speaking ability without language; the two are inseparable.

The purpose of this book is to help the beginning professional nursing student to develop knowledge and skill in the process of diagnosis and its application in practice. It is expected that the student will begin to use this book in the first course dealing with nursing process; as clinical experiences with clients begin, the student should again refer to the sections on process and application. Repeated self-evaluation and feedback on clinical judgments are critical for developing expertise in this component of practice.

The approach to the discussion of nursing diagnosis is based on four assumptions. The first and most important is that nursing diagnosis is an integral part of nursing process. Diagnoses are made for purposes of planning care; therefore the student will find diagnosis discussed in this context.

The second assumption is that nursing diagnoses are not made in isolation. Many professionals interact in care delivery and each has to appreciate the others' focus of practice. Although nursing diagnosis is emphasized in this book, the student will gain a broad perspective on clinical diagnosis in the health professions.

A third underlying assumption is that understanding facilitates the development of clinical reasoning and diagnostic judgment. Being aware of the logical operations that are involved in processing assessment data facilitates the development of diagnostic skills throughout a professional career. Thus the student will find an emphasis on cognitive aspects of the diagnostic process. Logical relationships among the following are clearly described: (1) a nursing framework and assessment format, (2) strategies for collecting and processing information, (3) diagnostic statements, and (4) use of diagnoses in care planning and other nursing activities. Questions are raised and discussed; examples can be grasped by the student who has completed preclinical arts and sciences.

The fourth assumption is that professional students will assume professional responsibilities. An appreciation must be gained of the issues surrounding classification system development and issues in nursing practice to which nursing diagnosis applies. Therefore the relevance of nursing diagnosis to quality assurance, reimbursement, staffing, and other care delivery issues will be discussed. The last chapter introduces the topics of classification system development and implementation.

Many individuals contributed to the development of this book. Early interest in the diagnostic process was stimulated by debates and deliberations with colleagues, especially Carol Soares-O'Hearn and Florence Smith-Milliot. Further work in this area was made possible by a 1970 National Institutes of Health fellowship for doctoral study (grant number 1F04-NU-27,282-01) and by two encouraging advisors, John Dacey and John Travers.

Nearly 10 years' association with the National Conference Group on Classification of Nursing Diagnoses sharpened my ideas about diagnostic nomenclature. My association with the Massachusetts Conference Group on Classification of Nursing Diagnoses prompted consideration of specialties other than my own and broader issues of implementation. For lively, intellectual discussions about diagnosis, I am particularly grateful to colleagues in these groups.

For raising questions that needed answers, I am especially grateful to graduate students. For all the times they listened, challenged, read, and reread drafts of this book, gratitude is extended to Joan Fitzmaurice and Ann McCourt. I am also indebted to the five baccalaureate students who reviewed this book: Nancy J. Caliguire, Ellen Dessureau, M. Fiascone, Maura L. Shea, and Patricia Twohig.

Deep gratitude is extended to friends for their support and encouragement. I am particularly grateful to Ardra Taylor and Winifred and Joe Hickman for providing encouragement and a refuge at critical times.

I am also indebted to Maura Shea, who provided humor as well as organization, and to Boston College secretarial and word processor staff members who assisted in manuscript preparation. Finally, David P. Carroll, the editor, deserves special thanks.

Marjory Gordon

CHAPTER 1

THE CONCEPT OF NURSING DIAGNOSIS

As a term, *nursing diagnosis* has had a relatively short history; as an act it goes back to the founding of modern nursing. Nightingale and her colleagues diagnosed nutritional deficits and other health problems in Crimean War casualties. On the basis of those nursing diagnoses, interventions were undertaken to correct the system of care in military hospitals. Today many of the same health problems exist in society, and nurses are being educated to contribute to their solution. Nursing diagnosis provides a clear focus for this contribution.

Nurses have always collected information to use as a basis for determining a client's[1] need for care. About three decades ago this process began to be called *nursing diagnosis*. The idea of nursing diagnosis broke the link between information collection and care planning. Clinical judgment was inserted as a recognized responsibility.

Stopping to make a judgment, or diagnosis, before determining the client's need for care revealed an important fact. Some of the information nurses were collecting signified health problems not described by the language of medicine, that is, disease names. New terms had to be created. These new terms described the judgments upon which nursing care was being based.

Implementation of nursing diagnosis in practice brought with it two realizations. One was that diagnostic skills had to be sharpened. The second was that nursing diagnosis was highly relevant to many current issues in practice.

An understanding of nursing diagnosis begins with its definition. In this chapter the concept will be isolated, defined, and described. A broader view will be given in Chapter 2, which contrasts and compares nursing diagnosis with other health professionals' use of diagnosis.

---

[1] The term *client* will be used to refer to individuals, families, and communities.

Description of the diagnostic process, examples, and exercises will acquaint the reader with current thinking about how to arrive at clinical judgments. Chapters 3, 4, 5, and 6 focus on the formulation of nursing diagnoses.

A grasp of nursing diagnosis and the diagnostic process will stimulate thinking about the use of diagnosis in direct client care. In Chapters 7 and 8 new views of somewhat old issues will be discussed. These issues include the relevance of nursing diagnosis to evaluation of care, staffing, and the development of the profession.

The degree of acceptance and implementation of nursing diagnosis is discussed in Chapter 9. Also included in Chapter 9 is information about the development of a nursing diagnosis classification system. This latter section is included with the belief that the reader will be enthusiastic about the concept of diagnosis and wish to influence the direction of classification development. In summary, this book will focus on *the area of practice described by nursing diagnoses*. It will deal with what a diagnosis is, the diagnostic process, and application in nursing practice.

DIAGNOSIS AS CATEGORY AND PROCESS

Some words people use to communicate their ideas have two or more definitions. The context in which the word is used clarifies the meaning. So it is with the term *nursing diagnosis*. It refers not only to the process of diagnosing but also to the diagnostic judgment reached and expressed in a category name.

The separation of diagnosis as category name and diagnosis as process is artificial; the two are actually interdependent. Yet it makes learning easier if initially they are considered separately.

Diagnosis as a Category

When a nurse describes a client's condition as "impaired mobility (level 2) related to decreased activity tolerance," a diagnostic category is being used. To help the reader understand the meaning of nursing diagnosis as a category, conceptual, structural, and contextual definitions will be explored.

Conceptual Definition A conceptual definition communicates the meaning of an idea. The following definition of nursing diagnosis has been proposed:

> Nursing diagnoses, or clinical diagnoses made by professional nurses, describe actual or potential health problems which nurses by virtue of their education and experience are capable and licensed to treat. (Gordon, 1976, p. 1299)

According to this definition there are two important characteristics of diagnostic categories: who uses them and what they describe.

The definition states that diagnoses are used by professional nurses. As will be discussed in Chapter 7, national standards of practice, educational preparation, and licensing laws support the use of diagnoses exclusively by professional nurses. Other nursing personnel may contribute information or carry out specified care, but registered nurses are responsible for making nursing diagnoses.

The second characteristic of nursing diagnoses stated in the definition is that they describe actual or potential health problems. An *actual problem* is an existing deviation from health. Dysfunctional grieving is an example. A client may be unable to progress through the grieving process after a loss, and this inability may influence many life activities. Sleep pattern disturbance is another example.

Nurses do more than treat conditions that have already occurred. They also identify risk factors that predispose individuals, families, or communities to health problems. When a set of risk factors is present, the condition is referred to as a *potential problem*, or high-risk state. Potential for injury and potential skin breakdown are two examples.

Traditionally, nursing has placed a high value on preventing health problems. One frequently sees anticipatory guidance and counseling used to help people maintain and promote good health and well-being. Thus, any listing or definition of nursing diagnoses has to include both actual and potential health problems. These are included in the currently identified diagnostic categories (Appendix A).

Some believe that limiting the scope of nursing diagnosis to actual and potential health problems (prevention and treatment) is too restrictive. They point out that nurses also deal with clients seeking enriched personal growth in areas such as parenting, health management, and self-development. As categories are identified in these areas, the definition of nursing diagnosis may expand beyond problematic or potentially problematic conditions.

Identification and use of nursing diagnoses requires a more specific definition than "describes health problems." This definition is too vague, as physicians and others also deal with health problems. What is needed is a conceptual focus to describe the scope of nursing. This will be discussed in Chapters 2 and 3. A second approach is to qualify the definition with a competency statement and a reference to the legal domain of nursing practice.

The previous definition supplies a qualifier; it states that nursing diagnoses describe only those health problems that nurses, by virtue of their education and experience, are capable and licensed to treat. Treatment is defined further:

> To treat, or the provision of treatment, refers to the initiation of accepted modes of therapy. . . . This definition thereby excludes health problems for which the accepted mode of therapy is prescription drugs, surgery, radiation, and other treatments that are defined legally as the practice of medicine. (Gordon, 1976, p. 1299)

Soares's statement that nursing diagnoses "can be alleviated by nursing actions" also is an attempt to clarify the domain of nursing diagnosis (Soares, 1978, p. 276).

Nurses are not educated to make treatment decisions for problems such as leukemia or congenital heart disease. Many nurses can diagnose a heart attack, but they do not assume accountability for its treatment. Yet accountability is assumed for the diagnosis and treatment of anxiety, independence-dependence conflict, knowledge deficits, and problems caused by decreased activity tolerance, all of which could accompany heart attack. Basic education prepares nurses to treat these problems, which are also within the scope of their licensing laws.[2]

---

[2] State laws govern the practice of nursing; they are referred to as *state nurse practice acts.*

Some may argue that clarifying domains of practice by using the qualifier *competency to treat* is inadequate. They argue that nurses do participate in the treatment of diseases. Nurses do, indeed, report observations and judgments, carry out physicians' orders that clients cannot carry out for themselves, and diagnose and treat diseases under physician supervision or protocols.[3] These activities of disease-related care are, in a sense, under the cognitive control of the physician. The nurse must anticipate what the physician would think and do (Hammond, 1966, p. 29). This is not the case with nursing diagnoses.

The important point is that diagnosis is merely an intellectual exercise unless followed by nursing care designed to resolve the problem. If a nurse is not *capable* of treating the problem judged to be present (whether the diagnosis is a nursing diagnosis or not), the client should be referred.

Saying that a nursing diagnosis is a health problem a nurse can treat does not mean that nonnursing consultants cannot be used. Aspects of treatment may require consultation with other specialized professions that emerged out of nursing. These include occupational therapy, physical therapy, social work, and respiratory therapy. Each offers specialized skills related to parts of the client's situation. Although aspects of a problem are referred, nurses are responsible for coordinating treatment of nursing diagnoses. Responsibility and accountability are important issues and will be considered further in other chapters.

In addition to a definition, positive and negative examples are always useful in clarifying a concept. Examples of what are and what are not considered acceptable diagnostic categories are helpful in drawing the boundaries. Positive examples of currently accepted diagnostic categories are contained in Appendix A. (As will be discussed later, some are marginal, given the definition previously proposed.) In an alphabetical classification, such as the one in Appendix A, only the problem statement of a diagnosis is entered. It is important to note that these diagnostic categories are not officially standardized, as are the disease names used by physicians. To say these diagnostic categories are *accepted* means that, in the opinion of the National Group for Classification of Nursing Diagnoses,[4] they are sufficiently developed for clinical testing.

Negative examples are also useful in clarifying an idea. The diagram in Figure 1-1 depicts entities that are *not* nursing diagnoses and are thus outside the boundary of the concept. Many are mentioned by Little and Carnevali (1976, p. 50).

The terms in Figure 1-1 deserve some comment. All are used in nursing practice, and it is not uncommon to confuse them with nursing diagnoses. Remember that a nursing diagnosis describes a client's health problem; it does not describe, for example, the "staff's problems in coping with clients" (Little and Carnevali, 1976, p. 50). That nurses and doctors react in stressful or frustrating situations has to be recognized, but *staff problems* should not be labeled as diagnostic judgments about the client.

---

[3]*Protocols* are guides for analyzing and treating a disease process or symptom complex. A protocol may be highly organized and directive or it may be more general and flexible; this will depend on the situation, education, and experience of those using the protocol, and the availability of physician support (Hudak, 1976).

[4]This national conference group is composed of nurses actively involved in the identification of a diagnostic nomenclature (system of names) and the development of a system for classifying nomenclature.

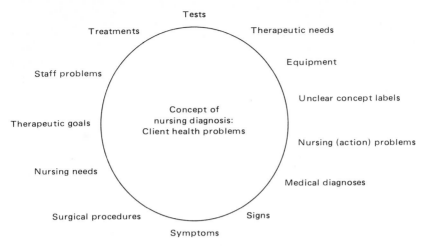

FIGURE 1-1
Concept of nursing diagnosis and terms excluded from the concept.

Therapeutic needs are not nursing diagnoses; they do not describe health problems or health states. For example, "needs emotional support" or "needs suctioning" has been a common way of describing needs for nursing care. These are therapeutic needs; the question arises as to why the client has these needs. In other words, what is the underlying health problem, the nursing diagnosis? Once a diagnosis is established, therapeutic goals and interventions can be determined, but not before.

As an example of the contrast between "needs" and diagnoses, imagine that a nurse says a client "needs emotional support." The client was observed (1) pacing the room during the day before surgery, (2) commenting about being unable to sit still, and (3) stating the wish that surgery was over. A nurse could rush in with emotional support, a diffuse nursing response. Yet in actuality the client may be having difficulty coping with the thought of disability from surgery. Perhaps a neighbor had the same surgery and suffered paralysis 2 days later. The client may be identifying with this situation although his risk for paralysis is extremely low. Diffuse emotional support would probably not assist this person in handling concerns; a problem-focused intervention is needed. Using therapeutic needs as diagnoses bypasses the problem formulation step in care planning.

The term *needs* is also commonly used in another context in nursing. When Maslow's needs hierarchy (Maslow, 1970), a nonnursing theory, is employed as a framework, physiological, safety, belonging, and other needs are stated. These are said to be needs of every human being. If unmet or conflicting, these needs are the *basis* for the development of health problems (Soares, 1978). To write "safety needs" on a chart communicates very little; everyone needs safety. So little information is contained in this statement that one is unable to infer what the problem may be.

Just as therapeutic need is not a nursing diagnosis, neither is a *therapeutic* nursing *goal*, such as "to maintain nutrition." Like "safety needs," this phrase transmits no information about the client's health problems. Everyone needs adequate nutrition. The question needs to be raised, Is there a potential or actual nutritional deficit?

The advantage of basing nursing intervention on a nursing diagnosis is the clear focus for care planning that the diagnosis provides. When a plan is based only on therapeutic goals, there is no way of knowing the client's health problem. In contrast, stating a nursing diagnosis clarifies the logical relationship that should exist between the client's problem and the proposed plan of care.

One *sign* or *symptom* is not a nursing diagnosis. For example, one sometimes sees "restlessness" as the nursing diagnosis. This could be a sign of pain, anxiety, or numerous other conditions. This sign is a totally inadequate base for planning treatment and may or may not be related to a problem nurses can treat. Similarly, a symptom, such as "fatigue," is not a nursing diagnosis. The presence of fatigue may be a predictor that the client will have a self-care deficit, impaired home-maintenance management, or other problems related to decreased energy. Isolated signs and symptoms do not identify the client's health problem. A nursing diagnosis describes a cluster of signs and symptoms.

The question sometimes arises, Is a nursing diagnosis the same as a *nursing problem*? The answer depends on how the term *nursing problem* is being used. If referring to a client's health problem that is amenable to nursing treatment, then *nursing problem* is synonymous with *nursing diagnosis*. *Nursing problem* or *medical problem* are terms used when care providers wish to specify who is treating a problem or wish to refer a client to the appropriate care provider.

The term *nursing problem* is not synonymous with a nursing diagnosis when used to refer to a problem in providing care. How to promote healing may be a nursing care problem, but the health problem is *decubitus ulcer*. A nursing diagnosis describes the client's problem, not the nurse's problem in designing and implementing care.

Little and Carnevali (1976, pp. 48-49) take issue with the use of *concept labels* as nursing diagnoses. Just using a conceptual term, such as *stress* or *maternal attachment*, does not indicate whether a problem exists. Yet not all signs and symptoms can be specified in the diagnostic label. If they were, the diagnosis would be lengthy and would not serve as a shorthand expression. The point Little and Carnevali (1976) make is that a diagnosis should adequately identify the problem for purposes of communication.

As seen in Figure 1-1 and as Little and Carnevali (1976) so clearly point out, nursing diagnoses do not describe *treatments, tests,* or *equipment*. For example, "catheter," "adrenalectomy," or "on heparin" are clearly not within the concept of nursing diagnosis. Treatments and tests do not represent health problems, nor do they represent a cluster of signs and symptoms. Possibly, further data collection will reveal a health problem and a need for nursing intervention.

The diagnosis of disease, or *medical diagnosis*, is not within the concept of nursing diagnosis. If a nurse makes a tentative judgment about a disease or a disease complication, this judgment is made for purposes of referral. These judgments are an important part of nursing practice but are not nursing diagnoses.

Some nurses argue that they are capable of making medical diagnoses, and indeed they are. It is not illegal to exercise one's intellectual capabilities. Yet if the diagnosis is communicated to the patient *and* if treatment, or lack of it, produces harm, it will probably be extremely difficult for the nurse who is responsible to present a substantive defense in court against a malpractice claim.

There are nursing roles in which additional educational preparation legally permits diagnosis and treatment of diseases under physician supervision or protocols. These roles are commonly practiced in ambulatory care or other community-based settings. The portion of the nurse's role that relates to medical diagnosis is similar to the performance of medical acts by a physician's assistant. Although not to the same extent as in ambulatory care, critical care nurses are also responsible for making disease-related judgments and providing treatment under protocols.

Judgments related to observations of disease manifestations or to treatments do not have to be labeled as nursing diagnoses. Disease terminology is perfectly adequate. It would seem ridiculous to relabel a disease with a nursing diagnosis when in fact it cannot be treated except under medical protocols. Clearly, not everything a nurse does will be labeled with a nursing diagnosis.

Although the diagnosis of diseases is never referred to as nursing diagnosis, there is a connection. A high probability exists that disease complications, surgical or other complex procedures, tests, and therapy can result in secondary health problems. Some of those problems may fall within the domain of nursing. As an example, think of a client who intends to follow a complex medication regimen consisting of several pills at different times of the day. The complexity of the regimen, coupled with the person's capabilities and situation, may suggest a risk for not adhering to the regimen. *Potential noncompliance* would be a nursing diagnosis that could serve to organize care. The nurse would use a preventive intervention, such as helping the client to develop a plan for taking the drugs. Nurses are competent to diagnose and treat this problem; in fact, many state nurse practice acts explicitly mandate health teaching.

Appendix A and the previous discussion provide examples of what are and what are not nursing diagnoses. In Chapter 3, diagnosis will be further clarified by examining the conceptual focus of nursing and, therefore, nursing diagnosis. At this point it is important to remember that the statement of a client's health problem should be formulated clearly and should facilitate nursing care planning. The following statements have appeared on clients' charts. Which of these are examples of nursing diagnoses upon which nursing care can be based?

1 Needs suctioning
2 Inadequate insight
3 Self-bathing deficit (level 2)
4 Backache
5 Alterations in parenting
6 Chronic lung disease
7 Difficulty taking medicine

It could be inferred that ineffective airway clearance is the problem in number 1, but we shall never know. The nurse has stated a need rather than a problem. Thus, needs suctioning is not a clinically useful diagnostic category. In number 2, the client's insight may be inadequate in some situations, but which ones and why? The modifier *inadequate* is too judgmental; what amount of insight is adequate? One would imagine there might be a health problem here, but it isn't well expressed. In contrast, number 3, self-bathing deficit, is a functional problem. It directs thinking about nursing care designed to help the client compensate for the deficit. (Level 2 means the person requires assistance or supervision.)

Backache, in number 4, is a symptom, not a diagnosis; it would cause the nurse to collect further information. Alterations in parenting, number 5, is an accepted diagnosis but is a rather broad category that requires further breakdown and definition. Although useful for the time being because it describes an area of concern to nurses, this diagnosis encompasses a number of distinct problems.

Chronic lung disease, number 6, is obviously a medical diagnosis. No doubt a client with this diagnosis has problems amenable to nursing therapy. Perhaps the nurse lacked the language to express nursing diagnoses, or chronic lung disease was the diagnosis used to organize the care ordered by the physician and was erroneously labeled as a nursing diagnosis. Number 7, difficulty taking medicine, is an observation, not a nursing diagnosis. It discloses nothing about the nature and cause of the difficulty. The trouble could be caused by the nurse's method of administration, the nature of the medication (pills versus liquid), or a number of other things.

Structural Definition   One of the simplest ways to grasp the concept of nursing diagnosis is to ask, How would I know one if I saw one? To build on the ideas already discussed, consider a structural definition and think how a nursing diagnosis may appear on various record forms. There are three essential components in a nursing diagnosis; they have been referred to as the *PES format* (Gordon, 1976). The three are the health problem (*P*), the etiology (*E*), and the defining cluster of signs and symptoms (*S*).

Problem Statement   The first component of the structural definition is illustrated by the diagnoses listed in Appendix A. Each of these describes a problem, or health state, of the individual, family, or community. The state of the client (problem) is expressed in clear, concise terms, preferably two or three words. For example, *ineffective family coping* and *noncompliance (specify)* are concise terms that represent a cluster of signs and symptoms.

The term *specify* used in this manner directs the user of the category to state the area in which the problem occurs. For example, noncompliance may be in the area of medication regimen, dietary prescription, or any other health management practices that the client had previously expressed the intention to carry out.

Etiological Factors   The second component of a nursing diagnosis is the etiology. This part of the statement identifies the probable factors causing or maintaining the client's health problem. The etiology can be behaviors of the client, factors in the environment, or an interaction of both. As an example, impaired reality testing may be a factor causing nutritional deficit in a client with psychosis who thinks food is poisoned. Another example is decreased activity tolerance acting as a causative factor in impaired home-maintenance management. Probable causes of a problem should be stated clearly and concisely, using a concise category name, if possible, to summarize the cluster of supporting data.

Etiological factors are subcategories of a diagnostic category, as may be seen in Figure 1-2. The factors that are predicted to be the primary reasons for the problem *and* the problem together constitute the focus of nursing therapy. For example, *noncompliance (low cholesterol diet) related to denial of illness* is a nursing diagnosis that would be used in planning care, as would *noncompliance (low cholesterol diet) related to knowledge deficit (food selection).*

Each etiological subcategory of a diagnostic category has a specific cluster of defining signs and symptoms. Clients may have the same problem but exhibit signs and symptoms indicating different etiologies. It is important to realize that a different diagnosis exists and different treatment is required when the etiology is different. Consider the following four diagnoses, each of which requires different nursing intervention:

1 Self-care deficit, level 4, related to decreased activity tolerance
2 Self-care deficit, level 4, related to uncompensated sensorimotor loss
3 Self-care deficit, level 4, related to autism
4 Self-care deficit, level 4, related to impaired reality testing

All four diagnoses share the common signs and symptoms of self-care deficit, level 4 (level 4 means the person is totally dependent and does not participate in self-care). Yet each has an additional set of signs and symptoms peculiar to the specified etiological factor.

When a self-care deficit, level 4, is judged to be present, a differentiation among possible reasons for the problem is required. This is an example of *differential diagnosis.* Differentiating among various etiologies is critically important because interventions differ, as is clear from the above examples, in which different modes of treatment obviously would be required. A person's ability to feed, bathe, dress, groom, and toilet is not going to improve with assistive devices if the cause is impaired reality testing. In fact, the problem may worsen if incorrect treatments are used.

Defining Signs and Symptoms   The third component of a nursing diagnosis is the cluster of critical, defining signs and symptoms. Each diagnostic category has a set of signs and symptoms that permit discriminations between health problems. These diagnoses, with their cluster of signs and symptoms, eventually will be standardized, nationally and internationally, and published. When a client manifests the critical

FIGURE 1-2
Examples of diagnostic categories and multiple etiological subcategories.

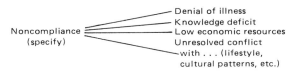

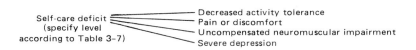

signs and symptoms that correspond to the defining signs and symptoms, then the use of the diagnostic category is appropriate.

Information is gathered, analyzed, and clustered in order to make a diagnostic judgment. The cluster of signs and symptoms used to make the nursing diagnosis should include the signs and symptoms that are typical of the category. This procedure is similar to any use of language. If each person who saw the same characteristics of a particular object called it by a different name, communication about the object would be impossible. As in medicine, or science in general, terms used in nursing diagnosis have specific definitions.

The definition of the medical diagnostic category *myocardial infarction* is standardized internationally so that in journals or other types of communication no erroneous interpretation will occur. It is the responsibility of the person using diagnostic terms to use them correctly. Most nurses contributing to the identification of diagnostic categories believe that identification of the critical defining characteristics (signs and symptoms) of accepted diagnoses needs a great deal of attention. Yet this identification cannot be completed until diagnoses are used clinically and the signs and symptoms most frequently present are described.

Diagnostic Concepts and Categories   Nursing diagnoses are abstractions. They summarize a cluster of signs, symptoms, and inferences. A mental grasp of a cluster of observations and their interrelationships is called a *concept*, in this case a *diagnostic concept*.

Throughout history nurses probably have had some level of understanding, or concept, of their clients' health problems before planning nursing care. What has been missing is a set of agreed upon diagnostic category names. This situation is being corrected by the current national effort to identify and name the health problems nurses treat (Appendix A). Naming and defining concepts is called *categorization* or *classification*. When concepts are identified, defined, and organized within a classification system of nursing diagnoses, they are called *diagnostic categories*.

It is important to appreciate the distinction between diagnostic concepts and diagnostic categories. A *concept* is a general idea or understanding. Important concepts are named and defined to prevent miscommunication. When a concept of a health problem is specifically defined and represents a division in a classification system of names for problems, it is called a diagnostic *category*. In nursing education students learn diagnostic concepts to describe health problems, each of which has a category name and definition. Stated differently, they learn the language of health care and the concepts the language describes. Then, in clinical practice, they grasp signs and symptoms manifested by a client and label them with the name of a previously learned diagnostic category.

In clinical practice diagnostic categories permit discrimination among different health problems. This enhances communication. Also, distinguishing one health problem from another permits nursing responses to be less generalized. As an example, nursing interventions for potential skin breakdown differ from those for decubitus ulcer. These two skin conditions are different health problems, the names are different, the names summarize different clusters of cues, and the two problems are treated differently.

Diagnostic categories are not only summaries of multiple cues, they are also generalizations. Humans are capable of making broad generalizations; they are also capable of extremely fine discrimination. Diagnostic categories are about midway between these extremes. They represent the *typical* signs and symptoms of a health problem. Diagnostic categories also provide a means for ordering and coding clinical data so that meaning can be derived. A family with a particular diagnosis, such as ineffective family coping, shares some common critical characteristics with all the other families in this diagnostic class. Classifying or categorizing signs and symptoms seems to be the only way of dealing with the tremendous diversity encountered in everyday practice.

To be clinically useful, diagnostic categories need to be sufficiently inclusive of individual variations. Yet overinclusiveness can result in undesirably broad classifications.[5] This breadth limits the development of diagnosis-specific interventions. At the other extreme, very fine discriminations limit the applicability of a category to clients who logically belong in the same diagnostic category even though their signs and symptoms are not absolutely identical.

If every client was considered to have a unique diagnosis, never seen before and never to be seen again, the mind would be overwhelmed with the complexity of practice. What is sought in developing diagnostic categories is some middle range between overgeneralization and overspecificity. Categories useful in practice have to be detailed and vivid enough to describe individual manifestations. Yet they have to be sufficiently general for applicability to groups of clients.

Diagnostic concepts should meet the criteria for scientific concepts. One of these criteria is that the reliable indicators of each concept should be identified. The indicators for diagnostic concepts are signs and symptoms that permit one to say with confidence, This is A and that is B. They are reliable in the sense of being well-defined descriptions of reality.

A knowledgeable clinician should be able to apply diagnostic labels consistently and without error from one client to the next. Also, other clinicians should be able to come to the same judgment from the clinical data. Actually, this is an ideal to be striven for. In the professions, in contrast to the basic sciences, it is not always reached. The currently listed nursing diagnoses are prescientific abstractions rather than scientific or theoretical concepts. Psychiatric nomenclature and some of the disease classifications share this state of development.

Do diagnostic categories describe real things? Yes and no. What exists is observable behavior. Intelligence sees relationships within a set of behaviors; observation confirms that these relationships occur repeatedly; logic sees meaning in the pattern; values say this pattern is desirable or not desirable. A generalization is made, and it is given a name and a clear definition. In this way a concept is created. To pursue whether the referents of the concept are real would take us into philosophy and the similar question of whether this book, as book, really exists.

This discourse on existence of diagnostic categories has a practical side. A diagnostic concept such as ineffective coping, arises from (1) reasoning and (2) generalizing (by induction) from experience. In turn, concepts and interrelations among concepts

---

[5]This is the problem with some current diagnoses; clinical testing will probably reveal two or more health problems (each of which is treated differently) within a single current diagnostic category. *Alterations in parenting* is an example.

are used to deal with the world of experience. They permit one to think of related ideas, such as the *meaning* of the particular diagnosis, the *consequences* that can occur, and the *interventions* that may help. An isolated cue, such as crying, cannot do this; a concept of a problem, such as ineffective coping, can.

The key is to be able to move back and forth when necessary between the typical characteristics represented by a diagnostic category and the unique characteristics manifested by the individual client. The former is the basis for diagnosis. The latter makes intervention more than a routine response to a diagnosis.

A second point to remember is that diagnostic categories *represent* a set of *real behaviors* observed to occur fairly frequently in a specific cluster. If a different but more useful way of viewing behaviors is found, categories are discarded or changed. Behaviors are real; people create categories to organize and deal with the world of health care.

Diagnosis as a Process

As previously stated, the word *diagnosis* has two meanings. It can refer to a category name in a classification system, the meaning explored in the previous section. The second meaning, a process leading to a judgment, is the topic introduced in this section.

It is important to appreciate the various cognitive operations involved in acquiring and using clinical information. Equally important is the appreciation that clinical information is acquired through nurse-client interaction. The quality of this interaction directly affects what information is obtained and, subsequently, what diagnostic judgment is made. Let us first consider some general characteristics of the diagnostic process, its components, and diagnostic strategies. The section will conclude with a proposed model of the process and some thoughts on common sense and critical reasoning in diagnosis.

The diagnostic process is, essentially, a process of determining a client's health state and evaluating the etiological factors influencing that state. Is it ever possible to truly know the state of another person, a family, or a community? Most philosophers who deal with questions such as this would say no. What the diagnostician seeks is sufficient understanding of clients and situations to evaluate health, predict future health, and provide assistance when needed. One definition of *diagnosis* is "an analysis of the nature of something" (Morris, 1978, p. 363). In clinical practice that "something" is a client's health status.

To diagnose is to distinguish or discriminate. As information is collected, the first discrimination that occurs is between indicators of a problem and indicators of health and well-being. This is a two-way discrimination task. If signs point toward a judgment of health, they are described and recognition is given to the client's health-promoting practices. Identifying and acknowledging healthful practices serves to support behavior that maintains health.

On the other hand, signs may point toward an actual or potential health problem. Search strategies and multiple discriminations are required to identify the problem clearly. Additionally, the cluster of signs and symptoms have to be labeled correctly with a diagnostic category. This process represents much more than a two-way differentiation between the presence and absence of health.

Diagnostic Process Components Within the diagnostic process are actions, and within these are other, more specific operations involving reasoning and judgment. In its broadest sense, diagnosis involves four activities:

1 Collecting information
2 Interpreting the information
3 Clustering the information
4 Naming the cluster

From this list it would appear that the four activities are a sequence of steps and that the diagnostician has only to collect all information available, analyze and arrange it, and apply category names to the health problems identified. If diagnosis were this uncomplicated, any nurse's aide could be taught the steps.

Instead, what occurs in the diagnostic process is a cycle of certain perceptual and cognitive activities. Observations lead to inferences and inferences lead to further observation. This cycle continues until the diagnostician feels confident to name the problem.

Information Collection The admission nursing history and examination are the beginning of information collection. (Actually, information collection never ends.) In adding a person, family, or community to his or her caseload, the nurse has two equally important goals. One is to obtain health-related information; the other is to begin to establish a therapeutic relationship.

Skillful collection of information, which is critically important in the diagnostic process, is influenced by clinical knowledge. One perceives what one expects to perceive. Clinical knowledge provides the expectations that make one sensitive to cues.[6] Knowing how to frame a question or measure a pulse is a basic skill. The judgment of *when* the question or measurement is appropriate is influenced by one's clinical knowledge.

Information Interpretation Collecting information is to no avail unless meaning is derived. Understanding and evaluating cues are the outcomes of interpretation. Interpreting clinical cues involves *inference*, which is the ability to make a judgment on the basis of information and to go beyond the information to predict or explain. Inferential reasoning permeates the entire diagnostic process.

Information Clustering In clinical practice nurses collecting and interpreting clinical information are heard to remark, "It fits the picture"; "I'm getting a picture of. . . "; or "No, that doesn't fit the picture." What seems to be occurring is the clustering of information in a meaningful way.

Nurses know "what goes with what." How do they know this? Probably, memory stores are searched for previously learned, meaningful ways of clustering clinical cues. The "picture" referred to is probably the memory cluster of signs and symptoms that defines a diagnostic category.

Naming the Cluster Information collection, interpretation, and clustering occur over and over during the diagnostic process. When observations seem to "fit" a diagnostic category, the category name is applied to the cluster of cues. Identification, or

[6]*Cue* is a word that will be used frequently. It is a term borrowed from cognitive psychology meaning a signal to action, initially a cognitive action. A client behavior exists; it becomes a cue if perceived and interpreted.

naming a health problem, is an act of judgment that says, It is *this* and not *that*. Diagnostic judgment is important because it is the basis for care planning.

The diagnostic process was previously described as a set of four activities. A deeper look will reveal that underlying these activities are decision making, inference, conceptualization, and judgment. Decisions have to be made about what information to collect. The information is then interpreted through inferential reasoning. If reasoning suggests that a problem is present, memory is searched for meaningful ways of conceptualizing the client's problem.

Judgment is used throughout the diagnostic process. Perceptual judgment is used to decide whether a sign is present or not present. Inferential judgment affirms that a relationship exists between the data that have been collected; interpretation of meaning is then possible. Finally, a judgment affirms that the cues in the cluster fit together and that the name of the cluster is the diagnosis.

Elements of Clinical Reasoning   The previously listed four components of the diagnostic process involve reasoning. Clinical reasoning is what enables one to collect pertinent information about the client, to interpret and organize the information, and finally to apply a diagnostic label.

Clinical reasoning has been viewed in various ways by psychologists. Some develop models that emphasize the element of judgment or the element of decision making; other psychologists emphasize inference, problem solving, or conceptual behavior. In this section each of these elements will be briefly reviewed. The main objective will be to acquaint the reader with terms and definitions of mental operations involved in clinical reasoning. Later chapters will explore how these elements of clinical reasoning are used in making nursing diagnoses.

The Clinical Inference Model   Some psychologists use a clinical inference model to represent the diagnostic process (Sarbin, Taft, and Bailey, 1960; Hammond, 1966). To help the reader understand clinical inference, formal and statistical inference, which are similar in form, will first be reviewed.

In *formal inference* (formal logic, Aristotelian logic) the inferential process is explicit; conclusions follow from premises, the truth of which is inconsequential, and terms have only one meaning. Reasoning is examined only for structure (it is the *form* of the argument that matters, not the content) and is expressed in a syllogism; a common example is:

> All men are mortal (premise).
> Socrates is a man (observation).
> Therefore, Socrates is mortal (conclusion).

Formal logic is a tool for analyzing the validity of a conclusion. It examines the structure of reasoning, not truth, and "describes how we think or should think" (Sarbin et al., 1960, p. 46).

Statistical inference is similar in structure but the truth-value of premises influence the accuracy of the inference drawn. Conclusions are probabilistic, referring to some portion of cases but not to the universal "all" of formal inference. An example follows:

> Ninety-three percent of a large random sample of American newborns weigh more than 5.5 pounds (premise based on observation).

Therefore, there is a high probability (93 percent) that American newborns weigh more than 5.5 pounds (conclusion).

In this form of inference the truth of the major proposition (first statement) is crucial. If the major premise is incorrect, all further reasoning is in error. To infer statistically is to draw probabilistic conclusions from probabilistic propositions.[7] When statistical conclusions from large-scale research are available, they can be applied in clinical inference.

In the *clinical inference* model of diagnosis, the diagnostician resembles the statistical decision maker, who works with probabilities. Also, reasoning approximates the formal syllogism, since diagnosticians employ clinical knowledge (premises or propositions) to interpret observations (clinical findings). The clinical inference model emphasizes the rational, intellectual quality of diagnosis and therefore provides guidelines for clear thinking. Is the model a prescription of how to reason, or a description of how reasoning is done? Probably both; it evolved from analyzing how *successful* diagnosticians reason.

Inferential reasoning employs major premises *constructed* from the clinician's experience, from theory, or from research (Sarbin et al., 1960, pp. 46–47). Propositions are usually used as if they were universally true; for example, a common premise in nursing is that preoperative patients are anxious. (This is in contrast to a statistical probability, such as, 80 percent of preoperative patients are anxious.) Applying this proposition to an individual would result in an inference: This preoperative patient is anxious. The accuracy of the inference is tested by observing the patient to see whether anxiety is present (as will be discussed later, this is how predictions are made and how hypotheses are generated as a guide for data collection).

The clinical inference model is useful for thinking about clinical reasoning in nursing. Kelly (1964), Aspinall (1976), and Fatzer (1979) have used an inference model in research about diagnosis and diagnostic skills. Davitz and Davitz (1980) have also used this model in a cross-cultural study of nurses' inferences of suffering.

Clinical inference may involve *intuitive knowing* (Hammond, 1966), what Polyani (1967) called *tacit inference*. These are terms used to describe the kind of comprehension in which the person who "knows" is unaware how the comprehension took place. Immediate insight, the "Aha!" or "Eureka!" experience, and the so-called intuitive leap are examples. A solution to a clinical problem or an understanding about a client may occur without the clinician's knowing how or why the intuition came about. The process is termed *nonanalytical inference* when the diagnostician cannot describe the propositions and derivations (the logical thought process) underlying the conclusion.

In regard to intuition and the great intuitive leaps in science, Caws (1969) says no mysterious concept, such as intuition, need be sought. Scientists inherit a wealth of knowledge and are trained to be keen observers. Some are able to perceive previously unknown relationships between phenomena. Sensitivity, or taking into account the necessary data, appears to be a sufficient explanation of intuition.

Greatly admired clinicians who reputedly can diagnose from a distance of 10 feet

---

[7]*Probabilistic* is an adjective used to indicate the likelihood of an event occurring. It refers to the possibility as opposed to the certainty of an occurrence. If expressed in numbers, probability is always less than 100. Note the definition, as the term will be used frequently to describe nursing situations.

are apt to be experienced, sensitive to cues, and in possession of a wealth of clinical knowledge. Intuitive inference is merely noncritical, nonanalytical thinking based on implicit, rather than explicit, assumptions (Henle, 1962; Sarbin et al., 1960, p. 40). It has its place, but a nurse who says, "I don't know what it is; he just doesn't look right," should recognize this as a signal to attend closely to cues and cue processing. Taking time and effort to bring data and propositions into conscious awareness may well remove the mystery from much so-called clinical intuition in nursing.

Usually included in a discussion of intuition is the idea of *empathy*. It is an aspect of social intelligence, presumably learned. Empathy involves predictive inferences about the feelings or intentions of another person by analogy with oneself. It is "standing in the shoes of another" for a moment and rests heavily on the assumption of similarity between the observer and the person perceived (Sarbin et al., 1960, pp. 40-42). Used as hypotheses to direct a search for cues, empathetic, intuitive inferences are useful; used as facts, they may lead to diagnostic errors.

The Clinical Judgment Model Some conceptual inferences require a complex strategy. Cues are probabilistic rather than absolute, and conflicting information is present that has to be weighed. If, in addition, some element of evaluation is involved, this type of inference is described as *clinical judgment*.

Is diagnosis a process of judgment, perhaps inferential judgment? In recent decades it seems to have been popular to think about diagnosis as clinical judgment. Numerous studies have employed clinical judgment as a model of diagnosis (Bieri, Atkins, Briar, Leaman, Miller, and Tripoldi, 1966; Newell, 1968, pp. 5-6; Kaplan and Schwartz, 1975; Feinstein, 1967; Elstein, Schulman, and Sprafka, 1978). Some authors make no distinction between judgment and inference, yet judgment implies careful evaluation and assertion of an opinion based on specialized knowledge. Inference does not have these implications, although terms such as *inferential judgment* or *intuitive judgment* are in popular use.

Newell (1968, pp. 5-6) sees judgment as an act; it concludes an extended process and involves identifying something. Diagnosis would be a categorical judgment (identification and naming) of the state of the client. Judgment is evaluative because norms (for example, a range of "normal" heart rate) are used to evaluate clinical observations. *Normative judgments* are made in conformity with social values about what is healthy and what is problematic.

Lonergan (1970) lists three levels in the judgment process: (1) perception of raw data that need to be understood, (2) understanding of what is emerging from the data and can be conceptualized, and (3) reflection that questions the accuracy of the formulations. With a philosopher's perspective on judgment, Lonergan states:

> The cognitional process is thus a cumulative process. Questions for intelligence presuppose something to be understood, that something is supplied by the initial level [the data]. Understanding grasps in given or imagined presentations [data and memory] an intelligible form emergent in the presentations. Conception formulates the grasped idea along with what is essential to the idea in the presentation. Reflection asks whether such understanding and formulation [problem identified] are correct. Judgment answers that they are or are not. (Lonergan, 1970, p. 275)

Philosophers deal with an additional dimension that is relevant to diagnosis. This dimension is responsibility. Rarely do we hear that one is responsible for one's infer-ences. But responsibility is implied in the notion of judgment. Lonergan comments explicitly on responsibility. He refers to the levels outlined above, particularly the third level of reflection and judgment:

> It is on this third level that there emerge the notions of truth and falsity, of certi-tude and the probability that is not a frequency but a quality of judgment. It is within this third level that there is involved the personal commitment that makes one responsible for one's judgments. It is from this third level that come utterances to express one's affirming or denying, asserting or disserting, agreeing or disagreeing. (Lonergan, 1970, p. 273)

Elstein, Shulman, and Sprafka (1978) used a clinical judgment model in their research on medical diagnosis. The physician's diagnostic process was described as data acquisition and interpretation, hypothesis generation and testing, and diagnostic judgment. Doona's (1976) description of clinical judgment in nursing specifies the steps of the process. Her outline is similar to, but more detailed than, Lonergan's three levels. Hornung (1956) and Kormorita (1963), two earlier writers on nursing diagnosis, also viewed diagnosis as a judgment process. Chambers (1962, p. 104) and Schaefer (1974) mention diagnostic judgment in their decision-making models of nursing process. Except for Doona, nursing authors do not specify the process of using clinical data in judgment.

The Clinical Decision-Making Model Is a judgment a decision? Is a decision a judgment? In the legal profession the two terms are synonymous. The "judgment of the court" is the legal decision. Aspinall (1979) viewed diagnosis as a decision-making process and studied the use of decision trees to improve diagnostic accuracy. Others have used the term *decision making* to denote such action as would be taken after a problem is identified (Grier, 1976; Janis and Mann, 1977). Schaefer (1974, p. 1852) also views decision making as an "act of choice following deliberation and judgment." The term *decision making* is more frequently used to refer to choice or therapeutic decision making than to the diagnostic process. This is not to negate the fact that judgments involve choice (decision), as will be elaborated in a later discussion of strategies.

The Clinical Problem-Solving Model Scandura (1977), Elstein and his colleagues (1978), and Newell and Simon (1972) use the term *problem solving* for identification of problems, of solutions, or of both. *Problem identification* is a better term for diagnosis than is *problem solving*; problem solution is part of therapy rather than of diagnosis. Clinical decision making and problem solving are more appropriate as models for the entire nursing process (Goodwin and Edwards, 1975) than as models just for the diagnostic component of the nursing process. Aspinall and Tanner (1981) provide an example of how clinical decision making and problem solving can be integrated into a description of the nursing process.

Broderick and Ammentorp (1979) studied cue-acquisition decisions; in their research they did not instruct nurses to make a diagnosis, but asked them just to collect the information they would need to intervene in a problem. These authors referred to the task as problem solving and inference, and called their research subjects "nurse judges," indicating the operations they perceived to be involved.

The Diagnostic-Concept Attainment Model   Diagnosis can also be thought of as concept attainment, that is, attainment of a concept of the state of the client (Gordon, 1980; Elstein et al., 1978). A large volume of literature exists on concept attainment and the strategies people use in forming concepts; the work of Bruner, Goodnow, and Austin (1956) is a classic. Whether or not the clinician consciously uses a strategy, the behavior that takes place during the process of diagnosing can be described as a strategy. The identification of strategies helps explain how information is collected and clustered.

Diagnostic concepts are much more complex than those used in psychological experiments. Complexity is evident in the number of cues that have to be put together, their probabilistic nature, and the strategies employed. Studies of nurses' (Gordon, 1972, 1980) and physicians' (Elstein et al., 1978) diagnostic concept attainment revealed similarities in the two groups' strategies for dealing with uncertainty in clinical information. The concept-attainment model appears to be useful for research about diagnostic behavior.

In summary, this discussion of models for the diagnostic process has provided a brief account of how diagnosis has been viewed. Inference, judgment, and concept attainment all end with an act of categorization. The category may or may not be labeled with a word (a name for that category). *Inference* emphasizes the structural process of clinical reasoning; *concept attainment* contributes the idea that information-processing strategies are used to attain a diagnostic concept of a health state. *Clinical judgment* emphasizes an evaluative component. All are useful for processing clinical information.

Diagnostic Strategies

The best way of getting an overview of the diagnostic process is to think of it as a strategy for collecting and using information. A *strategy* is an approach, a way of doing something. It requires thought and skill. A *diagnostic strategy* is a way of determining a client's health status.

The diagnostician does not learn the health status of a client in an instant. Arriving at the diagnosis requires a series of decisions about what questions to ask and what observations to make. The pattern of sequential decisions in acquiring, retaining, and using information constitutes a strategy (Bruner et al., 1956, p. 51).

No claim is made that expert clinicians are conscious of their strategies. Nor can it be said that they deliberately plan each decision and action. Yet observations indicate that they have developed successful *ways of proceeding.* Success results when strategies are well suited to the demands of diagnostic situations (Bruner et al., 1956; Gordon, 1980).

Diagnostic strategies employed by clinicians can be viewed as a *set of hypothesis-testing procedures.* An example from everyday life will clarify this way of thinking about the diagnostic process:

Imagine you are on the street of some wealthy suburb. You have a particular interest in automobiles because you are going to buy your first car! In your long-term memory stores are many cognitive categories for classifying automobiles. Each category has a set of defining characteristics; body shape, grillwork, and so forth.

Your attention turns to an object on the street. Immediate scanning classifies it as an automobile, but the model is not clear. Motivated to make a specific identi-fication you say to yourself: "Is that a Chevrolet? Maybe it's an Oldsmobile? It could be the new Ford?" Each question is a hypothesis.

Still wanting to know, you test each hypothesis. This requires a long, close look guided by your memory stores of the defining characteristics of automobiles. First the grillwork is examined. This may rule out one of the three hypotheses. Testing continues until you feel satisfied about the probability that your categorization is accurate. You may get an opportunity to validate your categorization. When the owner returns, you may ask the make and model of the car.

As this example illustrates, hypothesis testing is not confined to diagnostic strategies. Both children and adults generate hypotheses, or possibilities, when trying to identify something not immediately perceptible. Studies of general concept attainment indicate that in any identification task, when a few important cues are obtained, tentative hypotheses are generated. This behavior is seen in everyday life (Gholson, Levine, and Phillips, 1972), in science, and in clinical practice (Gordon, 1972, 1980; Elstein et al., 1978).

Models usually fail to capture the complexity of what they represent. Such is the case with models of the diagnostic process. Each focuses on different aspects but not on the complexity of the whole. The following model will be used in this book.

Diagnostic Process Model in Nursing

The purpose of the diagnostic process in nursing is to identify actual or potential health problems amenable to nursing therapy. The process is complex and involves a pattern of sequential decisions about what information to collect and how to use it. The procedure for making this series of decisions is a decision-making strategy (Bruner et al., 1956), or a diagnostic strategy.

A diagnostic strategy guides collection of information that is used to evaluate and describe a client's functional health patterns. Within a strategy, inferences are made by combining information about the client and clinical knowledge. Until validated, infer-ences are treated as hypotheses (possibilities) about what is perceived, the meaning of cues, or relationships among cues. Hypotheses are also used to direct the search for cues and to predict events.

By abstraction, information is clustered and a concept attained. At some subjective confidence level, a diagnostic category name (nursing diagnosis) is employed to rep-resent the cluster of clinical data.

Judgment permeates the diagnostic process. It begins with perception; something is judged to be *this* and not *that*. Judgment is used when a behavior or pattern of behavior is evaluated as expected or unexpected, normal or abnormal. Judgment is involved when hypotheses are selected, when they are held or discarded, and when they are affirmed. An inferential judgment is made when a diagnostic hypothesis is viewed as the most probable representation of a health state. A category name, judged to be descriptive of the state, is then applied.

Nursing diagnoses represent responsible judgments of the moment. Recognized as necessarily based in part on uncertain data, they are always open to challenge by new information.

One may ask whether this model is intended as descriptive or prescriptive. A descriptive model describes *what is*; a prescriptive model, *what should be*. Research describing the process of nursing diagnosis has not been done. Perhaps it cannot be done until diagnosis is integral to practice. Prescription can easily be done; it depends on opinion and judgment. The ideas in this book are based on (1) logical reasoning about the nature of the diagnostic task, (2) cognitive theory and research, and (3) minimal, nonrepresentative nursing and medical research about clinical judgment.

Common Sense and Critical Reasoning

The goal in health evaluation and diagnosis is correct and reliable judgments. Attaining this goal requires refinement of the commonsense approach that serves so well in everyday living. Refinement proceeds in a particular direction, toward an attitude of critical reflection and curiosity. This attitude increases the reliability of diagnostic judgments and differentiates professional expertise from the layperson's commonsense approach.

Common sense is based on *things as they appear*. It is used for *practical judgments and immediate, concrete actions of daily living*. Common sense is common in that it is shared through tradition and cumulative experience. When ideas work, they are considered true (Lonergan, 1970, pp. 289-299).

A caring parent, noticing that a child is irritable in the morning, infers illness and takes the child's temperature. If fever is present, certain actions will be required. This is sound, practical common sense, habitual and adapted as experience in child care accumulates.

The nurse caring for an irritable child before taking the temperature applies nursing knowledge and generates some possibilities. Caring, comforting, and precise description of the child and situation are the first task. Measuring body temperature may be appropriate, but this is determined by logical analysis of the initial information. Actions are not habitual, as they frequently are when common sense is used. Rather, they are derived from disciplined reasoning.

The term *disciplined reasoning* describes a pattern of thinking that withstands professional scrutiny. Disciplined reasoning, combined with critical self-reflection, provides an error-correcting process. Both lead to increased reliability of judgments.

A professional tries to refine commonsense ways of thinking to achieve more accurate and reliable judgments. This requires a specialized body of knowledge and an approach similar to scientific thinking. Deeper explanations are sought for "appearances" grasped by common sense. *Description is precise, analysis is logical, and standards and criteria exist for the explanations put forth.* Answers are sought to explain why things appear as they do, and reasoning is subjected to critical reflection. When ideas work, the scientific attitude asks why (Lonergan, 1970, pp. 289-299).

To make correct and reliable clinical judgments and to improve judgment continuously, curiosity is also required. Curiosity leads to questions and questions lead to further information. When the inadequacy of professional knowledge is revealed by unanswered questions, research is undertaken.

CONTEXTUAL DEFINITION OF DIAGNOSIS

Sometimes a concept becomes clearer if it is viewed in the context of related ideas rather than in isolation. In this section nursing diagnosis will be examined in its rightful place, within nursing process. The important understanding to be gained is that the purpose of diagnosis is to provide a focus for nursing care planning and evaluation.

Nursing process will be examined in its own right, then in the context of nursing practice that consists of more than just treating nursing diagnoses. Next, a look at the broader context of health care delivery will provide an understanding of the need for collaboration among health professionals, particularly in the treatment of the client's diagnoses. The major appreciation to be gained is that nursing diagnoses are not made in isolation.

Nursing Diagnosis in Nursing Process

Client care is the central focus of nursing. Caring for, about, and with clients are the scientific and humanistic elements. These elements of clinical practice describe a helping relationship actualized through nursing process.

Nursing process is a method of problem identification and problem solving.[8] Although derived from the supposedly objective scientific method, nursing process is not applied in an objective, value-free way. Human values influence both problem identification and problem solving.

The components of nursing process discussed in textbooks vary but generally include assessment, diagnosis, outcome projection, planning, intervention, and outcome evaluation. Having the key components spelled out encourages deliberation, organization, and thought as opposed to haphazard care planning. This is important when *human beings* are the recipients of care.

The six components named above only specify the activities to be done. How these activities are done requires a conceptual framework. A *conceptual framework* is a set of concepts that guide general decisions about *what* to assess and diagnose, *how* to intervene, and *what* to evaluate. In a later chapter a few selected frameworks will be discussed. The objective at this point is just to define diagnosis in the context of nursing process. The discussion here will be brief and introductory.

Nursing process begins with the problem identification phase. In the first contact with a client a nursing history and examination are done. This information-collection process is referred to as *assessment*. During assessment actual or potential health problems may be revealed. Nursing diagnoses are used to describe these problems.

It is important to understand that problem identification contains elements of uncertainty. One rarely is 100 percent certain that a diagnosis is valid. This is not peculiar to nursing; all health care providers are faced with the same situation. In a later chapter, methods for dealing with this lack of certainty will be discussed.

When a cluster of signs and symptoms is categorized using a nursing diagnosis, clinical knowledge stored in memory can be retrieved. This knowledge facilitates

---

[8] Most authors use the term *problem solving* to encompass both identification of the problem and its solution. To emphasize the two components, in this text they will be stated explicitly.

problem solving or problem prevention. It is then, in the intervention phase of nursing process, that diagnosis proves its worth.

The diagnosis, or problem identified, provides a focus for problem-solving activities. These include outcome projection, care planning, intervention, and outcome evaluation.

The first step in helping a client solve or prevent a problem is to identify clearly the outcome desired. An *outcome* is measurable behavior indicating problem resolution or progress toward resolution. For example, if the diagnosis is potential skin breakdown, the desired outcome is intact skin. Did you notice what just occurred? The diagnosis was used as a focus for projecting the outcome.

Having determined the desired health outcome, the nurse can now stop and think about what nursing care is needed to reach the specified outcome when the specified nursing diagnosis is present. Factors in the client's situation are also considered in decision making. Taking them into account serves to individualize care planning. During intervention there is continual assessment and evaluation of the problem, the effectiveness of care, and the progress toward outcome attainment.

This brief overview indicates how nursing diagnoses are used in nursing process. Diagnoses provide a distinct focus for establishing desired outcomes of nursing care and for making decisions about what care is needed. A diagnosis also provides a focus for daily evaluation of a client's progress and for any necessary revision of the care plan. For all these reasons nursing diagnoses make nursing care delivery easier. Further appreciation of this point will be gained when more specific guidelines and examples are provided in a later chapter.

Nursing Diagnosis in Nursing Practice

A broader view is necessary before nursing diagnosis can be thought of in the context of nursing practice. In this section we will see that nursing practice may include more than the treatment of nursing diagnoses. If clients have medical problems, nurses help them to carry out medical treatments (i.e., to follow their doctor's orders). It is important to grasp the difference. In one case, nursing diagnoses, the nurse is responsible for determining the care plan; in the other case, medical diagnoses, the responsibility is to see that the client is helped to carry out the care plan designed by the physician.

Aside from the issue of responsibility, in practice the separation is artificial. Clients have health problems. Physicians and nurses work together to help them overcome these problems. The issue that concerns many nurses is, What is the essence of *nursing* in practice, and is sufficient emphasis given to this?

A very interesting thing occurs when a group of nurses from various nursing specialties discuss the nursing diagnoses they encounter in their practice. It is obvious that the currently accepted diagnoses (Appendix A) occur in every specialty. Perhaps the incidence and the etiological factors are different, but the problems described by nursing diagnoses are the same. Self-care deficits, fear, disturbances in self-concept, potential for injury, and certain others seem to constitute a core of nursing practice irrespective of the setting and specialty.

Yet nursing diagnoses do not describe the whole of nursing practice. Clients have other health problems, as was previously stated, that are of concern to nurses. For a moment think of the whole of your practice as contained in a circle, such as that illustrated in Figure 1-3. Think of this whole as 100 percent of the time you spend in direct client care activities (ignore administrative tasks for the moment.)

A line has been drawn arbitrarily to section off the circle in a 50:50 ratio. Is this perhaps a description of time allocation in acute care? Where shall we move the line for intensive care? Some would claim the distribution is 10 percent nursing and 90 percent other. In ambulatory care would it be about 75 percent nursing and 25 percent other? In long-term care and rehabilitation the line may need to be moved to section off 90 percent as nursing and 10 percent as other. The line is movable, as is the emphasis nurses and administrators place on various aspects of practice.

The diagram is useful in conveying the information that nursing diagnosis is used in that aspect of practice unique to nursing. No one else is educated to perform this aspect of care. The diagram also helps clarify that nurses do not intend to ignore medical treatment orders or the client's disease; to do so would not be compatible with a holistic approach. It is imporant to notice also that disease-related nursing care

FIGURE 1-3
Time spent in direct care activities of nursing practice.

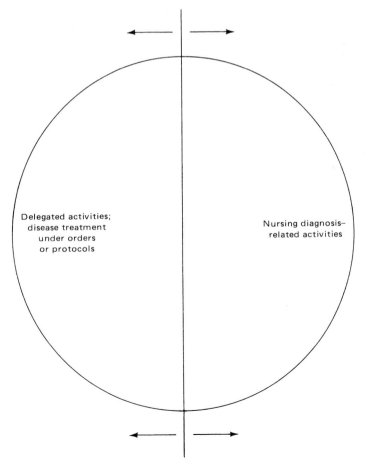

Delegated activities; disease treatment under orders or protocols

Nursing diagnosis–related activities

is not considered "nonnursing" activity. The current emphasis on nursing diagnoses has come about because this aspect of practice (diagnosis) has not been described; the others have.

Clinical judgments in nursing practice are not confined to nursing diagnosis. Nurses diagnose actual and potential problems (1) related to clients' health perceptions and health management practices and (2) occurring secondary to illness, therapy, developmental changes, and life situations. Generally, these health problems are in the realm of nursing.

Nurses also make diagnostic judgments about actual or potential problems (1) for purposes of referral and (2) under protocols or medical supervision. Words for describing problems in these two areas are available in medical textbooks and classification systems.

The four areas just named, in which nurses make diagnostic judgments, require at least a brief discussion. This is because three options exist after a judgment is made. The nurse could develop a treatment plan, refer the problem to a member of another profession, or treat the problem under protocols. It is important to know which action to take.

Most health problems diagnosed in the area of individual, family, or community health maintenance and management are within the scope of nursing diagnosis and treatment. Clients' responses secondary to illness, medical therapy, developmental changes, or life situations are also in this realm. In both of these areas are the actual and potential problems (nursing diagnoses) nurses currently are attempting to describe and classify.

Nurses also tentatively diagnose disease or disease complications for purpose of referral. Perhaps it is stretching the term to call this activity diagnosis. Nevertheless, it is impossible to make judgments about referral, or "calling the doctor," if the problem is not tentatively formulated. Early recognition of disease complications in acute care settings requires this. Similarly, in other settings a tentative diagnostic judgment is the basis for referral to a physician. In addition, nurses are legally responsible for observation, interpretation, and judgment regarding referral for health problems that are in the domain of medical care.

Diagnostic judgments made for purposes of referral are not within the realm of nursing diagnosis. This is because nurses are neither educated nor licensed to *treat* diseases; that is the practice of medicine. This is not to argue that the nurse does not assist the patient in activities related to disease treatment. In acute care settings patients depend on nurses to monitor their diseases and to assist them in obtaining the recommended medicines and carrying out therapies. These activities do not have to be labeled nursing diagnoses.

Some diagnoses accepted for clinical testing (see Appendix A)—decreased cardiac output, fluid volume deficit, altered tissue perfusion, impaired gas exchange, and ineffective breathing patterns—are conditions probably requiring referral to a physician. Examination of the defining signs and symptoms of these categories supports this conclusion (Kim and Moritz, 1981). Furthermore, most nurses would agree that if *they* developed these conditions they would seek a medical opinion about treatment.

The diagnosis, treatment, or long-term care of noncomplex disease conditions *under protocols* (prepared guidelines) is another aspect of current nursing practice. In recent decades nurses have been increasing their knowledge and skills related to diagnosis and treatment of diseases. Nurse practice acts have been changed to permit diagnosis and treatment under protocols. The conditions may range from simple upper respiratory infections to stable diabetes mellitus or other chronic diseases.

This aspect of nursing practice is characteristic of primary care delivery where the client is ambulatory and relatively stable physiologically and psychologically. The nurse assumes responsibility for total health care and uses physician consultation for medical problems as needed. Protocols provide the direction for diagnosis and treatment.

The clinical nurse specialists and nurse practitioners practicing in this role are expected to be competent in diagnostic and therapeutic skills. Their diagnosis of medical conditions is not considered nursing diagnosis because protocols, as well as physician supervision, are required.

In this discussion of nursing practice, comparisons have been made among nursing diagnosis, tentative diagnosis for purposes of referral, and diagnosis under protocols. The medical nomenclature, such as names for diseases, syndromes, and symptom complexes, is sufficient for the latter two types of diagnoses. There is no need to spend precious time relabeling these conditions from a nursing perspective. Rather, time and effort should be expended in identifying and naming health-related conditions in the realm of nursing diagnosis.

Nursing Diagnosis in Health Care Delivery

In this section we will take a broader view that encompasses nursing process and nursing practice. Health care delivery is the combined objective of many groups: physicians, nurses, administrators, agencies of the federal government, and others. Basic health services are delivered by two professions, nursing and medicine. These basic services to the consumer are supplemented as necessary by a number of other health care providers. For example, when clients' health problems warrant, referrals can be made to social workers, physical therapists, or psychologists.

Figure 1-4 symbolizes the components of coordinated care when only a nurse, a physician, and a consultant are involved in providing services. Although the interactions and outcome shown by the arrows do not always take place, coordination represented by arrows toward a central focus is a realistic goal.

Clients' contributions to the coordination of their health care management include (1) their personal perceptions of their health state, (2) their plans, and (3) their health practices. They have expectations that the "specialists" in health will offer information, recommendations, and the required care. Health professionals formalize clients' health concerns with diagnoses and treatment plans, as the diagram indicates. Thus the major elements are present for joint planning by the client, nurse, and physician.

Coordinated care as illustrated in Figure 1-4 is not a new idea; it can be found in textbooks dating back 30 or more years. Yet the challenge to implement this coordination is still present for the next generation of clinicians in the health professions.

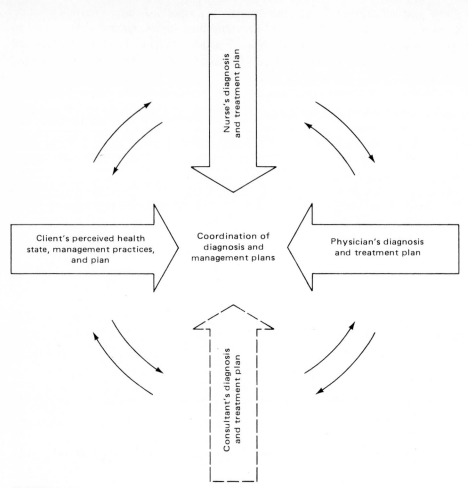

FIGURE 1-4
Components of coordinated health care delivery.

Figure 1-5 illustrates the current situation in many institutions devoted to health care, "part and parcel care delivery." The professions operate rather separately and each offers its own "parcel" to the consumer. Nursing has not clearly understood what its own contribution is, and consequently has not been able to clarify this matter for consumers. The language used in health care circles is not just one of actions and doing. It deals with what the problem is and what can be offered, a rather logical stance.

If health care is to go from the situation in Figure 1-5 to that in Figure 1-4, the *first* step is for nurses to share, in some clear and concise way, their conceptions of clients' current functional health states and nursing care needs. Nursing diagnoses provide a method for synthesizing and communicating nurses' observations. As later chapters will show, the ability to communicate health needs of clients can influence funding of preventive and comprehensive health care services.

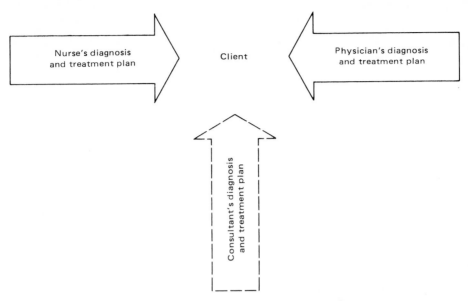

FIGURE 1-5
Independent (uncoordinated) components of current health care delivery.

SUMMARY

Interest in and enthusiasm about nursing diagnosis is widespread. In the United States and other countries nurses are recognizing the implications for nursing practice, education, and research. In particular, those providing direct care to clients view nursing diagnosis as a way to improve nursing care. As one nurse said, "Nursing diagnosis helps me to define what I do and feel good about how I do it."

In this chapter, nursing diagnosis and the diagnostic process were introduced. It was noted that the term *diagnosis* is used to refer both to a category name for a health problem and to a process of identifying health problems. Diagnosis as a category was explained by contrasting what diagnosis is with what it is not. Leaving other conceptual distinctions for a later chapter, a nursing diagnosis was defined as an actual or potential health problem amenable to nursing intervention.

Diagnosis as a process was seen to include collection, analysis, and synthesis of health-related information. Various models exist for thinking about this process, each with a slightly different emphasis. Combining these ideas, a clinical judgment model of the diagnostic process was described. A brief overview indicated that a clinical judgment about the health status of an individual, family, or community encompasses actions and cognitive operations. Diagnosis as process and diagnosis as category were isolated for purposes of discussion, but were then described as inseparable when used in practice.

Nursing diagnosis was examined in the context of nursing process in order to establish its essential and practical meaning. An important point of that discussion was that a diagnosis provides the focus for health-problem prevention and for problem solving, two important aspects of the helping relationship established with clients.

It was recognized that practicing nurses make many types of clinical judgments. Those judgments that pertain to nursing diagnoses have a particular characteristic that distinguishes them from nursing judgments related to disease or disease complications; when nursing diagnoses are made, responsibility and accountability exist for *determining* the care plan, as opposed to implementing the plans of physicians or others.

An examination of health care delivery demonstrated that a variety of professionals make diagnoses and develop treatment plans. Not to be overlooked are clients' perceptions of their health or their health management plans. Ideally, coordinated health care takes all of these into account. There were two important implications for nursing discussed. One was that nursing diagnoses represent a clear focus for nursing participation in coordinated planning. The second was that nurses, physicians, consultants, and clients (insofar as their condition permits) have to pool their conceptions of health problems and treatment plans in order to coordinate activities.

Because nursing diagnoses are not made in isolation and because nurses need to increase their participation in joint planning, an appreciation of other professions is needed. When participating in a joint care planning conference it is important to know the perspectives of other professions (just as they need to understand the perspective of nursing). Chapter 2 will provide information on this subject. It will also provide an opportunity to see how nursing's perspective and the focus of diagnosis evolved.

BIBLIOGRAPHY

Aspinall, M. J. Use of a decision tree to improve diagnostic accuracy. *Nursing Research*, May–June 1979, *28*, 182–185.

Aspinall, M. J., & Tanner, C. A. *Decision-making for patient care: Applying the nursing process.* New York: Appleton-Century-Crofts, 1981.

Bieri, J., Atkins, A. L., Briar, S., Leaman, R. L., Miller, H., & Tripoldi, T. *Clinical and social judgment.* New York: Wiley, 1966.

Broderick, M. E., & Ammentorp, W. Information structures: An analysis of nursing performance. *Nursing Research*, March–April 1979, *28*, 106–110.

Bruner, J. S., Goodnow, J. J., & Austin, G. A. *A study of thinking.* New York: Wiley, 1956.

Caws, P. The structure of scientific discovery. *Science*, December 12, 1969, *166*, 1375–1380.

Chambers, W. Nursing diagnosis. *American Journal of Nursing*, November 1962, *62*, 102–104.

Davitz, L., & Davitz, J. *Inference of patients' pain and psychological distress.* New York: Springer, 1980.

Doona, M. E. The judgment process in nursing. *Image*, June 1976, *225*, 82–90.

Elstein, A. S., Shulman, L. S. & Sprafka, S. A. *Medical problem solving: An analysis of clinical reasoning.* Cambridge, Mass.: Harvard University Press, 1978.

Feinstein, A. R. *Clinical judgment.* Huntington, N.Y.: Robert E. Krieger, 1976. (Originally published, 1967.)

Fratzer, C. Relationship between logical reasoning and nursing diagnosis. In *Nursing Diagnosis Monograph*. Denton, Tex.: Texas Women's University College of Nursing, Fall 1979.

Gholson, B., Levine, M., & Phillips, S. Hypotheses, strategies, and stereotypes in discrimination learning. *Journal of Experimental Child Psychology*, 1972, *13*, 423-446.

Goodwin, J. O., & Edwards, B. S. Developing a computer program to assist the nursing process: Phase 1–From systems analysis to an expandable program. *Nursing Research*, July-August 1975, *24*, 299-305.

Gordon, M. Predictive strategies in diagnostic tasks. *Nursing Research*, January-February 1980, *29*, 39-45.

Gordon, M. *Probabilistic concept attainment: A study of nursing diagnosis*. Unpublished doctoral dissertation, Boston College, 1972.

Gordon, M. Nursing diagnosis and the diagnostic process. *American Journal of Nursing*, August 1976, *76*, 1298-1300.

Grier, M. R. Decision making about patient care. *Nursing Research*, March-April 1976, *25*, 105-110.

Hammond, K. R. Clinical inference in nursing: II. A psychologist's viewpoint. *Nursing Research*, Winter 1966, *15*, 27-38.

Henle, M. On the relation between logic and thinking. *Psychological Review*, 1962, *69*, 366-378.

Hornung, G. J. Nursing diagnosis: An exercise in judgment. *Nursing Outlook*, 1956, *4*, 29-30.

Hudak, C. M. *Clinical protocols: A guide for nurses and physicians*. Philadelphia: Lippincott, 1976.

Janis, I. L., & Mann, L. *Decision making: Psychological analysis of conflict, choice, and commitment*. New York: Free Press, Macmillon, 1977.

Kaplan, M. F., & Schwartz, S. *Human judgment and decision processes*. New York: Academic Press, 1975.

Kelly, K. J. An approach to the study of clinical inference in nursing: Part 1, Introduction to the study of clinical inference in nursing. *Nursing Research*, Fall 1964, *13*, 314-322.

Komorita, N. I. Nursing diagnosis. *American Journal of Nursing*, 1963, *63*, 83-86.

Little, D., & Carnevali, D. The diagnostic statement: The problem defined. In B. Walter, P. Pardee, & D. M. Molbo (Eds.), *Dynamics of problem-oriented approaches: Patient care and documentation*. New York: Lippincott, 1976.

Lonergan, B. J. F. *Insight: A study of human understanding* (3d ed.). New York: Philosophical Library, 1970.

Maslow, A. *Motivation and personality*. New York, Harper and Row, 1970.

Morris, W. (Ed.). *American heritage dictionary of the English language*. Boston, Houghton Mifflin, 1978.

Newell, A. Judgment and its representation: An introduction. In B. Kleinmuntz (Ed.), *Formal representation of human judgment*. New York: Wiley, 1968.

Newell, A., & Simon, H. A. *Human problem solving*. Englewood Cliffs, N.J.: Prentice-Hall, 1972.

Polyani, M. *The tacit dimension*. New York: Anchor Books, Doubleday, 1967.

Rosch, E., & Lloyd, B. B. (Eds.). *Cognition and categorization*. Hillsdale, N.J., Lawrence Erlbaum Associates, 1978.

Sarbin, T. B., Taft, R. B., & Bailey, D. E. Clinical inference and cognitive theory. New York: Holt, Rinehart, and Winston, 1960.

Scandura, J. *Problem solving: A structural process approach with instructional implications.* New York: Academic Press, 1977.

Schaefer, J. Interrelatedness of decision making and the nursing process. *American Journal of Nursing,* October 1974, *74,* 1852–1855.

Soares, C. A. Nursing and medical diagnoses: Comparison of variant and essential features. In N. L. Chaska (Ed.), *The nursing profession: Views through the mist.* New York: McGraw-Hill, 1978.

CHAPTER 2

CLINICAL DIAGNOSIS IN THE HEALTH PROFESSIONS

Placing the adjective *nursing* before the term *diagnosis* merely identifies the area of health care problems being addressed. Just as nurses use the term *nursing diagnosis* to refer to health problems within their scope of practice, physicians use the term *medical diagnosis* and social workers, *casework diagnosis*.

The client problems addressed by the various professions differ. Yet the overall method of identifying and using diagnostic categories is the same.[1] Appreciating these similarities and differences should enhance interprofessional communication as well as clarify some issues in nursing diagnosis. Usually, we can better understand our own domain of practice when it is viewed in the context of overall professional health care delivery.

In this chapter clinical diagnosis in nursing, medicine, and social work will be examined. Each profession will be considered separately in terms of its professional focus, conceptual frameworks, concept of causality, classification systems, and diagnostic process. These five elements cannot be separated, because one influences the others.

Professional focus is the structure and purpose, or social mandate, of a profession. The focus of a profession influences its conceptual framework of practice. A *conceptual framework* is a set of general ideas, or concepts, that are logically interrelated. One concept that will be examined here is the professional's conceptual model of the client. This model is what guides the naming of diagnostic categories and provides a perspective for the profession.

---

[1] In the profession of medicine, *clinical diagnosis* is used to refer to diagnosis based on a patient's history and examination. Supplementary laboratory or other types of tests are generally employed before a final judgment is reached.

Each person views the world from some cognitive perspective, and this viewpoint affects the way the person explains and predicts events. Similarly, in the professions the focus of concern in practice is described and explained from a particular perspective or frame of reference.

A conceptual model is a simplification, a cognitive construction that ignores as irrelevant some aspects of the phenomenon being considered. It narrows attention to the area of concern and purpose. For example, some psychologists find a game theory model useful in describing interpersonal relations; the model helps explain and predict one phenomenon of concern—human interaction—although (perhaps *because*) it disregards some factors to focus on others.

It is important to understand that the conceptual models of the client to be discussed in the following sections are merely approximations of reality. They currently provide practitioners with a useful way of thinking about clients. If knowledge, purpose, or values change in the profession, the models are subject to change.

In addition to professional focus and conceptual models, each profession's *concept of causality* will be examined. *Causality* here means probable reasons for a health problem; the word *etiology* is commonly used to denote these reasons.

The way each profession names and classifies health problems will also be considered in a section on *classification systems*. It will be emphasized that the profession's purpose, focus, and conceptual models of the client are logically related to the phenomena named and classified. Lastly, each profession's *diagnostic process* will be discussed, with an emphasis on diagnostic skills.

NURSING

The nursing profession arose out of needs associated with human suffering. First seen as a religious calling to care for the injured, ill, or infirm, nursing was practiced within religious orders. Today religious nursing orders exist, but the majority of practitioners are secular.

Nursing has passed through historical phases parallel to those of social or religious movements. Similar to western society in general, nursing had its "dark ages" coinciding with periods of general social neglect of human suffering. "Renaissance" periods paralleled periods of humanitarianism and social reform. In contemporary society nursing has taken an increasingly active role in health care policy formation and health care delivery.

Public attitudes and values sanctioned the nursing profession in its early days and are still favorable, even in the general atmosphere of criticism of health care that currently prevails. Sometimes, in striving for ideals, nurses are more critical of nursing than the public is. In a Maryland legal association's study of a representative sample of households, nursing was held in highest regard among eight established professions in society ("Maryland Public," 1979, p. 2094).[2] Society sanctions a profession through state licensing laws. In the last 10 years these laws have expanded or clarified nurses'

---

[2] The professions included dentistry, medicine, law, teaching, and others.

social responsibility in health care. In many states, laws include statements about nursing diagnosis as a professional function. Delegated medical diagnosis and treatment is also permitted under some degree of supervision of the physician (V. C. Hall, 1975).

Nightingale's concept of nursing was formulated when she founded the profession; it is still current (1949). It emphasized helping both the sick and the well to perform activities that contribute to health and recovery. A definition of contemporary nursing is found in the American Nurses' Association Model Practice Act:

> The practice of nursing means the performance for compensation of professional services requiring substantial specialized knowledge of the biological, physical, behavioral, psychological, and sociological sciences and nursing theory as the basis for assessment, diagnosis, planning, intervention, and evaluation in the promotion and maintenance of health; the casefinding and management of illness, injury, or infirmity; the restoration of optimum function; or the achievement of a dignified death. Nursing practice includes but is not limited to administration, teaching, counseling, supervision, delegation, and evaluation of practice and execution of the medical regimen. . . . (American Nurses' Association, 1980a)

As generalists or specialists, nurses are involved in all levels of health care. These levels include (1) primary care, focusing on health maintenance and preventive care in clinics or community settings; (2) secondary care, which may or may not require hospitalization for common illnesses; and (3) tertiary care, requiring the sophisticated technology of specialized units.[3] In each level the focus is on individuals and families. Primary care may also include the health of communities. Recognized areas in which nurses specialize include (1) settings, such as community health; (2) age groups, such as geriatrics and child health; and (3) health problems, or health states, such as maternal, medical-surgical, and psychiatric–mental-health specialties.

Some nurses have private practices. This is most common in the psychiatric–mental-health specialty. Reimbursement to clients through insurance payments may increase private practice in this and other specialties in the future. Most nurses are employees of health care institutions. This arrangement can sometimes present a dilemma to the practitioners because of conflicts between institutional and professional values. In fact, this conflict is experienced to some extent by members of all the health professions.

Professional Focus

All health professions are concerned with human behavior. Differences exist in the way health problems are conceptualized and labeled and the level of understanding sought. For example, medicine's predominant focus is on human biological phenomena, conceptualized as disease states. Understanding is sought at the cellular or subcellular level.

Historically, the focus of nursing has been individual, family, or community needs relevant to health and welfare. These needs have ranged broadly, from sanitation in a community to energy conservation in an individual. Generalizing across specialties

---

[3] These are levels of care required by clients as opposed to primary, secondary, and tertiary *preventive intervention*, which is a model of intervention.

and practice settings, the concern has consistently been humans' optimal function in their environment.

Although expressed in various terms, the specific phenomena nursing addresses are potential or actual functional problems. Potential problems can result from health-related practices and may predictably contribute to future illness of an individual, family, or community. Actual problems occur in association with illness or with social, occupational, or maturational changes.

Each of the professions seeks a certain level of understanding of the phenomena with which it deals. As new knowledge becomes available, the level may change. For example, a few decades ago physicists sought to understand the nature of matter at the atomic level; today, as a result of advances in knowledge and theory, subatomic particles are the level of interest.

Nurses seek to understand health-related behavior at the level of human organism-environment interaction. Clinical problems are viewed as holistic, or whole-person, expressions of this interaction, and diagnosis and intervention are performed within this holistic model. As we shall see in a later chapter, nursing theorists deal in different ways with the inherent complexity of this focus.

Underlying and supporting the focus of a profession is the art and science of practice. Theories, concepts, principles, and methods of treatment compose the science of a profession. The art is the way knowledge is used, especially in human interactions, and reflects attitudes, beliefs, and values. Yet there can never be a clear separation of art and science. Attitudes, beliefs, and values, whether internal or external to the profession, influence its science—particularly in the selection of methods, focus, and interpretations. Some interesting historical examples of the influence of changing beliefs and values on the naming and interpretation of diagnostic entities will be discussed in regard to medicine.

As would be expected in a profession with such a diverse practice focus and broad, holistic perspective, the body of clinical knowledge in nursing is extensive. Nursing science, as Rogers (1970) states, is only beginning to be identified. Currently the knowledge base for practice rests to a large extent on the application of biological, psychological, and social science theory. Extension of this knowledge in a way that is relevant to nursing concerns will develop the science of nursing.

The body of knowledge in a profession has to be descriptive, explanatory, and predictive. Increasing emphasis on clinical research in recent years has served to increase the science base of practice. Nursing diagnoses, because they isolate phenomena of concern to the profession, provide direction and focus for research and the development of nursing science.

Conceptual Frameworks of Practice

As stated previously, different professions have different perspectives that are expressed in their conceptual frameworks for guiding practice. One component of a framework is the conceptual model of the client which guides assessment and diagnosis. A brief consideration of the historical models of the client will help the reader understand the background of contemporary frameworks for nursing.

Out of the belief that gods, demons, or evil spirits caused suffering arose the sana-
toriums of ancient Greece. The priest-physicians and attendants of these temples of
healing were the forerunners of the religious nursing orders that arose when Christian-
ity spread through the world. From Kalisch and Kalisch's (1978) review of nursing
history, it appears that nursing and Christian charity were interwoven. The "client"
was seen as a "child of God," whether aged, infirm, orphaned, a casualty of war, or
lacking relatives and friends to provide care. Devotion to religion motivated men and
women of the Middle Ages to nurse the helpless in an evidently excellent manner
(Tappert and Lehman, 1976, p. 296).

Industrialization and urbanization in the eighteenth and nineteenth centuries were
accompanied by crowded living conditions, poverty, and devastating epidemics. The
capacity of the religious hospitals and asylums was strained, and secular nursing began.

In the eighteenth and nineteenth centuries, both in America and Europe, the
religious, devotional model of client care was lost in the public hospitals. Nurses were
hired attendants who used alcohol and snuff as a means of psychological escape from
the poor conditions. They were portrayed in all their depravity by Dickens's description of Sairy Gamp in mid-nineteenth–century England (Dickens, 1910, pp. 312-313).
The physicians of that day were not much better. In America, "a common saying was
that 'a boy who's unfit for anything else must become a doctor'" (Kalisch and Kalisch,
1978, p. 25). Interestingly, war provided the impetus for change.

The internationally recognized contributions of Florence Nightingale to the improvement of British military hospitals during the Crimean War and the postwar
humanitarian concern in Europe combined to change these conditions. In America
the Civil War brought about great changes in nursing. The changes of the late nineteenth and early twentieth centuries occurred in a social context: reform; women's
rights; and advances in health care, particularly asepsis and beginning control of
infectious disease. It must be remembered that these were the days where "common
law and biblical tradition bound women to an inferior status" (Kalisch and Kalisch,
1978, p. 71).

When modern nursing began, illness was believed to be nature's *remedy* for removing
the effects of conditions interfering with health. Neither nurses nor physicians "cured";
that was nature's realm. Out of Nightingale's experience with horrendous conditions
in the Crimean hospitals, the idea began to be expressed that a person had to be
considered in interaction with the environment (Nightingale, 1949, p. 26). Nature
could not cure if sanitation, diet, and living conditions were not improved.

The emphasis within the client-environment model was clearly on the environment.
The person was viewed from the perspective of a "dependency model." This perspective seemed logical when common practice dictated that the sick or injured were put
to bed. The rationale was to conserve "vital power" (Nightingale, 1859, p. 6); rest
and good living conditions were the major therapy for *all* illnesses. Ideally, the "rest
cure" was provided at home. It was the poor and uneducated of the cities, the travelers,
and the casualties from the battlefields who were brought to the hospital.

Clara Weeks Shaw, a contemporary of Nightingale, stressed the dependency model
of the client and the complementary "maternity model of nursing": The "sick person
is, for the time being, as a child and looks to his nurse for a mother's care" (Shaw,

1855, p. 19). This conception of nursing emphasized personal care, environmental comfort, and cleanliness.

Changes occurred in the first half of the present century. The dependency model was beginning to wane, influenced by society's focus on education of the masses, the mental hygiene movement, and advances in medical treatment. Nursing's participation and leadership in the public health movement of the late nineteenth century was also influential.

The nursing literature began to place stress on clients' regaining independence; this emphasis was reflected in discussions about learning hygienic practices, preventing illness, and using available community resources (Frederick and Northam, 1938, p. 3). This self-responsibility theme was further extended by Henderson (Harmer, 1955, p. 4; 1966). She wrote of the individual's physical strength, will, or knowledge to perform activities related to health and recovery; nursing was required when these factors were *absent*.

From the textbooks of the time it appears that the biomedical model of the human being, used by medicine, was adopted by nursing. There were nurses who independently determined the nursing care needed, but generally the doctor was responsible for identifying problems (medical problems). Nurses were supposed to know how to provide comfort, observe for disease complications, and report observations. The frequent mention in the literature of "needs" and "needs-for-help" suggests that a human needs model of the client predominated around midcentury.

Orlando (1961) published a model of practice referred to as the dynamic nurse-patient relationship. Included was a distress-coping model of the client. Her method of assisting and of judging the client's need for help had a great impact and is still pertinent today. Orlando's model, and later Orem's self-care model (1959, pp. 5-6; 1971) emphasized self-direction and individual responsibility. Nursing was to do only what the person and his or her resources could not do unaided.

One can see the increased complexity of the nursing model for practice that was evolving in the twentieth century. If people were to learn resonsibility for self-care and prevention of illness, nurses had to do more than carry out physicians' orders and administer routine personal care. They had to make judgments about what was needed and what was not.

Lydia Hall (1955, pp. 212-213) used the term *nursing process* in the early 1950s, and through the years her approach has evolved into the accepted method of delivering nursing care. The basic tenets of the Nightingale model—client-environment interaction, religious traditions of wholeness, self-direction, and will—were retained in twentieth-century nursing (Orem, 1959, pp. 5-6; Harmer, 1955, p. 4).

At midcentury the term *nursing diagnosis* appeared in the literature (McManus, 1950). Bonney and Rothberg (1963) employed the term *nursing diagnosis* in a client evaluation instrument to predict needs for nursing service. The objective was to use clients' nursing diagnoses as predictors of nurse staffing needs in long-term care facilities. Their report defined diagnoses as a "listing of factors" which affected the client's condition. The list was divided into strengths and liabilities. Lists rather than problems were formulated, yet this contributed to shifting the focus of description from nursing actions to client conditions.

In 1980 the American Nurses' Association published a social policy statement that identified the "phenomena of concern" to nurses as "human responses to actual or potential health problems" (1980b p. 9). Human responses were viewed as:

1 reactions of individuals and groups to actual problems (health-restoring responses), such as the impact of illness-effects upon the self, family, and related self-care needs; and

2 concerns of individuals and groups about potential problems (health-supporting responses), such as monitoring and teaching in populations or communities at risk in which educative needs for information, skill development, health oriented attitudes, and related behavioral change arise. (American Nurses' Association, 1980b, pp. 9–10)

These two areas of human responses are similar to the focus of nursing diagnosis previously identified in Chapter 1: problems in health management and problems secondary to illness, medical therapy, developmental changes, or life situations. The social policy statement reflects the current focus on clients' conditions (rather than nurses' actions) and the social responsibility for "diagnosis and treatment of human reponses" (American Nurses' Association, 1980b, p. 9).

In the last two decades many nursing theorists have proposed conceptual models to guide nursing diagnosis and treatment. Essentially, these models retain the client-environment focus (Newman, 1979, pp. 16-18). A few current conceptual models of practice will be reviewed in detail in Chapter 3.

Concept of Causality

A profession's concept of causality is the way its members view the cause-and-effect relationships existing between health problems and the factors that interact to produce them. Some philosophers argue that the concept of causality should be abandoned; others say it is so implicit in human thinking that it cannot be discarded. The notion of causality in nursing practice is rarely addressed, although Field (1979) has provided a review of this concept in science. This is not to suggest that the idea is not used in nursing. Clinically, one hears explanations of the causes of clients' problems that range from single to multiple factors. Simple reasons and single causes may be valued for their noncomplexity. Yet when asked to explain the cause of a patient's clinical problem, nurses tend to respond with explanations that include complex, multifactor chains of events. In Chapter 3 the subject of causality is discussed further and etiologic factors are considered.

Classification Systems

Diagnosis and systems for classifying the health problems addressed by nurses did not receive widespread attention in nursing until the 1970s. Considering the way modern nursing evolved, this may be difficult to understand. During the Crimean War Florence Nightingale, 24 nuns, and 14 other women diagnosed and treated health problems so effectively that the mortality rate in British military hospitals showed an overall drop from 42 percent to 2.2 percent (Kalisch and Kalisch, 1978, p. 42). Well before this, in the twelfth century, when women studied nursing and obstetrics at the University of Salerno, the famous treatise *Tortula on the Cure of Diseases of Women* was written by a midwife (Kalisch and Kalisch, 1978, p. 5).

At the end of the first century of modern nursing, concepts of practice emphasized procedures, tasks, and nursing functions. The first classification of nursing problems was for the purpose of education. A subcommittee of the National League for Nursing, while revising student record forms, perceived the need to describe generic nursing practice in terms of a patient-centered, as opposed to task-centered, focus. From a survey of more than 40 schools of nursing, the first classification—of 21 problems—was completed (Abdellah, 1959, pp. 83–88). As Table 2-1 shows, these now-famous "problems" were therapeutic goals of nursing. This was consistent with the emphasis at the time on client needs (therapeutic needs) and nursing problems (therapeutic problems).

Nursing was commonly described as a set of functions. In fact the numerous

TABLE 2-1
NURSING PROBLEMS CLASSIFICATION ACCORDING TO ABDELLAH, 1959

Master List of Nursing Problems Presented by Clients
To facilitate the maintenance of oxygen to all body cells
To facilitate the maintenance of nutrition of all body cells
To facilitate the maintenance of elimination
To facilitate the maintenance of fluid and electrolyte balance
To promote safety through the prevention of accident, injury, or other trauma and through the prevention of the spread of infection
To facilitate the maintenance of regulatory mechanisms or functions
To facilitate the maintenance of sensory function
To promote optimal activity: exercise, rest, and sleep
To maintain good body mechanics and prevent and correct deformities
To maintain good hygiene and physical comfort
To recognize the physiological responses of the body to disease conditions—pathological and compensatory
To identify and accept interrelatedness of emotions and organic illness
To identify and accept positive and negative expressions, feelings, and reactions
To facilitate the maintenance of effective verbal and nonverbal communication
To promote the development of productive interpersonal relationships
To facilitate progress toward achievement of personal spiritual goals
To accept the optimum possible goals in the light of limitations, physical and emotional
To use community resources as an aid in resolving problems arising from illness
To create or maintain a therapeutic environment
To understand the role of social problems as influencing factors in the cause of illness
To facilitate awareness of self as an individual with varying physical, emotional, and developmental needs

Source: Abdellah, 1959, pp. 83–88.

studies of nurses and nurses' functions caused Abdellah to comment that "as valuable as such studies are, they portray what the nurse is doing, not why she is doing what she is, nor if she should be doing what she is" (Abdellah, 1959, p. 74). Fifteen years would elapse before a change in the focus of nursing diagnosis would begin to provide answers to the questions she posed.

In 1966 Henderson identified a list of 14 basic human needs that comprised the components, or functions, of nursing. This formulation further supported the functional needs approach. These basic needs, listed in Table 2-2, address not health problems of the client but areas in which actual or potential problems could occur. Both Abdellah's and Henderson's lists were widely used in education and practice. Their contributions stimulated nurses to go beyond routine functions and tasks to identify therapeutic problems. This shift in focus set the stage for the next step—nursing diagnoses, or client problems as the focus of care.

The shift from care organized around therapeutic problems, such as "to facilitate the maintenance of effective verbal communication," to care organized around client problems, such as "impaired verbal communication," began in the early 1970s. This change was facilitated by the First National Conference on Classification of Nursing Diagnoses in 1973. The conference provided a beginning language with which to express judgments and to organize nursing care.

National conferences have been held approximately every 2 years since 1973. Hundreds of nurses have participated in the conference objective, to develop diagnostic nomenclature (a system of category names) and classify nursing diagnosis. The evolu-

TABLE 2-2
BASIC NEEDS CLASSIFICATION ACCORDING TO HENDERSON, 1966

Fourteen Basic Needs
Breathing normally
Eat and drink adequately
Eliminate body wastes
Move and maintain desirable postures
Sleep and rest
Suitable clothes—dress and undress
Maintain body temperature within normal range by adjusting clothing and modifying the environment
Keep body clean and well groomed and protect the integument
Avoid dangers in the environment and avoid injuring others
Communicate with others in expressing emotions, needs, fears, or opinions
Worship according to one's faith
Work in such a way that there is a sense of accomplishment
Play or participate in various forms of recreation
Learn, discover, or satisfy the curiosity that leads to normal development and health and use the available health facilities

Source: Henderson, 1966, pp. 16–17.

tion of the current classification system may be seen in Appendix F, which shows the changes, deletions, and additions that occurred in diagnostic categories in 1973, 1975, 1978, and 1980.

One could ask, What are nurses classifying? An examination of 1980 category names (Appendix A) would suggest that alterations in functions or functional patterns predominate. Ineffective, impaired, or altered human functions occur frequently in the listing. There is nearly a balance between physiological areas and psychosocial-spiritual areas. This division, of course, is invalid, since the signs and symptoms defining each category in many cases are biopsychosocial (Kim and Moritz, 1981).

A developing classification system requires some conceptual focus to ensure consistency in classifying so that, for example, *apples, dogs,* and *chairs* do not get classified together. Consistency among the diagnoses classified is provided by the conceptual focus or framework. The development of a classification system will be addressed in a later chapter. It is sufficient at this time to point out that several frameworks are available in nursing. Which shall be chosen? The decision of the conference group has been to identify what nurses say they treat, irrespective of the framework they employ.

Roy (1975, pp. 92-93) suggests that conceptual frameworks in the current nursing literature provide a basis for logically deducing diagnostic categories. The problem with this approach, as she notes, is how to choose among frameworks and how to resolve the disparate perspectives of the client reflected in the frameworks. Yet, she argues, the development of a diagnostic classification system is an urgent task in the profession. A number of nursing theorists are working with the national conference group to develop a conceptual framework to guide diagnostic category development.

This discussion of the evolving classification system illustrates the relationship between the conceptual focus of a profession and its system of classifying client conditions: The latter flows from the former. If a profession has multiple frameworks, must it also have multiple diagnostic "languages"? One hopes not; that would result in chaos.

Should a classification system reflect the traditional beliefs and values of a profession? Absolutely, when these values are still relevant in contemporary practice. Thus it is appropriate to ask, Does this evolving classification system (Appendix A) reflect both (1) nursing's concept of the client-environment interaction and (2) the philosophical and theological roots of nursing that have led to concern for wholeness, self-direction, and will? Some would say, Yes, as long as nurses implement care within this system of values and beliefs. Others would say, No, there is not an adequate reflection of holism.

Diagnostic Process

The diagnostic process as such has not been widely discussed in the nursing literature. Basic textbooks rarely mentioned nursing diagnosis or the process of diagnosing to any great extent before the 1970s. Yet assessment, with emphasis on information collection, has had widespread attention in the literature of the last 15 years.

Nurses assumed responsibility for noticing the effects of illness and the needs it produced. As nursing practice became more clearly defined, assessment became important for determining clients' needs for nursing care. Today diagnostic process skills are recognized as critical if clinical practice is to be maintained at an acceptable professional level. Professional standards mandate that nursing diagnoses be derived from health status data (American Nurses' Association, 1973).

Information collection and problem identification are viewed as the steps that make up the diagnostic, or assessment, process in nursing. Assessment for purposes of diagnosis requires history taking as well as examination of the client. Skill in observation and clinical interviewing are stressed as basic to adequate assessment. Stuart and Sundeen (1976, pp. 8-9) have presented a good overview of problem formulation, including the need for analysis, synthesis, and logical reasoning. Preciseness, specificity, conciseness, and neutrality of the diagnostic statement are emphasized by Little and Carnevali (1976, pp. 58-64). Gordon (1976) stresses (1) the complexity of diagnostic judgments in nursing, (2) error avoidance, and (3) the probabilistic nature of judgments. Doona (1976) also emphasizes the importance of the cognitive skill of judgment in nursing.

Little research (College of Nursing, Texas Women's University, 1979; Aspinall, 1976; Gordon, 1972, 1980) has been done on the diagnostic process actually used by nurses, but it may be expected to adhere to general principles of cognition and problem identification. One major problem, noted by Bloch (1974), is the lack of agreement on definitions of crucial terms within the profession, such as *assessment* and *diagnosis*.

Nurses are just beginning to make conscious applications of conceptual models of the client in their clinical activities. As this application progresses, one should see a logical relationship among the conceptual model utilized, the assessment data collected, and the types of problems diagnosed. The diagnostic process can then be more systematically applied.

MEDICINE

Medicine's view of diagnosis is of interest here because of the many myths that surround disease and because of the interrelatedness of nursing and medical care, especially in acute care settings. Background information about the profession will provide a context for viewing physicians' assumptions, concepts, and practices in regard to diagnosis.

People naturally seek explanations for experiences that have an impact on their lives. So it has been with illness and disease. When people explained illness as being caused by evil spirits, they called upon the medicine man for therapy. When illness was viewed as the result of transgressions against the gods, the priest acted as physician; medicine and theology were one. When people themselves and the environment began to be implicated in disease and illness, medicine began to emerge as a science and healing became a profession.

Medicine has been a highly influential health profession during most of this century, although it also has had its "dark ages" (Duffy, 1967, p. 136). Although physicians are fewer in number than some other groups of health professionals, society has looked to physicians for direction in health care and related policies. As a result, they share both the adulation of society, for health care advances, and the scorn for current deficiencies in health care provision. Physicians traditionally have assumed responsibility and authority in health care matters. They have been protective of their professional boundaries and have been seen by many as pursuing a paternalistic role toward other health professionals.

Clinical medicine is concerned with the diagnosis and treatment of disease. Practice is based largely on knowledge from biomedical sciences. These sciences seek to describe, explain, predict, and control events associated with pathophysiology or psychopathology. Understanding of illness is sought at the molecular level. For example, medical researchers in the area of congestive heart failure are attempting to describe chemical and physical derangements in the metabolic process of failing myocardial cells, and biochemical changes in the brain are being studied as a means of understanding psychiatric disorders.

High value is placed on scientific explanation in medicine. Scientific generalizations about patterns of disease and general responses to treatments are being sought. These generalizations from medical research have to be applied to individuals so they may be used in the clinical care of patients; this is the task of the medical practitioner. The ideal practitioner is described as one who can combine the scientific aspects of medicine with compassion and understanding of the individuality of human beings (Tumulty, 1973, p. 66).

Diagnosis is an accepted part of the clinical practice of medicine. Both physicians and the public place high value on avoidance of diagnostic error. The consequences of error may be death, disability, or unwarranted expense. Society has high expectations of physicians, as is attested by the frequency of malpractice claims and the size of compensations awarded. When "injury" in the legal sense results from poor judgment, carelessness, or ignorance, society awards compensation through the judicial system (Cassell, 1977). Thus the physician, in making a diagnosis and determining treatment, is faced with a moral and humanitarian concern for the individual patient as well as concern about personal legal liability.

The value placed on diagnostic expertise within the medical profession is reflected in the clinical training of medical students. Repeated experiences are given in diagnosis and treatment planning, review of decisions, and case conferences. Practicing physicians are expected to expand their diagnostic skills continually. Opportunities are provided in hospital rounds and conferences for colleague review.

In medicine it is assumed that one never ceases being a student. This attitude is reflected in the following passage from a medical textbook:

> A fine method of continuing education is to place one's self in a situation where he will be continuously checked on, where his diagnoses are questioned daily and his treatments frequently modified. This is done best in a teaching hospital where young physicians and old mutually teach and learn. It takes courage and it takes humility for the established practitioner to do this, but it pays tremendous rewards. The physician who is afraid to have his opinions scrutinized is already out of date. (Keefer and Wilkins, 1970, p. 1051)

Professional Focus

The professional focus of medicine is diagnosis and treatment of disease. Since late in the eighteenth century physicians have studied and labeled pathophysiological and psychopathological phenomena. Disease has been conceptualized as a lesion. Predisposing factors, the historical course, morbidity, and mortality of disease have been studied extensively.

Challenges to the concept of disease as a lesion have arisen. Obesity is an example; it is a deviation from a statistical norm, not a disease per se. In fact, in many instances it is considered a behavioral problem similar to drug addiction or alcoholism. With medicine's professional focus on disease and its conception of disease as a lesion, what shall be done with these conditions?

Blaxter (1978) observes a contemporary trend toward widening the boundaries of medicine into social, psychological, and behavioral fields; she notes that this appears to be a return to the Hippocratic idea of "the whole person in his environment." Card and Good, medical educators, have broadened the definition of disease to "displacement from the normal state of dynamic, self-regulating system" (1974, p. 60).

The observations of these British authors possibly reflect the large and well-established family practice component of British medical care. Many of the health problems encountered by physicians in family practice are psychosocial. On the other hand, even American medical literature is beginning to reflect the need for a broader professional focus. It will be interesting to note whether this broader focus becomes a reality in practice. If medicine expands its current professional and diagnostic focus, will it be expanding into other professions such as nursing or social work?

Conceptual Frameworks of Practice

As was stated earlier, a conceptual model or framework for practice is a mental construction. It is used to derive meaning and understanding, that is, to make sense out of phenomena that are puzzling or disturbing. In addition, conceptual models of practice in the professions reflect the culture and milieu of the times. Early medicine, in particular, had strong ties to philosophy and theology.

Throughout history people have observed in themselves and others deviations that produce discomfort or disability. These deviations have been explained and treated in various ways. In primitive times few differences existed between medicine, magic, and religion (Rivers, 1927; R. L. Engle, Jr., 1963). Illness was thought to be produced by sorcery or a higher power such as a deity. Something was in the body that did not belong, or something had been removed! This simple dichotomous model was associated with a logical approach: The diagnostic problem was to find the seat of disease. The model guided the search for the demon possessing the person, the sin committed, or the witch involved.

Rational elements in thinking existed side by side with the magical in primitive times. The idea that symptoms occurred in combinations (anticipating the present-day notion of symptom clusters, or syndromes) was deduced from observations of people experiencing illness. However, it was thought that the symptoms, for example, fever, *were* the disease.

Scientific medicine began in ancient Greece. Hippocrates, who is considered the father of modern medicine, and his students and followers at Cos believed illness was due to a state of disequilibrium. Health was a condition of perfect equilibrium. The model for practice within the Hippocratic school emphasized the wholeness of the person, as opposed to the mind-body dualism (separation) that arose later. Habits, lifestyle, pursuits, thoughts, sleep, and dreams were all of concern (Blaxter, 1978). This model was consistent with the philosophy of the times; the Greeks believed equilibrium and harmony with nature were fundamental to life.

The medical scholars of ancient Greece developed the humoral model to guide medical practice. Instead of a consequence of sin or demonic possession, illness was seen as a disequilibrium in the humors: blood, black bile, yellow bile, and phlegm. For example, in discussing convulsions (which were referred to as the "sacred disease" and associated with divine visitation), Hippocrates described the symptom cluster of inability to speak, choking, foaming at the mouth, clenching of the teeth, and convulsive movements. These symptoms, he thought, came about because the normal flow of phlegm from the brain to the mouth was blocked and phlegm consequently entered the blood vessels (King, 1971). Although this explanation of grand mal epilepsy sounds primitive today, it represented a dramatic departure from the previous explanatory model that combined theological and medical thought. One of the Hippocratic school's major influences on models for the practice of medicine was the idea that disease could be explained by natural causes such as the "humors" rather than supernatural or magical forces.

Building on the work of the Hippocratic school and influenced by Aristotelian philosophy, Galen introduced in the second century the idea that nature was a dynamic, active process directed toward the restoration of health. Interestingly, this is the root of the commonsense notion of the "healing power of nature." The Galenic concept of vitalism was based on a model of purposeful, goal-directed activity inherent in humans and attributed to a psyche, soul, or life-force (King, 1971, p. 13; Ruesch, 1963). The search for the cause and cure of disease was beginning to move from a focus on outside influences to one on factors within the person and the environment.

In the fifth and sixth centuries there were few challenges to the accepted explanations of events or to models of disease and medical practice. Most medical care continued to be based largely on models of mysticism, magic, and a few scientific elements. Like other disciplines, the fledgling science of medicine almost disappeared during the Dark Ages.

In contrast to the marked influence of theology and philosophy in earlier times, after the Renaissance biological and physical science influenced medical thought and models of practice. Scientific investigation of disease processes predominated. Use of the scientific method led to rational rather than magical thinking about illness. The alliance between medicine and the biological sciences became firmly established and formed the basis for the biomedical model used in medical practice today. In part, this alliance was the result of theological influences.

The influential Christian church of the fifteenth century supported a mind-body dualism in regard to the study of humans. This position, in response to physicians' and scientists' anatomical dissections, mandated that the investigation of physical and mental processes should be undertaken by two different groups. The body was viewed as "a weak and imperfect vessel for the transfer of the soul from this world to the next" (G. L. Engel, 1977), and therefore, in Christian thought, it could be objectively studied as a machine and subjected to scientific and medical investigation. The mind and soul were left to the philosophers or theologians, who used noninvasive study techniques. The assumption was that the whole human could be understood as a sum of the parts (G. L. Engel, 1977, p. 131). An implicit agreement existed between the church and those wishing to perform dissection to increase medical and biological knowledge: The mind and the soul would be ignored. According to Engel's (1977) analysis, this agreement was largely responsible for the anatomical and structural model upon which western scientific medicine was to evolve.

Medicine is committed to advancing knowledge of disease and treatment. It employs the scientific method, which has procedural rules for concept formation, the conduct of experiments, and validation of hypotheses by observations and experimentation. The less manageable behavioral or psychosocial dimensions of disease are generally ignored (psychiatry is an exception) so that observations can meet the standards of objectivity required by the scientific method.

The current biomedical model combines this dualistic separation of mind and body with a mechanistic model. Clients' diseases are viewed from the perspective of biophysical or biochemical processes. Thus in the biomedical model the body is conceptualized as a machine; disease represents breakdown of the machine, and treatment consists of repair of the machine (G. L. Engel, 1977).

The reader may wonder whether a pure scientific approach to clinical care is possible, since physicians deal with people rather than inanimate objects or machines. What probably occurs is that the clinician considers the disease an entity in itself; in a sense, it is abstracted from the person with the disease. Other implicit models of psychosocial behavior are probably used to interpret the *behavior* of the person and to plan therapy.

The components, or subsystems, of the biomedical systems model are listed in Table 2-3. Except in psychiatry, the personal and social system is generally limited to structural factors such as the patient's place in the family network and the number of siblings. This segregation and limitation is typical of the dualistic framework employed during diagnosis, which separates the biological from the psychosocial.

Shortcomings of this conceptual focus on biological (physiological) systems have been described by G. L. Engel (1977, pp. 129-136), who argues that full understanding of the patient requires additional concepts and models. McWhinney (1972) has pre-

TABLE 2-3
COMPONENTS OF THE BIOMEDICAL SYSTEMS MODEL

Cardiovascular system

Respiratory system

Gastrointestinal system

Genitourinary system

Neuromuscular system

Endocrine system

Reproductive system

Integumentary system

Personal and social system

sented essentially the same arguments. He recommends a general systems theory approach which would deal with different levels of organization, such as molecular, organ, system, person, and family levels. This, he argues, would provide a more holistic way of viewing the phenomena of concern in medical practice.

The current biomedical model of the client narrows the body of knowledge with which the physician has to deal. This narrowing permits the clinician to focus on the already vast knowledge in biomedical diagnosis and therapy and to use a relatively commonsense approach to the psychosocial aspects of disease.

The secondary position given to human psychosocial behavior in medical diagnosis has produced controversy, particularly in medical specialties such as psychiatry and family practice. According to Lazare (1973), psychiatry in fact frequently uses a combination of conceptual models, although the combination remains implicit. Lazare describes the biomedical model, psychological model, behavioral model, and social model. He concludes that all of medicine utilizes a multidimensional model of human behavior although not always in a conscious manner.

Concept of Causality

Various explanations of disease have dominated medical thinking down through the centuries. Ruesch comments that notions about what causes illness have remained relatively simple. Only five origins of illness are mentioned in the medical literature:

 1 Coercive intrusion into the organism of evil spirits, foreign objects, bacteria, or viruses.
 2 Deficient, excessive, or faulty intake of food, fluid, gases, poisons, or information.
 3 Deficient, excessive, or faulty output as it occurs in disordered elimination, excessive work and strain, inability to express feelings and thoughts, atrophy or hypertrophy of certain physical structures, or one-sided development of social and psychological functions.
 4 Loss of, or deficiency in, essential parts, for example, mental deficiency, castration, abortion, sensory defects, mutilation, loss of love objects, or loss of hope.
 5 Disintegration of orderly structures as in cancer, toxic states, senile psychoses, or breakdown of social relations and patterns of communication. (Ruesch, 1963, pp. 506–507)

The search for causation of disease has always been based on the need to understand, prevent, and treat. Indeed, there have been historical relationships between the prevailing notion of cause and the methods of treatment. A good example is the "removing" of disease by bleeding and purging the patient, which a generation later was supplanted by "building up" the patient with iron and diet (Berman, 1954).

In general the etiology of disease (the theory of causation) and the effect (disease state) have been viewed as having a linear, or direct, relationship. The doctrine has been that one basic main cause, known or unknown, existed for each disease. This single-causation hypothesis has dominated scientific medicine since the demonstration that a particular microorganism caused a particular infection. The goal has been to find the one cause for each disease entity. When cause is known, control can be instituted.

Science, in general, has moved to multicausation (many interacting causal factors) hypotheses. Multicausation is currently under discussion by physicians but not fully accepted in medical practice. Walter states that "the doctrine of one cause for one disease has certainly failed to be a profitable concept in the search for the etiology of many common diseases, such as cancer, arteriosclerosis, emphysema, and chronic bronchitis" (Walter, 1977, p. 3). According to Thomas (1978, p. 462), the multi-factorial approach to the cause of human illness is now "in fashion"; infectious diseases are the exception. He groups current notions of causality into two classes, environ-ment and lifestyle. Facetiously he describes the ultimate unified theory of causality that would appeal to the entire "political" spectrum:

> At the further right, it is attractive to hear that the individual, the good old free-standing, free-enterprising American citizen, is responsible for his own health and when things go wrong it is his own damn fault for smoking and drinking and living wrong (and he can jolly well pay for it). On the other hand, at the left, it is nice to be told that all our health problems, including dying, are caused by failure of the community to bring up its members to live properly, and if you really want to improve the health of the people, research is not the answer; you should upheave the present society and invent a better one. At either end you can't lose. (Thomas, 1978, p. 463)

In clinical practice, everyday thinking probably ignores the possibility of multi-factorial causes. The simplified view prevails, that there is one cause of disease, whether that cause is known or unknown. Contributing or predisposing factors such as lifestyle may be considered but tend not to receive as much attention as metabolic derange-ments. Vaisrub describes the current divergent viewpoints this way:

> Suspended between the polarities of the known and completely unknown, multi-factorial etiology can be interpreted in two ways. It can be regarded as a combina-tion of factors, each contributing its share to the causation of a disease. Although one or more of these factors predominate in an individual case, none can be re-garded as a single, specific cause. In fact, it can be assumed tacitly or explicitly that no single specific cause exists, and the pursuit of such cause would be futile.
>
> On the other hand, multifactorial etiology can be viewed as a temporary ad hoc concept, which will do until a specific cause, *the* cause, will be discovered. Pre-senting this view, Thomas (1978) cites tuberculosis as an example of a disease that might have been easily consigned to a multifactorial etiology before the tubercle bacillus was identified as its cause. Like cancer, tuberculosis involves many organs and is influenced by environmental factors. Fortunately, the causa-tive organism was discovered, and the disease escaped the multifactorial label before it was invented. (Vaisrub, 1979, p. 830)

Classification Systems

Discrimination among types of illnesses existed in primitive spiritual medicine; names were assigned to such conditions as loss of consciousness and convulsions. Many of the present labels for diseases are inherited from Greek and Roman civilizations (Fejos, 1963, pp. 52–53).

The beliefs and values of a society influence societal concepts of what shall be classified as health and illness. Leavitt and Numbers (1978, p. 13) comment, "Ideas, like individuals and institutions, have their own histories and concepts of sickness and health are no exception. What one generation of Americans may have considered an illness, another regarded as perfectly normal." Normality, they point out, is socially defined and in part rests upon familiarity.

The more familiar a condition is, the less likely it is to be labeled abnormal. For example, childbirth and malaria, once considered normal, now are generally thought to require medical attention. On the basis of social beliefs and values, some conditions have shifted from sin to sickness and from sickness to normality.

Masturbation has had quite a history; once it was classified as sin, then it was considered a sickness, and now it is thought of as normal (Englehardt, 1978). Alcoholism, drug addiction, and obesity, at one time crimes and vices, are now considered illnesses (Leavitt and Numbers, 1978, p. 13). "Nervousness," hysteria, and other so-called self-indulgent female maladies were legitimized as illnesses when labeled *neurasthenia.* Neurasthenia also provided a reasonably respectable label to apply to the symptoms when they were experienced by men. The relabeling of neurasthenia served to establish a clientele for the new specialty of neurology in the early twentieth century (Sickerman, 1978).

Nosography, the systematic description and classification of diseases, began in the eighteenth century. Nosography arose because of a need to analyze the causes of death in the population. A model for classification existed; 100 years earlier botany had established its taxonomy (classification). By the year 1893, an international classification system for mortality statistics was developed. It had 161 diagnostic titles and was referred to as the *International Classification of Diseases* (ICD).

Today this classification contains 1040 categories and is the official international code for reporting morbidity and mortality statistics. Its periodic review is sponsored by the World Health Organization (1977). The American *Hospital Adaptation of International Classification of Diseases–Adapted* is the official code in the United States. It is used for discharge analysis of hospital records by the Committee for Professional and Hospital Activities of the Joint Committee on Accreditation of Hospitals.

In the specialty of psychiatry, mental disorders are classified in the *Diagnostic and Statistical Manual of Mental Disorders (DSM III)*, developed by the American Psychiatric Association. This manual "contains a multiaxial system emphasizing psychosocial factors" (Talbott, 1980, p. 25). The manual presents the first classification system that codes five client dimensions: mental disorders, personality and developmental disorders, physical disorders, psychosocial stress severity, and highest level of adaptive function in the last year. It is suggested that some axes will also be relevant to evaluations done by activity therapists, social workers, nurses, psychologists, and others.

A number of psychiatric classifications have been based on intensive study of single client cases in a prescientific era. This historical fact led to criticism of the American

Psychiatric Association's *DSM II*, particularly because of the overlap in various diagnostic classifications. There is generally thought to be little support for specific clinical diagnoses, such as *paranoid schizophrenia* or *anxiety reaction*, and only general support for broad categories, such as *functional psychosis, psychoneurosis,* or *organic psychosis.* The recently published *DSM III* addresses some of the previous concerns.

Many other classification systems are in use in medicine and medical specialties. They vary depending on their purpose. As Engle and Davis have observed (1963, p. 517), problems exist because there is no unified concept of disease that could be used as an organizing principle. Disease and diagnosis may be based on "gross anatomical defects, microscopic changes, so-called specific etiological agents, specific deficiencies, genetic aberrations, physiologic or biochemical abnormalities, constellations of clinical symptoms and signs, organ and system involvement, and even just description of abnormalities" (Engle and Davis, 1963, p. 517). Another problem is that diagnoses are not always well defined, often lacking specific etiologies.

Vague definitions of diagnostic categories decrease accuracy and reliability. As understanding of diseases improves, the uncertainty about using categories decreases. Engle and Davis (1963, pp. 517-519) describe four levels of certainty associated with the use of various medical diagnoses. The levels of certainty are reflected in (1) category definition, (2) clarity of etiology, and (3) variances in the clinical picture (from person to person, or environment to environment). Sickle cell anemia (abnormal hemoglobin) is at the first level of certainty. The collagen diseases are ambiguous and are classed at the fifth, or lowest and most uncertain, level.

Diagnostic Process

In medicine, diagnostic skills are highly valued. Accordingly, much attention has been directed toward understanding and teaching the diagnostic process. Here it will suffice to consider briefly the elements of the process as it is used in clinical medicine.

The physician's purpose during diagnosis is to observe for any manifestations of illness and, secondly, to conceptualize the manifestations in terms of diagnostic categories. The information physicians collect during the medical history and physical examination is standardized. Each physician uses essentially the same format, which leads to consistency in the clinical data base and consistency among physicians.

Interpretation, analysis, and utilization of the information is facilitated because classifications of diseases correspond to the history and examination categories. For instance, one category of the history format relates to the gastrointestinal system. A physical examination of organs within this system is also done. Correspondingly, a set of gastrointestinal disease categories exist. From a cognitive perspective, clustering information according to an area of concern facilitates diagnosing disease of that area if such a disease is present.

Additionally, the basic information to be collected in each category is delineated in the standard data base. For instance, during the history a client is asked about the following gastrointestinal functions: appetite, digestion, nausea, vomiting, hematemesis, abdominal pain, food idiosyncrasies, jaundice, bowel habits, constipation, diarrhea, stools, hemorrhoids, hernia, and use of cathartics. These inquiries screen for the major diseases of the system. If the client's complaint suggests pathology, further review of symptoms is done. Laboratory tests may be used to supplement the clinical data.

This rather detailed description serves two purposes. First, it provides an overview of the process of collecting information in medicine. Second, it provides an example of a system that conserves cognitive capacity and facilitates information processing. We will return to these points in a later chapter.

Physicians use a hypothetico-deductive method in diagnosis (Elstein, Schulman, and Sprafka, 1978). This is an effective method, according to research findings about how human beings attain concepts. Hypothetico-deductive thinking involves careful observation and generation of diagnostic hypotheses about what early clinical data indicate. By deduction it is reasoned that if a hypothesis is true then certain cues should be present. Information is collected to test the hypothesis. On the basis of the information collected, diagnostic hypotheses are retained, discarded, or altered.

The emphasis placed on clinical reasoning and diagnosis in medicine has provided a fertile field for research by psychologists. Traditionally, "bedside diagnosis" has been considered an art involving a large component of clinical intuition. In recent years there has been more acceptance of the fact that this "intuition" is a logical process that can be taught, not a mysterious skill that is absorbed in apprenticeship training.

SOCIAL WORK

Social work, in comparison to medicine and nursing, has had a relatively short history. It arose out of the nineteenth-century Charitable Societies, which were designed to relieve poverty and suffering, reform the maladjusted, and, especially, relieve the community of the burden and unpleasantness of poverty (Robinson, 1978, p. 36).

The profession's traditions lie in social causes and a concern for the helpless of society. Its practitioners have been influential in the formulation of social policy at governmental levels by focusing attention on social conditions that influence the quality of life (Morris, 1977, p. 353). Social work has been referred to as the conscience of society, prodding it to recognize and deal with social problems (Cooper, 1977, p. 361). Through the social services it delivers, it is also the profession that reflects and implements contemporary social attitudes and values (Dean, 1977).

This twofold purpose can present a dilemma to the practitioner of social work, especially if he or she is employed by a public social welfare agency. In one sense the social worker is an agent of society, obliged to carry out its public programs and enforce conformity to the existing social environment, attitudes, and values. On the other hand the profession is committed to improving social services, the social environment, and the quality of life; these objectives may not always be consistent with current values or financial commitments.

As may be expected from the diversity of social problems within different age groups, social work deals with a variety of problems in a variety of settings. The unifying factor in the profession is its primary commitment to people, to society, and to the interrelationships between people and society. Differing viewpoints of professional purposes either emphasize the individual in interaction with society or focus upon the society and its impact on people (Simm, 1977, p. 394).

These viewpoints are reflected in the diverse areas of practice in which social workers engage. A large number are involved in social planning activities, but approximately 52 percent of social workers deliver direct care to individuals and families (Morales, 1977, p. 392). One example of practitioners who focus on the individual are the clinical caseworkers who provide psychotherapy through private practice or on mental health teams. Others who develop, modify, or administer social service programs focus on the society and its impact on people. Carroll (1977) has developed a three-dimensional model to encompass all the diverse areas of social work practice. As may be seen in Figure 2-1, the model incorporates the phenomena that are of concern, that is, social problems; the units that are of concern, from individuals to societies; and the technologies characteristic of social work practice, such as family therapy or social planning (Carroll, 1977, p. 431).

Currently, social workers are seeking licensure by the states in which they practice; a few states have licensure for clinical activities (nonmedical psychotherapy) (Morales, 1977, p. 390). A clear definition of social work practice is specified in the National Association of Social Workers Model Licensing Act. It defines social work practice as

. . . service and action to effect changes in human behavior, a person's or persons' emotional responses, and the social conditions of individuals, families, groups, organizations, and communities, which are influenced by the interaction of social, cultural, political, and economic systems. (Morales, 1977, p. 390)

It is within these areas of practice that the social caseworker, who treats individuals and families, interacts most frequently with physicians and nurses. Thus we will examine this area of practice most closely.

The typical pattern of casework practice in health care institutions (hospitals, clinics, and community health care agencies) is to assist clients and families with social problems referred by nurses or physicians. For example, a patient with a medical illness may have a problem, such as unsatisfactory living conditions, which contributes to the illness. Referral to the medical social worker in the social service department of

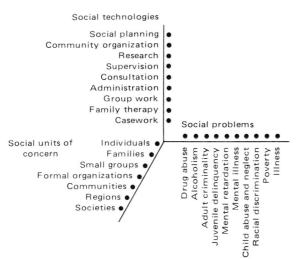

FIGURE 2-1
A three-dimensional model of social work practice. (*Adapted from Carroll, 1977, p. 431. Used with permission.*)

the institution can bring assistance to the patient and specialized knowledge of community resources.

In another situation, a multiproblem family may require coordination of social services in the community, such as child care, vocational counseling, and welfare. The social worker can coordinate these services on a long-term basis and help the family learn how to deal with their problems. Through client contacts, the need for programs may also become evident to a worker in the community and efforts may be made to engage the community in developing services, such as social programs for the elderly.

Professional Focus

In contrast to medicine, which seeks to understand clinical problems of clients at the molecular or physiochemical level, social casework emphasizes the intrapsychic, interpersonal, and social level of understanding. It draws heavily on psychological, psychiatric, and sociological theory in its practice.

The social problems addressed by the profession, according to Reid (1977, p. 374), are "social" in two senses: (1) the problematic behavior has social consequences for the individual or family, or (2) the problem is troubling society. Reid identifies broad problem areas, such as mental illness and emotional distress, difficulties in interpersonal relationships, dysfunctional and deviant behavior, and inadequate resources (unsuitable living arrangements, insufficient income, lack of health care, and the like).

Diagnosis was introduced into the practice of social work in its early years and influenced the development of casework. Also influential was an alliance with psychiatry and psychoanalytic thought (Germaine, 1970, p. 13). Today, consistent with the profession's modern focus, diagnoses describe problems, or social dilemmas, in the context of the client's interaction with the world.

Some schools of thought within the profession do not rely heavily on diagnostic categorization of clients' problems but do use a narrative type of problem identification as part of practice. Each of the four major approaches to casework (psychosocial, functional, problem-solving, and behavioral) defines the concept of *social problem* differently (Roberts and Nee, 1970, pp. 33-218). Some suggest that the diversity in practice negates a unified approach. They argue that a uniform conceptualization of the problems addressed by social work is needed to clarify professional objectives (Reid, 1977, p. 374).

Conceptual Models of Practice

It seems that as long as human beings form relationships in groups or societies, problems will arise. In noncomplex societies these problems are usually handled within families, tribal communities, or religious groups. When societies undergo rapid social and technological changes, as did western society with the advent of the Industrial Age, social problems arise that overtax the known ways of handling them. This was the situation in the nineteenth century when changes caused by industrialization produced stresses in the social order.

Charitable associations began to supplement the efforts of families and religious groups; "friendly visitors," the volunteers of these organizations, were dispatched to the homes of the poor. As an example, in Boston in 1884 there were 600 who visited "drunkards and their families and the poor widows with dependent children" (Robinson, 1978, p. 36). To relieve the conditions of poverty, they used advice, persuasion, and exhortation, as was dictated by the *Handbook for Friendly Visitors of the New York Society* ("Handbook," 1883).

The model for practice at that time, if it can be called such, rested firmly on the society's belief that hard work, thrift, and a belief in the Almighty would lead to individual success, thereby eliminating poverty and degradation (Robinson, 1978, p. 36). In the early twentieth century the voluntary charity workers, as well as the associations for which they worked, became organized and the newly paid workers began to seek professional status. That was the beginning of the social work profession and the beginning of the development of conceptual models for practice. In order for these new workers to differentiate themselves from nurses in institutions, and in order to implement the scientific commitment inherited from the philanthropy movement, caseworkers adopted the medical process: study, diagnose, treat (Germaine, 1970, pp. 16-22).

Richmond greatly influenced this new profession with a book on social diagnosis (Richmond, 1917). It emphasized the "scientific" collection of information about the person as a basis for diagnosis. The approach to practice that utilized Richmond's ideas was referred to as the diagnostic school of thought.

Conceptual models were borrowed from medicine, particularly psychiatry, and from psychoanalytic theory, probably because of the events of that era. Caseworkers were needed to handle not only the demands of the poor in society but also the large numbers of emotional problems of veterans and their families after World War I. The birth of the mental health movement in the second decade of the twentieth century also influenced the practice models that developed in social casework (Germaine, 1970, p. 16).

The model for practice during the 30s and beyond was derived from personality theory, particularly Freudian. Patients' conscious, preconscious, and unconscious thoughts were examined in order to understand problematic behavior (Germaine, 1970, p. 18). The use of the medical process model and psychoanalytic theory brought with it an emphasis on problems of the individual. This focus on individuals represented a change from the earlier emphasis on social problems and social causes. It produced controversy in the profession for many years, and the issue is still debated.

Today some conceptual models of social work practice emphasize the *service* aspect and focus upon the therapeutic *method* of practice, that is, what social workers do in handling clients' problems. In contrast, the diagnostic model (now referred to as the psychosocial model of practice) still strongly advocates the need for diagnostic classification, particularly clinical diagnosis (Hollis, 1970, p. 53).

With the increased development of knowledge in sociology, particularly role theory, the psychosocial model has broadened from the conception proposed by Richmond in 1917 and the personality focus. Theoretical constructs are derived from the behavioral sciences and include anthropological and cultural theories. The theories from these behavioral sciences in addition to theories developed in the profession are used to conceptualize the problems of clients, such as character disorders, alcoholism, and drug addiction. Traditionally, medical and psychiatric caseworkers have used the psychosocial model.

Within this model of practice the client is viewed from a systems perspective and diagnosis is directed toward the "person-situation gestalt" (Hollis, 1970, pp. 33–76). This client model includes both the individual and the social environment as the entity of concern. Included in the concept of the social environment are social roles (family, work, social groups), the educational milieu, and other social systems.

Consistent with a systems theory approach, it is assumed that changes in one part of the mutual interaction between person and social environment, such as a role change, changes the entire system's equilibrium. In the use of this model, the phenomena of concern to the social caseworker are interadaptational problems. These include problems that arise in the subsystems of the client-situation complex, that is, the individual, the situation, or the interaction between individual and social environment. These problems of equilibrium or adaptation of the person-situation complex are the focus for social intervention in the psychosocial approach to casework (Hollis, 1970, pp. 50-51).

Other conceptual models of social casework either bypass the diagnostic step in the clinical process or have a different conception and utilization of diagnosis. In some approaches diagnosis is seen as part of treatment, with treatment conceived as the client-therapist relationship process. This viewpoint results in an emphasis on diagnosis as a *process* for specifying the problem, rather than a basis for categorization prior to treatment. For example, the *functional approach to casework,*[5] as described by Smalley (1970, pp. 77-128), uses the term *diagnosis* but views it as an insight the client arrives at in relation to his or her problem. The "diagnosis" constantly changes as the client progresses during the relationship.

The *problem-solving model* of casework uses the term *diagnosis* to refer to the specification of the problem to be worked on at a particular time; diagnosis is an ongoing process as the client and caseworker together define the client's perception of the objective problem and subjective involvement in the problem. In this model the caseworker identifies the client's motivation and ability to solve the problem and the social means or resources available to the client (Perlman, 1970, pp. 129-180). As the name of the model implies, the focus is on guiding the client in problem solving. The social problem is not of maximum concern but, rather, the person's problem-solving motivation and ability.

All models for practice include a diagnostic statement although some do not label it as such. Due to the lack of agreed-upon nomenclature to summarize the clinical assessment, or due to the low value placed on specific problem identification and diagnostic classification, usually the caseworker writes a paragraph or more narrating the problem(s). There is no generally accepted structure and format for the diagnostic statement.

---

[5] The functional approach is characterized by its focus on objectives and function of the social agency, which are viewed as directly influencing the worker's role. The agency is seen as a system that may be the object of change as well as the instrument for social change (Germaine, 1970, p. 17).

Concept of Causality

At the turn of the century, under the influence of the mechanistic physics of Newton, cause and effect were viewed as directly related. Each effect had one cause. It was believed that if the cause of a social problem could be found, the cure would be obvious (Germaine, 1970, pp. 10-11).

Today the high degree of complexity of social problems is recognized in the profession. Within the model of person-situation complex, the cause of a problem can reside in the *person* or in the *situation.* Actually, it is more likely to be found in the *relationship pattern* or transaction between the two (Germaine, 1970, p. 29). Thus these three main elements have to be considered when determining causality, and multicausation is usually found.

In addition, all three aspects of the person-situation complex demonstrate growth, change, and potentiality. *Potentiality* refers to emergent capabilities such as new behaviors. Germaine suggests that to be "in accord with the modern scientific viewpoint, this requires that casework view and handle phenomena in terms of directions, flow, action and transaction, rather than in terms of cause" (Germaine, 1970, p. 29). This idea will become clearer when addressed in more detail in Chapter 3 in relation to a conception of causality used in nursing.

Classification Systems

In social work, as stated earlier, there is no generally accepted typology, or classification, of social problems. An attempt was made early in the history of the profession to specify the domain of problems addressed. With Richmond's concept of social diagnosis (Richmond, 1917) as a stimulus, in 1929 an alphabetical listing of casework problems was developed. The problems ranged from alcoholism to vagrancy (American Association of Social Workers, 1929).

Recent authors addressing the subject of a diagnostic classification system appear to agree with Reid's argument:

> The compelling advantage of formulating social work's objectives in terms of the problems it seeks to solve is that this formulation provides a clear basis for organizing and interpreting professional efforts, a basis that can be precisely explained and generally understood. (Reid, 1977, p. 376)

Classifications cited in the literature (Ackerman, 1958, p. 329; Ripple and Alexander, 1956, pp. 38-54) are specific for certain problem areas, for example, family therapy. Reid (1977, p. 374) proposes four areas of social work practice that could guide the conceptualization of specific problems: intrapersonal, interpersonal, personal-environmental, and environmental. Lowenberg (1977, pp. 53-54) specifies a set of three: interpersonal relationships, formal relationships, and role transaction. The examples given within these typologies range from symptoms to broad problem areas.

It is obvious from the literature in this field that a number of issues have to be resolved before a diagnostic classification system can be developed. The need for decisions about the domain of practice, a theoretical system to organize diagnostic categories, and determination of the unit of classification (individual, family, or community) are stressed by authors who advocated a classification system (Selby, 1958, pp. 341–349; Finestone, 1960, pp. 139–154).

Irrespective of whether the social work profession will undertake development of a classification system, the value of doing so has been recognized. Finestone (1960, p. 139) views this task as providing rich rewards for systematic theory building, for organizing knowledge for teaching, and for making practice more effective.

Diagnostic Process

As may be recalled from the discussion of other professions' diagnostic processes, information collection, analysis, and synthesis are broad common steps necessary to arrive at a concept of the state of the client and to label that state for purposes of treatment. In all the conceptual models of practice in social work, the collection of information is stressed as an important clinical activity. It is viewed as a means of understanding the client's problem and is an ongoing process. The information-collection process is referred to as casework assessment; it incorporates history taking.

All the models of practice emphasize the dual purpose served by information collection—the simultaneous establishment of a relationship with the client and acquisition of useful clinical information. Both of these purposes are probably of crucial importance in this profession, considering the focus of concern—social problems —and the psychosocial nature of the clinical data required. It is logical to expect that only after the caseworker has established trust and communicated empathic concern will the client share this type of personal information.

Some practice models stress to a great extent that treatment begins immediately. No doubt this is true. In the collection of psychosocial information, listening is required. Therapeutic outcomes may result as clients verbalize feelings and perceptions, the clinical data. In addition, clients may gain insights by relating a problem to another person. For all these reasons, social casework emphasizes the importance of the initial phase of interaction with the client in which assessment and problem identification occur.

Hollis (1970), who advocates the psychosocial approach to casework, states that the purpose of assessment is to deduce, from the information available and background knowledge of human behavior or social situations, the client's problem and what contributes to it. This deduction can then be used to determine the need and focus for change as well as the casework methods to be applied.

The data-collection method that is advocated is consistent with the psychosocial model. Hollis (1970, p. 51) states that assessment focuses on the client-situation complex, which "must be viewed repeatedly against a series of approximate norms of average expectancies 1) concerning behavior of the client and others, 2) concerning pertinent aspects of his social situation, and 3) concerning concrete realities."

The client-situation complex is viewed from sociological and psychological perspectives in order to collect information in problematic areas and to identify the scope of etiological factors involved (Hollis, 1970, p. 52). No one generally agreed upon systematic format (history form) for collecting a clinical data base is used in casework.

In social work, as in other professions, *analysis* of clinical data is emphasized. In order to make a decision about treatment, the caseworker must have an accurate and precise understanding of the problem(s). Hollis (1970, p. 52) recommends that alternative conceptions of the client and his or her situation be considered by examining the clinical data from various frames of reference. Middleman and Goldberg (1974, pp. 88–89) suggest to social workers three areas for analysis: (1) patterns of interaction in the client's various social roles, (2) content themes that point to areas of concern, and (3) metamessages (usually nonverbal) underlying overt expressions.

Caution is suggested in case analyses to avoid (1) stereotyping, which results from faulty deductive thinking; (2) overgeneralization from experiences that may not be representative; and (3) oversimplification of cause, such as single-focused explanations. The last two represent faulty inductive thinking (Lowenberg, 1977, p. 261). Any of these three practices can lead to diagnostic errors.

Concise diagnostic classification is not generally found in social work except when terms borrowed from psychiatry can be used. This situation exists even among caseworkers using the psychosocial (diagnostic) approach. Hollis, in her review of this model of practice, states that three types of diagnostic inferences are employed:

> These inferences will be mainly of three types: dynamic, etiological and classificatory. (1) In the *dynamic* diagnosis we examine, among other things, how different aspects of the client's personality interact to produce his total functioning. We look at the interplay between the client and other people and at other systems and the interactions within them to understand how change in one part of a system may affect another. The dynamics of family interaction are particularly important here and form a large part of what is often referred to as a family diagnosis. (2) *Etiological* factors are looked for, whether these lie in the current interactions or in preceding events which still actively affect the present and are among the causes of the client's dilemma. Usually, causation is seen as the convergence of a multiplicity of factors in the person-situation configuration. The dynamic and etiological aspects of the diagnosis together provide both a "linear" and an interactional or "transactional" view of causation. Where antecedents exist they are noted; they are usually seen as multiple. At the same time the continuous action between and among the various causative components in the transactional sense is an integral part of understanding the nature of the client-situation gestalt. (3) Effort is made to *classify* various aspects of the client's functioning, including, where pertinent and possible, a clinical diagnosis. (Hollis, 1970, p. 51–52)

SUMMARY

Neither nursing diagnosis nor client care is done in isolation. Nurses, physicians, social workers, and others have to collaborate if clients are to receive coordinated care. Understanding one's own and others' viewpoints is the first step toward collaborative practice. To take this first step was one of the purposes of this chapter.

The second purpose was to help the reader further define nursing diagnosis. Various concepts of diagnosis were compared and contrasted to promote understanding. The discussion pointed out that nursing traditionally has been concerned with individuals, families, and communities. Social work and medicine also have this broad area of concern. Actually, three professions evolved because of needs individuals, families, or society could not meet by themselves. Needs are expressed as societal mandates to the professions.

Although each profession follows essentially the same process for determining clients' needs, the information processed differs. Nurses, physicians, and social workers determine the need for professional services by collecting information and defining problems. Good judgment is valued in each profession and each sees itself as a helping profession. The three groups' distinctiveness lies in their social mandates and the models of practice developed from those.

Nursing, in contrast to the other two professions, has traditionally taken a holistic view of clients and their situations. Nurses are concerned with the broad range of human functional responses to life situations. Both physicians and social workers specialize in *areas* of the client's situation—disease and social problems, respectively.

Each profession uses conceptual frameworks for practice that are consistent with its mandate and concerns. If psychosocial problems are the focus of concern, then logically the model of the client should promote the collection of psychosocial information; if disease is the phenomenon of interest, then attention is directed toward pathophysiological or psychopathological manifestations. The focusing of attention leads to the naming and classification of conditions the profession can address. Thus there is consistency between a profession's focus and its classification systems.

Essentially the same cognitive processes are applied by each profession, but the focus for their application differs. The information collected, concepts used to interpret information, and the problems addressed vary. Generally, these differences are reflected in professional care.

The reader may not be sure that a clear understanding of *nursing's* focus has been attained. General aspects of a belief system have been emphasized but the topic of specific conceptual frameworks for diagnosis has been skirted. The next chapter will be devoted to this topic; as previously stated, a specific conceptual focus for diagnosis is crucial for its definition.

BIBLIOGRAPHY

Abdellah, F. G. Improving the teaching of nursing through research in patient care. In L. E. Heidgerken (Ed.), *Improvement of nursing through research.* Washington, D.C.: Catholic University of America Press, 1959.

Ackerman, N. W. *Psychodynamics of family life.* New York: Basic Books, 1958.

American Association of Social Workers. *The Milford conference report.* New York: American Association of Social Workers, 1929.

American Nurses' Association. *Standards of nursing practice.* Kansas City, Mo.: American Nurses' Association, 1973.

American Nurses' Association. *The nursing practice act: Suggested state legislation.* Kansas City, Mo.: American Nurses' Association, 1980. (a)

American Nurses' Association. *A social policy statement.* Kansas City, Mo.: American Nurses' Association, 1980. (b)

Aspinall, M. J. Nursing diagnosis—The weak link. *American Journal of Nursing,* July 1976, *24,* 433–437.

Berman, A. The heroic approach in 19th century therapeutics. *Bulletin of the American Society of Hospital Pharmacists,* 1954, *11,* 320–327.

Blaxter, M. Diagnosis as category and process: The case of alcoholism. *Social Science and Medicine*, 1978, *12*, 10.

Bloch, D. Some crucial terms in nursing—What do they really mean? *Nursing Outlook*, November 1974, *22*, 689–694.

Bonney, V., & Rothberg, J. *Nursing diagnosis and therapy*. New York: National League for Nursing, 1963.

Briar, S. Social work's function. *Social Work*, March 1976, *21*, 90.

Card, W. I., & Good, I. J. A logical analysis of medicine. In R. Passamore (Ed.), *A companion to medical studies*. London: Blackwell Scientific Publishers, 1974, vol. 3, sec. 60.

Carroll, N. K. Three dimensional model of social work practice. *Social Work*, September 1977, *22*, 428–432.

Cassell, E. J. Error in medicine. In H. T. Englehardt & D. Callahan (Eds.), *Knowledge, value and belief*. New York: The Hastings Center, 1977.

College of Nursing, Texas Woman's University. *Nursing Diagnosis Monograph*. Denton, Tex.: Texas Woman's University, Fall 1979.

Cooper, S. Social work: A dissenting profession. *Social Work*, September 1977, *22*, 361.

Dean, W. R. Back to activism. *Social Work*, September 1977, *22*, 369–373.

Dickens, C. *Martin Chuzzlewit*. New York: Macmillan, 1910.

Doona, M. E. The judgment process in nursing. *Image*, June 1976, *8*, 27–29.

Duffy, U. The changing image of the American physician. *Journal of the American Medical Association*, 1967, *200*, 136–140.

Elstein, A. S., Schulman, L. S., & Sprafka, S. A. *Medical problem solving:* An analysis of clinical reasoning. Cambridge, Mass.: Harvard University Press, 1978.

Engel, G. L. The need for a new medical model: A challenge for biomedicine. *Science*, April 1977, *196*, 129–196.

Engle, R. L., Jr., & Davis, B. J. Medical diagnosis: Present, past, and future: I. Present concepts of the meaning and limitations of medical diagnosis. *Archives of Internal Medicine*, October 1963, *112*, 512–519.

Engle, R. L., Jr. Medical diagnosis: Present, past, and future: II. Philosophical foundations and historical development of our concepts of health, disease and diagnosis. *Archives of Internal Medicine*, October 1963, *112*, 521–529.

Englehardt, T., Jr. The disease of masturbation: Values and the concept of disease. In J. W. Leavitt & R. L. Numbers (Eds.), *Sickness and health in America*. Madison, Wis.: University of Wisconsin Press, 1978.

Fejos, P. Magic, witchcraft and medical theory in primitive cultures. In I. Galdston (Ed.), *Man's image in medicine and anthropology*. New York: International Universities Press, 1963.

Field, M. Causal inferences in behavioral research. *Advances in Nursing Science*, October 1979, *2*, 81–93.

Finestone, S. Issues involved in developing diagnostic classifications for casework. In *Casework papers, 1960*. Papers presented at the 87th Annual Forum, National Conference on Social Welfare, Atlantic City, June 5–10, 1960. New York: Family Service Association of America, 1960, pp. 139–154.

Frederick, H. K., & Northam, E. *A textbook of nursing practice* (2d ed.). New York: Macmillan, 1938.

Germaine, C. Casework and science: A historical encounter. In R. W. Roberts & R. H. Nee (Eds.), *Theories of social casework*, Chicago: University of Chicago Press, 1970.

Gordon, M. Predictive strategies in diagnostic tasks. *Nursing Research*, January–February 1980, *29*, 39–45.

Gordon, M. *Probabilistic concept attainment: A study of nursing diagnosis.* Unpublished doctoral dissertation, Boston College, 1972.

Gordon, M. Nursing diagnosis and the diagnostic process. *American Journal of Nursing*, August 1976, *76*, 1300.

Hall, L. Quality of nursing care. *Public Health News*. N.J.: State Department of Health, June 1955, *36*, 212–213.

Hall, V. C. *Statutory regulation of the scope of nursing practice.* Chicago, Ill.: National Joint Practice Commission, 1975.

Handbook for Friendly Visitors among the Poor, Compiled by the Charity Organization Society of the City of New York, 1883.

Harmer, B. *Textbook of the principles and practice of nursing* (5th ed.) (Revised by V. Henderson). New York: Macmillan, 1955.

Henderson, V. *The nature of nursing.* New York: Macmillan, 1966.

Hollis, F. The psychosocial approach to casework. In R. W. Roberts & R. H. Nee (Eds.), *Theories of social casework.* Chicago: University of Chicago Press, 1970.

Kalisch, P. A., & Kalisch, B. J. *The advance of American nursing.* Boston: Little, Brown, 1978.

Keefer, C. S. and Wilkins, R. W. *Medicine: Essentials of clinical practice.* Boston: Little, Brown, 1970.

Kim, M. J., & Moritz, D. A. *Classification of nursing diagnoses: Proceedings of the 3rd and 4th National Conference on Classification of Nursing Diagnoses.* New York: McGraw-Hill, 1981.

King, L. S. (Ed.). *A history of medicine: Selected readings.* Baltimore, Md.: Penguin Books, 1971.

Lazare, A. Hidden conceptual models in clinical psychiatry. *New England Journal of Medicine*, February 15, 1973, *288*, 346–353.

Leavitt, J. W., & R. L. Numbers (Eds.). *Sickness and health in America: Readings in the history of medicine and public health.* Madison, Wis.: University of Wisconsin Press, 1978.

Little, D., & Carnevali, D. The diagnostic statement: The problem defined. In J. B. Walter, G. P. Pardee, & D. M. Molbo (Eds.), *Dynamics of problem-oriented approaches: Patient care and documentation.* New York: Lippincott, 1976.

Lowenberg, F. M. *Fundamentals of social intervention.* New York: Columbia University Press, 1977.

Maryland public rates nursing high in survey. *American Journal of Nursing*, December 1979, *79*, 2094.

McManus, L. Assumptions of functions of nursing. In Teachers College Division of Nursing Education, *Regional planning for nursing and nursing education.* New York: Teachers College Press, 1950.

McWhinney, I. R. Beyond diagnosis: An approach to the integration of behavioral science and clinical medicine. *New England Journal of Medicine*, August 24, 1972, *287*, 384–387.

Middleman, R. R., & Goldberg, G. *Social service delivery: A structural approach to social work practice.* New York: Columbia University Press, 1974.

Morales, A. Beyond traditional conceptual frameworks. *Social Work*, September 1977, *22*, 392.

Morris, R. Caring for vs. caring about people. *Social Work*, September 1977, *22*, 353.

Newman, M. *Theory development in nursing.* Philadelphia: Davis, 1979.

Nightingale, F. *Notes on nursing: What it is and what it is not.* London: Harrison, 1859.

Nightingale, F. Sick nursing and health nursing. In I. Hampton (Ed.), *Nursing of the sick, 1893.* New York: McGraw-Hill, 1949.

Nunehan, A., and Pincus, A. Conceptual framework for social work practice. *Social Work*, September 1977, *22*, 346.

Orem, D. E. *Guides for developing curricula for the education of practical nurses.* Washington, D.C.: Government Printing Office, 1959.

Orem, D. E. *Nursing: Concepts of practice.* New York: McGraw-Hill, 1971.

Orlando, I. J. *The dynamic nurse patient relationship.* New York: Putnam, 1961.

Perlman, H. H. The problem-solving model in casework practice. In R. W. Roberts & R. H. Nee (Eds.), *Theories of social casework.* Chicago: University of Chicago Press, 1970.

Reid, W. J. Social work for social problems. *Social Work*, September 1977, *22*, 374.

Richmond, M. *Social diagnosis.* New York: Russell Sage, 1917.

Ripple, L., and Alexander, E. Motivation, capacity, and opportunity as related to the use of casework service: Nature of the client's problem. *Social Service Review*, 1956, *30*, 38–54.

Rivers, W. H. R. *Medicine, magic, and religion.* New York: Harcourt, Brace, and World, 1927.

Roberts, R. W., & Nee, R. H. *Theories of social casework.* Chicago: University of Chicago Press, 1970.

Robinson, V. P. Changing psychology in social casework. In V. P. Robinson (Ed.), *Development of a professional self: Teaching and learning in professional helping processes: Selected writings 1930-1968.* AMS Press, New York, 1978

Rogers, M. *Introduction to the theoretical basis of nursing.* New York: Davis, 1970.

Roy, C. A diagnostic classification system for nursing. *Nursing Outlock*, February 1975, *74*, 91.

Ruesch, J. The helping traditions: Some assumptions made by physicians. In I. Galdston (Ed.), *Man's image in medicine and anthropology.* New York: International Universities Press, 1963.

Selby, L. G. Typologies for caseworkers: Some considerations and problems. *Social Service Review*, 1958, *32*, 341–349.

Shaw, C. S. W. *A textbook of nursing.* New York: Appleton, 1855.

Sickerman, B. The uses of diagnosis: Doctors, patients and neurasthenia. In J. W. Leavitt & R. L. Numbers (Eds.), *Sickness and health in America*, Madison, Wis.: University of Wisconsin Press, 1978.

Simm, B. K. Diversity and unity in the social work profession. *Social Work*, September 1977, *22*, 394.

Smalley, R. E. The functional approach to casework practice. In R. W. Roberts & R. H. Nee (Eds.), *Theories of social casework.* Chicago: University of Chicago Press, 1970.

Stuart, G. W., and Sundeen, S. J. The nursing process. In S. J. Sundeen, G. W. Stuart, E. D Rankin, & S. P. Cohen (Eds.), *Nurse client interaction: Implementing the nursing process.* St. Louis: Mosby, 1976.

Subcommittee on the Working Definition of Social Work Practice for the Commission on Social Work Practice, National Association of Social Workers. "Working definition of social work practice." In H. R. Bartlett, Toward clarification and improvement of social work practice. *Social Work,* April 1958, *3*, 3–9.

Talbott, J. An in-depth look at DSM III: An interview with Robert Spitzer. *Hospital and Community Psychiatry*, January 1980, *31*, 25–32.

Tappert, T. G. (Ed.). *Luther's works*. Philadelphia: Fortress Press, 1967, vol. 54.

Thomas, L. Notes of a biology watcher: On magic in medicine. *New England Journal of Medicine*, August 31, 1978, *299,* 462.

Tumulty, P. A. What is a clinician and what does he do? In R. T. Bulger (Ed.), *Hippocrates revisited: A search for meaning*. New York: MEDCOM Press, 1973.

Vaisrub, S. Groping for causation. *Journal of the American Medical Association*, February 23, 1979, *241*, 830.

Walter, J. B. *An introduction to the principles of disease*. Philadelphia: Saunders, 1977.

World Health Organization. *International classification of diseases*. Geneva: World Health Organization, 1977.

CHAPTER 3

FRAMEWORKS FOR THE DIAGNOSTIC PROCESS

The diagnostic process begins with the collection of information and ends with an evaluative judgment about a client's health status. To carry out this process in nursing, one must make decisions about what information to collect and in what areas responsibility exists for diagnostic judgments. A conceptual framework provides the basis for these decisions.

As the term implies, a *conceptual framework* is a framework of interrelated concepts. The concepts are abstract ways of looking at the *client, nursing goal*, and *nursing intervention*. To be applicable in many diverse nursing situations, the concepts must be abstract and must provide a useful perspective for practice.

Concepts within a framework provide a conceptual focus for nursing process. In this chapter, four conceptual frameworks will be reviewed. Discussion will be limited to concepts related to the client, the nursing goal, and the view of diagnosis within each framework.

One purpose for reviewing selected conceptual frameworks here is to find what to assess and why. One's conceptual perspective on clients and on nursing's goals strongly determines what kinds of things one assesses. Everyone has a perspective, whether in conscious awareness or not. Problems can arise if the perspective "in the head" is inconsistent with the actions taken during assessment. Information collection has to be logically related to one's view of nursing.

A second purpose for reviewing selected frameworks is to further define nursing diagnosis. Conceptual frameworks specify the focus of nursing and thus of nursing diagnosis. For example, one framework specifies that nursing diagnoses are actual or potential self-care deficits; another specifies maladaptations as the problems of concern to nurses.

The two concepts in a framework that have relevance to the diagnostic phase of nursing process are the concept of the client and the concept of nursing goal. The concept of the client provides guidelines for logical deduction of what is to be assessed; the concept of goal describes the overall purpose of nursing that assessment, diagnosis, and care planning are to achieve.

All nursing frameworks specify optimal health as the goal of nursing, but perspectives on health differ. Concepts of the client also differ, but they all focus on health-related behavior. The conceptual view of the client and of the goal of nursing are logically related;[1] a review of a few frameworks will demonstrate this.[2]

To be useful in all nursing situations, frameworks have to be abstract. Yet concrete guidelines for assessment are also necessary. This chapter will present a set of health patterns which, it is proposed, specify areas in which basic information must be collected no matter what framework is being used. The objective of that section of the chapter will be to explain the concept of functional health patterns and the definitions of the 11 patterns proposed, and to help the reader consider how these patterns can provide a basic data base for nursing diagnosis, irrespective of which framework is employed.

CONCEPTUAL FRAMEWORKS

There are a number of ways to arrive at a concept of nursing that provides guidelines for information collection (assessment) and for diagnostic judgments. One approach is to start with the abstract question, What is nursing?, and then try to reason "down" to the clinical level. A number of frameworks that have been proposed by nursing theorists can be used to do this. A *deductive process* of reasoning is involved, beginning with assumptions and beliefs and ending with applications to specific situations.

A second way of deciding what is to be assessed is to examine the assessment formats in current use. In nursing there is no lack of proposed assessment tools; they are numerous in the literature. A review of these would show how items could be grouped into broad categories for guiding information collection. This would be an *inductive process* of reasoning, from particular to general areas. The assumptions of persons constructing these tools influence the end products—the assessment data—that result from use of the tools.

There is still another approach to determining what information to collect: *Why not look at the clients themselves?* What health problems amenable to nursing intervention do they have? A list of these problems could be turned into broad assessment categories. Again it is true that the nurses doing the "looking" have assumptions that influence what they pay attention to in the situation. These assumptions influence the end product.

A related method is to ask clients one simple question: Which health problem could nurses assist you with? Asking this of many clients would provide items to categorize. What has been done is to shift the assumptions to the client. Now, clients' assumptions

---

[1] This logical relationship between the goal and client focus (also intervention focus) is referred to as the *internal consistency* of a conceptual framework.

[2] Frameworks will not be comprehensively discussed; certain concepts have been selected because of their pertinence to diagnosis. The reader is encouraged to read the original work and the reviews listed in the bibliography at the end of this chapter.

about nursing and what nurses do will influence the end product of the assessment process.

All these methods are encompassed to some extent in the conceptual frameworks of nursing that have appeared in the literature. Theorists who developed these frameworks are nurses, and their beliefs and experiences in nursing are incorporated. During the following discussion of selected frameworks, the reader may wonder why nursing has more than one way of viewing the client. We will return to this question; at this point the reader needs to know that philosophical differences exist, that there are strong vested interests, and that many are reticent to close off development of ideas at too early a point.

Life Process Model

A framework encompassing the whole of the life process is proposed by Martha Rogers (1970). Life is viewed as a creative, formative process. It is characterized by the human species' evolution toward greater diversity and innovation. Nursing promotes the attainment of these emerging potentialities by its focus on the means to this end of continuing development: maximum health potential. Individuals, families, and communities are conceptualized as energy fields that have pattern, organization, and openness to constant transaction with the environment.

The life process is a transaction between the human energy field and the environmental field. Both fields are characterized by wholeness of life pattern, and both are continuously and simultaneously repatterned as person and environment transact (Rogers, 1970, p. 53). This means that nursing focuses on the whole person-environment complex, not the sum of the psychological, biological, or social parts. Further, it means that the client and environment are continuously affecting each other.

With simultaneous and continuous client-environment interaction, new life patterns emerge. Nursing seeks to help the client maintain a pattern of living that coordinates, rather than conflicts, with the emerging pattern. Although assessment and diagnosis focus on the life process at a particular point in time, the probability that new behaviors will emerge has to be considered.

The ideas in this model need to be carefully considered from a broad, world-view perspective. For example, do you think new human and world patterns are developing? Is this happening sequentially, such that the human race is never what it was, only what it is becoming? Is emergence goal-directed? Is life pattern and organization getting more complex? Are the changes innovative and spiral (something like the Slinky toy with its cyclic spirals)? Is there order to evolutionary development?

If you answer yes to the above questions, you share the same assumptions about human beings as Rogers:

1 Man is a unified whole possessing his own integrity and manifesting characteristics that are more than and different from the sum of his parts.

2 Man and environment are continuously exchanging matter and energy with one another.

3 The life process evolves irreversibly and unidirectionally along the space-time continuum.

4 Pattern and organization identify man and reflect his innovative wholeness.

5 Man is characterized by the capacity for abstraction, imagery, language, thought, sensation, and emotion. (Rogers, 1970, pp. 43–77)

Nursing Goal Nursing can promote a client's progress toward his or her maximum health potential by (1) strengthening the mutual interaction of the human and environmental pattern, (2) recognizing the potentialities of the client and the environment, and (3) helping the client to use conscious personal choice in goal-seeking. Is change orderly? Yes. Is it predictable, that is, can we ever predict client health outcomes? Yes, but only in terms of probabilities and only by looking at the holistic, rhythmical pattern of the person and the environment (Rogers, 1970, pp. 89–102.) Needless to say, highly probable predictions are few and far between unless the most influencing factors are identified. This, Rogers would say, requires research in nursing science.

Client Focus Rogers's conceptual model of the client is *unitary man* and particularly, the *life process* of man. The individual is thought of as an electrical energy field which extends into space. Part of the field, the body, is visible. Pattern and organization of life (1) provide personal integrity, individuality, and wholeness and (2) reflect the life process, which is creative, formative, and evolving. The person and the environment affect each other's pattern, organization, and creative-formative evolution. The life process model, therefore, represents a holistic concept of the unity of person-environment. Neither the client nor the environment can be understood separately.

To understand the holistic life pattern, one must consider a configuration of events both within and external to the person's awareness. Examples would be client-other interactions (some of which are perceptible) and radiation levels in the environment (imperceptible) (Rogers, 1970).

In assessment of the client life pattern, the holistic concept must be at the forefront. At a point in time, the nurse describes the extent to which the client is emerging toward maximum health potential. This emergence is assessed by (1) observing the pattern and organization of the creative, formative process (life process) and (2) determining the degree to which the environment permits achievement of maximum health potential. More specifically, the nurse assesses the (1) client and environment pattern and organization and (2) preceding patterns (configuration of events) leading up to the present.

Behavioral manifestations of unified human functioning are the assessment data (Rogers, 1970, pp. 124–127). This is the extent to which Rogers's publications specify what to assess. Data are synthesized to reveal a view of the client's life process (creative, formative). The life process model does not include a set of categories for guiding assessment of behavior or of patterns; only principles are delineated (Rogers, 1970). Nurses using the life process model have the challenge of developing holistic assessment parameters.

Theorist's View of Diagnosis Rogers states, "The total pattern of events at any given point in space-time provides the data for nursing diagnosis." She refers to *the* "diagnostic pattern" and adds that "nursing diagnosis encompasses the man-environment relationship and seeks to identify sequential cross sectional patterning in the life process" (Rogers, 1970, p. 125). Health problems have multiple causes, and relationships between cause and effect are always probabilistic rather than absolute.

In summary, the concept of the client in Rogers' life process model is unitary man. Diagnosis focuses on the pattern of client-environment interaction. The goal of nursing is to help clients repattern toward healthful behaviors in order to realize the potentialities of the creative-formative process.

Adaptation Model

Roy (1976) and her colleagues (Roy and Roberts, 1981) have proposed that an adaptation model provides a useful way of thinking about nursing. Adaptation is seen as a process necessary to (1) maintain human integrity and (2) free energy for healing and for attaining higher levels of wellness. This conceptual framework utilizes Helson's model, which views adaptation as a state of dynamic equilibrium (Roy and Roberts, 1981, p. 84).

Nursing Goal Within this framework the goal of nursing is to promote responses that lead to adaptation. In turn, adaptation is a "response to the environment which promotes the person's general goals including survival, growth, reproduction, self-mastery, and self-actualization" (Roy and Roberts, 1981, p. 53). *Adaptation* is a term that refers to both a process and a state: the client may be either in the process of effectively coping with stressors or in the adapted state that results from effective coping.

Client Focus Consistent with the goal of nursing, the client is viewed as an open, adaptive system. The adaptation level reflects the system's ability to cope with environmental interaction. Coping may be adaptive or ineffective in maintaining human integrity. Ineffective coping behaviors require nursing attention.

Two coping mechanisms are identified: the cognator and the regulator. The cognator mechanism consists of (1) perceptual information processing, (2) learning, (3) judgment, and (4) emotion (Roy and Roberts, 1981, p. 60). Coping with stressors also occurs through the regulator mechanism, which has "1) neural, 2) endocrine and 3) perception-psychomotor" processes (Roy and Roberts, 1981, p. 60).

The processes of the cognator and regulator are manifested in four modes of adaptive behavior: the physiologic, self-concept, role function, and interdependence modes. These are defined in Table 3–1.

The four adaptive modes provide a format for nursing assessment. In each mode behaviors are assessed and any stressors in the client-environment interaction are identified. Behaviors may be judged to be "adaptive or ineffective" relative to (1) the client's goals and (2) the maintenance of human integrity (Roy and Roberts, 1981, p. 57).

Theorist's View of Diagnosis In the adaptation framework, a nursing diagnosis is

TABLE 3-1
FOUR ADAPTATION MODES IDENTIFIED BY ROY

Physiologic mode	Role-function mode
Exercise/rest	Expressive/instrumental
Nutrition	Role identity
Elimination	Role expectations
Fluids and electrolytes	Role interactions
Oxygen and circulation	**Interdependence mode**
Regulation of temperature	Cognitive/affective,
Regulation of senses	parameters in relation
Regulation of endocrine system	to independency-
Self-concept mode	dependency needs:
Physical self	Affection achievement
Personal self	(love, support)

Source: Adapted from C. Roy and S. L. Roberts, *Theory construction in nursing: An adaptation model.* Englewood Cliffs, N.J.: Prentice-Hall, 1981, pp. 71–283.

defined as a "judgment about ineffective or potentially ineffective behavior within a mode and identification of the most relevant influencing factors" causing the behavior (Roy and Roberts, 1981, p. 286). It is suggested that influencing, or etiological, factors can be *focal stimuli* (stressors) or *ineffective cognator and regulator processes.* The latter is discussed in relation to cross-modal diagnoses (Roy and Roberts, 1981, pp. 286-287).

This notion of etiology raises the question of whether intervention is facilitated by (1) specifying the stressor producing ineffective adaptation or by (2) describing the client's ineffective, or maladaptive, response to the stressor. If the nursing goal is to promote adaptation, identification of maladaptive responses appears more useful for directing intervention. It is important in diagnosis that it be clear whether (1) the coping response to the stimulus or (2) the stimulus itself is specified as the cause of the problem. The former would dictate a typology of maladaptive coping responses (cognator and regulator processes) and the latter, a typology of stressors and the needs or deficits they produce. This issue may be resolved as the adaptation model is further developed and tested in practice.

In summary, the adaptation model provides four categories (Table 3-1) and two coping mechanisms (cognator and regulator) as a framework for assessment. Diagnoses are viewed as problems in adaptation due to stressors or responses to stressors occurring during client-environment interaction. The goal of nursing is to promote adaptive responses so that higher levels of wellness can be attained.

Behavioral Systems Model

The behavioral systems model was initially proposed by Dorothy Johnson (1968). In recent years it has been extended by Grubbs (1980).[3] Although the framework

---

[3] This review relies mainly on the presentation and extension of Johnson's theory by Grubbs (1980).

contains the term *systems*, the focus is different from the focus of the biomedical systems framework used in medicine.

Nursing Goal   Health, the goal of nursing, in the behavioral systems framework is viewed as behavioral balance or stability. This stability is seen as the ability to adjust and change but still maintain purposeful, orderly, predictable behavior (Grubbs, 1980).

Client Focus   Using the behavioral systems model, the nurse would view the client as an organized, interrelated *complex of interacting subsystems*. Each subsystem, for example, affiliation, has a pattern. Patterns that the client develops determine and limit interaction with the environment (Grubbs, 1980).

Development of efficient and effective behavioral patterns requires the "sustenal imperatives" of protection, nurturance, and stimulation (Grubbs, 1980, pp. 231-234). Drives explain goal-directed behavior, choice, predispositions to act, and the repertoire of actions developed to sustain each subsystem. Interrelationships among the subsystems are monitored and controlled by biophysiologic, psychologic, and sociocultural mechanisms (Grubbs, 1980, p. 235).

Stress can disturb the client's patterns and lead to disequilibrium. Factors that cause disturbances in regularity and orderliness of behavior patterns threaten the integrity and function of the entire behavioral system. Disturbances may be due to (1) inadequate drive satisfaction, (2) inadequate fulfillment of the functional requirements of the subsystems, and (3) fluctuations in environmental conditions which exceed the system's capacity to adjust (Grubbs, 1980, p. 224). Stress can also result from changes in sustenal imperatives (protection, nurturance, stimulation). As may be obvious from deductive reasoning, if the client is viewed as a system with behavioral subsystems, then these are assessed in order to determine health status.

Assessment focuses on (1) behavioral patterns, (2) interrelations, and (3) sustenal imperatives. Questions that direct the assessment of subsystems may be, Is there an actual or perceived threat to loss of pattern stability? Are there changes in behavioral patterns? Are there sufficient "sustenal imperatives"? What are the abilities of the client to adapt? Problematic subsystem behavior, if identified, is further assessed in order to plan intervention; nine areas of problem analysis have been identified and include client actions, predispositions, and choice (Grubbs, 1980, pp. 239-240). The behavioral subsystems that lend structure to assessment when this model is used are listed in Table 3-2. The goal is behavioral stability; therefore, present behavior is compared to past behavior so that one may judge whether change has occurred and evaluate the contribution of the change toward stability.

Theorist's View of Diagnosis   Within this model, the meaning of diagnosis is to determine "underlying dynamics of the patient's problematic behaviors in a situation" (Grubbs, 1980, p. 240). A problem is defined as actual or potential instability in the system. As will be discussed below, the problem may be either functional or structural. Problem, etiology, and problem source are all included in the statement of the diagnosis. Problem source is stated as an adjective that classifies the problem.

Diagnostically, a health problem originating in one subsystem is classified as an *insufficiency* or a *discrepancy* relative to the subsystem goal. *Incompatibility* and

TABLE 3-2
EIGHT BEHAVIORAL SUBSYSTEMS OF JOHNSON'S FRAMEWORK

Achievement subsystem—to master or control oneself or one's environment:; to achieve mastery and control
Affiliative subsystem—to relate or belong to something or someone other than oneself; to achieve intimacy and inclusion
Aggressive/protective subsystem—to protect self or others from real or imagined threatening objects, persons, or ideas; to achieve self-protection and self-assertion
Dependency subsystem—to maintain environmental resources needed for obtaining help, assistance, attention, permission, reassurance, and security; to gain trust and reliance
Eliminative subsystem—to expel biologic wastes; to externalize the internal biologic environment
Ingestive subsystem—to take in needed resources from the environment to maintain the integrity of the organism or to achieve a state of pleasure; to internalize the external environment
Restorative subsystem—to relieve fatigue and/or achieve a state of equilibrium by reestablishing or replenishing the energy distribution among the other subsystems; to redistribute energy
Sexual subsystem—to procreate, to gratify or attract, to fulfill expectations associated with one's sex; to care for others and be cared about by them

Source: Grubbs (1980, p. 228).

dominance are the two classifications for multisubsystem problems. These classes are defined in Table 3-3 and help identify intervention, according to Grubbs. Grief is an example of a problem or behavioral pattern instability. The problem source is classified as insufficiency in the affiliative subsystem. Cause, or etiology, of the instability in the subsystem pattern may be either internal or external stress. In addition, the client may be an active or passive participant in the etiology (Grubbs, 1980, p. 241). Etiological classification is done on the basis of two possible causes: *structural stress* and *functional stress*. These are defined in Table 3-4. Grubb's classification places the source of structural stress within the subsystems (client). Functional stress is most often caused by factors in the external environment.

The active or passive participation of the client, as the cause of stress, rests on the assumption in the model that the client has a choice of alternative behaviors. An example of an etiology of structural stress is given: "deliberate avoidance of achievement situations" (Grubbs, 1980, p. 241); the cause is within the person and, more specifically, within the achievement subsystem. The goal of the subsystem is to master and control, but the behavior chosen is not meeting this goal. Thus, the etiology lies in the client's behavior: choosing not to achieve.

Grubbs compares the above example to functional stress. The etiology could be "lack of achievement opportunities." Grubbs says that in this case "the patient is essentially a passive victim of his environmental situation" (Grubbs, 1980, p. 241). Note the dichotomous judgment the diagnostician has to make regarding internal or external stressors when using this classification. The dichotomy will not appeal to those who support the concept of multicausality or those believing that problems result from the *interaction* between the person and environment.

The author states that identifying whether the stress is structural or functional is

TABLE 3-3
DIAGNOSTIC CLASSIFICATIONS OF DISORDERS IN THE BEHAVIORAL SYSTEMS MODEL

Single-subsystem disorder	*Insufficiency* This exists when a particular subsystem is not functioning or developed to its fullest capacity due to inadequacy of functional requirements
	Discrepancy This exists when a behavior does not meet the intended goal
Multi-subsystem disorder	*Incompatibility* The goals or behaviors of the two subsystems in the same situation conflict with each other to the detriment of the individual
	Dominance The behavior in one subsystem is used more than any other subsystem regardless of the situation or to the detriment of the other subsystem

Source: Adapted from Grubbs (1980, pp. 240–241).

TABLE 3-4
ETIOLOGICAL CLASSIFICATION IN THE BEHAVIORAL SYSTEMS MODEL

Etiology of health problem	Definition of etiological type
Structural stress	Refers to that which occurs within the subsystems; involves internal control mechanisms and reflects inconsistencies between the goal, set, choice, or action
Functional stress	Refers to overload or insufficiency of any of the sustenal imperatives and results in functional disorders; usually arises externally from the environment

Source: Adapted from Grubbs (1980, p. 241).

helpful for diagnostic purposes. Even if this dichotomy of probable sources of stress is accepted, caution would be needed to avoid value-laden statements (with or without sufficient clinical data). In Grubbs's example, the term *deliberate avoidance* has a negative connotation. Secondly, it does not seem that with this level of formulation "the intervention course becomes clear" (Grubbs, 1980, p. 241). A nurse who *thinks* "avoidance" is "deliberate" when the clinical assessment data are analyzed surely needs to go on to further understand why this is so.

The specification of etiology requires an in-depth assessment. It also requires analysis of clinical data to gain an understanding of the probable factor(s) that precipitate or maintain the less-than-optimal state. Explanatory concepts (etiology) are helpful in care planning if they are formulated at a level that suggests nursing interventions. For diagnostic purposes, if one accepts the dichotomy implied in this concept of etiology, then Table 3–4 is useful as a structure to organize thinking. It may ensure that neither the client's behavior nor external circumstances and events are ignored in understanding the probable contributing, predisposing, or precipitating factors.

In summary, the behavioral systems model views the client as having a set of interrelated behavioral subsystems. These subsystems are the framework for the diagnostic process. Each subsystem is assessed and problems of instability diagnosed. A number of guidelines are offered for identifying problems and their etiologies.

Self-Care Agency Model

Client self-care abilities and operations are the phenomena of nursing concern in Orem's (1980) self-care model. Emphasis is placed on the capacities of clients to manage their own health and that of their dependents, such as children. Nurses help them to do this.

Client Focus   People are viewed as having universal, developmental, and health deviation *self-care requisites*. The *universal* requisites are described as follows:

> Universal self-care requisites are common to all human beings during all stages of the life cycle, adjusted to age, developmental state, and environmental and other factors. They are associated with life processes and with the maintenance of the integrity of human structure and functioning. (Orem, 1980, p. 42)

Universal self-care requisites include sufficient intake of air, water, and food; elimination; a balance between activity and rest and between solitude and social interaction; prevention of hazards; and the promotion of human functioning and development relative to potentialities (Orem, 1980, p. 42).

Developmental self-care requisites vary with age or with condition, such as pregnancy. Two categories of developmental requisites are identified:

> The bringing about and maintenance of living conditions that support life processes and promote the processes of development, that is, human progress toward higher levels of the organization of human structures and functions and toward maturation . . . [and] provision of care either to prevent the occurrence of deleterious effects of conditions that can affect human development . . . or to mitigate or overcome these effects. (Orem, 1980, p. 47)

Like universal self-care requisites, these developmental needs are met either through one's own abilities (if one is an able adult) or by another (as in case of dependent children).

In the third area of clients' self-care needs, *health deviation* self-care requisites, Orem identifies six categories and summarizes them as follows:

> Health deviation self-care requisites are associated with genetic constitutional defects, human structural and functional deviations and their effects, and medical diagnosis and treatment. (Orem, 1980, p. 41)

From these areas the total "therapeutic self-care demand" of any individual can be determined. Also, self-care actions can be examined for their "therapeutic value" (Orem, 1980, pp. 39–40). If therapeutic, the person's actions contribute to "(1) support of life processes and promotion of normal functioning; (2) maintenance of normal growth, development, and maturation; (3) prevention, control, or cure of disease processes and injuries; and (4) prevention of, or compensation for, disability" (Orem, 1980, p. 40).

When self-care is not done or is done in a nontherapeutic manner, deficits exist. Self-care deficits are determined by examining (1) an individual's therapeutic demands (required actions) in the universal, developmental, and health deviation areas; (2) the self-care actions currently being done; and (3) the therapeutic value of current actions. In addition, potential decreases in self-care abilities or increases in demands can be predicted.

Nursing Goal In discussing the goal of health care, Orem uses a comprehensive definition of health: "Health signifies human functional and structural integrity, absence of genetic defects, and progressive integrated development of a human being as an individual unity moving toward higher and higher levels of integration" (Orem, 1980, p. 121). Within the overall goal of the health professions, which is to bring about health, nursing defines its role. The goal of nursing is independent, responsible self-care on the part of clients. Self-care is considered to be present when the client's actions (in regard to self and dependents) regulate "internal and external conditions necessary to maintain life processes and environmental conditions supportive of life processes, integrity of human structure and functioning, and human developmental processes" (Orem, 1980, p. 24).

As may be evident, Orem's underlying view of clients is that they are responsible and engage in deliberate choice and action. In accordance with this view, clients are expected to be socially responsible agents of their own self-care and the care of their dependents. Deficits or limitations in self-care actions, relative to requisites, require nursing attention.

Theorist's View of Diagnosis It clearly follows from this model of the client that the focus of nursing diagnosis is deficits in self-care agency (abilities). These may be due to the client's lack of knowledge or skill, limitations in capacity (transitory or permanent), or lack of resources (Orem, 1980, p. 141). The diagnostic judgment of deficits or limitations is related to (1) universal self-care requisites and the quality and type of present self-care activities and (2) actual or predicted developmental or health deviation demands relative to present or predicted abilities or actions. Essentially, diagnosis involves a *comparison* of current actions and potential for action with actual or potential demands. If deficiencies are found, a problem in self-care agency is diagnosed.

Orem does not discuss a concept of etiology explicitly. Comments are made about the underlying cause of inability to perform self-care actions, such as nonuse of a fractured leg. It is stated that limitations in self-care "may be caused by the effects of the disease process, the therapy used, the lack of necessary knowledge and skills, or a lack of resources" (Orem, 1980, p. 141). In addition, lack of motivation to alter self-care actions can also cause limitations in therapeutic self-care or care of dependents (Orem, 1980, p. 62).

In summary, Orem's framework views the client as a self-care agent. The goal of nursing is the client's independence in self-care actions. As a framework for the diagnostic process this model would direct assessment toward data related to self-care demands and self-care capabilities. Self-care agency deficits, actual or potential, would be the focus of diagnosis.

The models reviewed above provide a sampling of various conceptualizations of the client from a nursing perspective. Recall that the purpose of reviewing these was to demonstrate that there are answers to the question of what information to collect and in what areas responsibility exists for diagnostic judgments.

TABLE 3-5
FOUR FRAMEWORKS FOR THE DIAGNOSTIC PROCESS

Framework	Assessment focus	Diagnostic focus	Causality
Rogers life process model	Behavioral manifestations of events in the human and environmental field Holistic patterns of functioning (total pattern of events at a given point in spacetime)	Pattern and organization of the life process which does not support maximum health potential and the creative-formative process (No diagnostic classification)	Multicausality found in human and environmental field interaction
Roy adaptation model	Adaptive responses to need deficits or excesses: Physiological mode 　Rest/exercise 　Nutrition 　Elimination 　Fluids and electrolytes 　Oxygen and circulation 　Regulation of temperature 　Regulation of senses 　Regulation of endocrine system Self-concept mode 　Physical self 　Personal self 　　Moral-ethical 　　Self-consistency 　　Self-ideal 　　Self-esteem	Potential problems in adaptation; actual maladaptation problems (Diagnostic classification according to 4 adaptation modes: physiological, self-concept, role function, and interdependence modes)	Causality lies in need deficits or excesses produced by stressors (focal stimulus) or in coping mechanisms (cognator and regulator) Multicausality concept, but intervention focus is on primary cause

| Johnson (Grubbs) behavioral system model | Role function mode
  Primary/secondary/
  tertiary roles
Expressive/instrumental:
  Role identity
  Role expectations
  Role interactions
Interdependence mode
  Cognitive/affective,
  parameters in relation
  to independency-
  dependency needs:
    Affection achievement
    (love, support)
Influencing factors: focal, con-
textual, and residual stimuli
Structural and functional level
of behavioral system and the
behavioral subsystem:
  Achievement
  Affiliative
  Agressive/protective
  Dependency
  Eliminative
  Ingestive
  Restorative
  Sexual
  Coping effectiveness | Instability in the system; be-
havior at variance with the
desired state; behavior that
does not maintain equilibrium:
  Intrasubsystem insufficiency
  Intrasubsystem discrepancy
  Intersubsystem
  incompatibility
  Intersubsystem dominance
  Inadequate coping/adaptation
(Diagnostic classification ac-
cording to 8 subsystems, intra-
subsystem or intersubsystem
problem) | Etiological classification ac-
cording to source of stress/
instability
Etiology used in singular sense |

TABLE 3-5
FOUR FRAMEWORKS FOR THE DIAGNOSTIC PROCESS (*continued*)

Framework	Assessment focus	Diagnostic focus	Causality
Orem self-care agency model	Eight universal self-care requisites, 2 developmental self-care requisites, and 6 health deviation self-care requisites (as well as interrelationships among these) Current repertoire of self-care practices (self and dependent): Degree of development Degree of operability Adequacy relative to demand	Presence of a deficit between existing powers of self-care agency and the demands on it Actual or potential deficits in type and quality (therapeutic value) of self-care actions (Diagnostic classification according to self-care needs in relation to (1) development, (2) health deviation), and (3) universal	Cause may be disease process; therapy used; or lack of knowledge, skills, resources, interest, or motivation

Source: Adapted from M. Rogers, *An introduction to the theoretical basis of nursing.* Philadelphia: Davis, 1970; C. Roy, *Introduction to nursing: An adaptation model.* Englewood Cliffs, N.J.: Prentice-Hall, 1981; D. Orem, *Nursing: Concepts of practice.* New York: McGraw-Hill, 1980; J. Grubbs, *The Johnson behavioral system model.* In J. P. Riehl & C. Roy (Eds.) *Conceptual models for nursing practice.* New York: Appleton-Century-Crofts, 1978.

In this discussion of frameworks for the diagnostic phase of nursing process, concepts of the client, diagnostic focus, and causality were of interest. For the conceptual frameworks reviewed, these ideas are summarized in Table 3-5. Although some overlapping can be seen, these are essentially different views based on different assumptions about clients.

To implement any framework for nursing process, the nurse must understand the entire model and its philosophical assumptions. The reader is encouraged to review a number of models and their interrelated concepts of client, intervention (nurse-client interaction), and nursing's goal. The bibliogrpahy at the end of this chapter contains references that pertain to the conceptual frameworks just discussed. Other nursing conceptual frameworks focus on human needs (Yura and Walsh 1978; Putt, 1978); needs, conservation, and adaptation (Levine, 1973, pp. 1-33); needs and distress (Orlando, 1961); needs and social systems (King, 1971); existential becoming (Patterson and Zderad, 1976); and stress (Neuman, 1980, pp. 119-134).

ACQUIRING AND USING A CONCEPTUAL MODEL

Now the question arises as to how to choose a model that can give purpose and direction to nursing process and, particularly, to diagnosis. For students, the conceptual framework of the curriculum should provide guidance. The framework includes the faculty's concept of the client, nursing goal, and nursing intervention.[4] For example, Roy's adaptation framework can guide a student to assess adaptation modes. Using the concepts underlying the curriculum organization as a framework for nursing process provides consistency between theoretical and clinical aspects and makes learning easier.

The reader who is currently practicing nursing is already assessing, diagnosing, intervening, and evaluating on the basis of some framework, possibly without full awareness of what that framework is. It can be an interesting experience to discover one's own professional point of view by reflecting on one's own practice. Examining personal assumptions about clients and about nursing will lead to consciousness raising.

Sometimes nurses find they are using a medical or social work model to guide *nursing* practice! Although this sounds illogical, it can occur. The aforementioned reviews and further reading about conceptual frameworks may assist in formulating a model for nursing practice.

Those who claim, "I don't need all that theoretical stuff to give nursing care" or "I don't need that, I just look at what the patients need or tell me they need," are deluding themselves. All nurses, including these, act on some of their observations and make referrals on the basis of others. Beneath these actions and referrals is a personal concept of nursing and some idea of what "should" receive attention.

Even implicit, unrecognized models influence perception and judgment. In the second statement quoted above, the nurse has a model but doesn't know it. A human needs model is obviously being used and probably just requires some conscious organization.

---

[4] The conceptual framework of a curriculum serves to organize the body of professional knowledge, skills, attitudes, and values. Its importance is reflected in the fact that one standard for national accreditation of colleges and schools of nursing is that the curriculum be organized within a conceptual framework (National League for Nursing, 1977).

Testing a Model in Practice

Conceptual models or frameworks of nursing can be elegant designs with logical relationships between the concepts specified. The crucial test, however, is whether a framework is workable in clinical practice. Does it provide a useful way of viewing clients? Does it capture the essence of the special contribution nursing makes to health care delivery? Does the concept of what nurses should do with and for clients (intervention concepts) seem realistic?

The only way to answer these questions about a model is to try it in one's practice. The concept of the client has to be used in assessment and diagnosis. One has to try stating and then evaluating client outcomes that are developed from the framework's concept of nursing's goal. The concept of intervention in the model has to be used as a guide for planning and implementing nursing care. After a number of months of this testing, the strengths, weaknesses, and areas needing further development become apparent. Undoubtedly the nursing theorist who developed the model would welcome a thoughtful critique and ideas for further development. These critiques and comments could be published in the nursing literature or relayed through personal communication. That is how conceptual models become refined. Clinicians have to test them in practice and identify their clinical usefulness.

Why the emphasis on models of the client? To reiterate, because *nursing diagnosis* cannot be done without a *nursing model* that provides clear guidelines for the collection of clinical information. It is as simple as that.

THE SEARCH FOR A UNIFIED MODEL

At this point, if not well before, the reader may be asking why nurses don't agree on just one model of the client. Riehl and Roy (1974, pp. 293-294) state that the advantage of having a single model would be facilitation of communication, development of a body of knowledge, and one common nursing approach to practice. On the other hand, they cite disadvantages and barriers: basic philosophical differences exist, frameworks have not been sufficiently tested, and there are strong vested interests. These authors note that with unification the question would arise as to *which* model to select. They point out that such a selection might inhibit creativity and close off new and more productive conceptualizations.

Although most theorists today would agree with the above list of advantages and disadvantages, Riehl and Roy now advocate a unified model of the client and goal (1980, pp. 390-403). They argue that this would still allow diversity in concepts of and approaches to nursing intervention. They synthesize various theorists' concepts of the client and nursing's goal under a systems model and suggest diversity be retained in the concept of nursing intervention.

Roy and Riehl (1980) are correct in saying there are areas of agreement among the theorists. Although, as Zerad (1978) has suggested, these would be more explicit if when a new model was proposed, similarities and differences were addressed. When conceptual models are published, it is rare for theorists to compare their perspective with previously published models.

The idea of a unified model is not foreign to other disciplines. In the general scientific community theories have been proposed to unify the sciences. For example, Miller proposed a living systems theory (1978). This, he suggests, could integrate the separate bodies of knowledge in all the sciences. Yet Miller's idea that interrelations among subsystems, for example biological, psychological, and social, lead to understanding human beings is contradictory to the holistic pattern in Rogers' life process model.

There is a problem in assuming that the search for unification of the sciences presupposes that nursing also move in this direction. Within many sciences, there is a great deal of knowledge from research that can be integrated by a unified model. Nursing science is just beginning.

For all the reasons discussed, it is unlikely that a unified model (client, goal, intervention) will be accepted in the near future. It might be well to examine what problems this presents for nursing diagnosis and if there are potential solutions.

For nurses who each day confront clients, students, or research data, the issue of a unified model of the client to guide assessment and diagnosis is not just an "ivory tower" idea. It has implications for nursing care delivery, nursing education, and research—and critical implications for developing commonly agreed upon diagnostic nomenclature. For example, diversity now exists among nursing care delivery settings: clients may have different aspects of their health status assessed, depending on the hospital they go to, the level of care they receive (primary, secondary, or tertiary), and the particular nurse they happen to encounter.

From the nurse's own perspective, every time there is a change in employment settings there usually is a different format for assessment. Similarly, it is not unusual for a student to be exposed to a different assessment tool with each different clinical instructor or area of practice. This variation certainly does not facilitate learning or the development of nursing practice expertise. Lastly, it does not facilitate clinical nursing research.

How can continuity of nursing care in various settings and with various nurses be provided if there is not a basic clinical assessment data base? How can there be studies of common health problems nurses treat? There is no assurance that assessment and diagnosis are comprehensively done. Nor can a consumer of nursing care be reasonably assured that all his or her actual or potential health problems have a high probability of being detected.

Components of nursing practice have been agreed upon and standardized nationally. From the consumer's perspective, it can be expected that nurses do assessment, diagnosis, intervention, and evaluation. This is the familiar nursing process that is incorporated into the *Standards for Nursing Practice* (American Nurses' Association, 1973).

About 20 to 30 years elapsed between the appearance in the literature of the term *nursing process* (Hall, 1955) and the national acceptance of this process as standard practice in 1973. Interestingly, nursing process, a set of steps, began to be described in the 1950s; in using nursing process, clinicians no doubt found that there was no framework to decide what to assess, diagnose, act upon, and evaluate. Perhaps the move toward a unified view of these *components* of practice stimulated the proliferation of conceptual models in the late 1960s and the 1970s.

Pressuring for unification at the abstract level of the *models*, which could remain diverse, may not be the solution. Maybe what is needed for practice, education, and research is a unification at the concrete level of *assessment* (information collection). Then more abstract concepts of nursing could be applied to the clinical data.

Unification of Assessment Structure

Could there be agreement, at a very concrete level, about the information needed for nursing assessment? Are there common *areas* of information about the client that are needed to implement *any* of the models of nursing? For example, irrespective of the model used in clinical practice, is every nursing clinician interested in information about dietary patterns? Remember that the focus of this discussion is on structural aspects of assessment, that is, *what* information to gather. Differences are expected in the way the information is interpreted and used.

Let us consider some of the models. Take, for example, the clinician who believes with Orem that the goal of nursing is to facilitate self-care agency. The nutritional pattern is decidedly an aspect of self-care, so nutritional patterns are assessed. The approach includes a nutritional pattern description, but emphasis is given to self-care actions underlying the pattern.

The nurse clinician who has adopted Roy's adaptation framework wants to know the basic nutritional pattern, also. This nurse will approach the analysis of clinical data by determining the person's or family's adaptation of nutritional patterns under certain situations.

The clinician concerned with patterns of living coordinated with environmental changes (Rogers's life process model) is interested in nutritional pattern changes related to other rhythm changes, for example, during hospitalization. Information about diet would be considered as (1) a behavioral manifestation and (2) specific data to be included in synthesizing a holistic view of the life process. The client's dietary pattern would be evaluated in terms of the goal of maximizing health for the creative-formative process of evolution (becoming).

Diversity in nursing models does not prevent standardization of assessment structure. Standardization does not imply a standardized interpersonal *approach* to assessment or to analysis and synthesis of clinical data. Neither does it suggest that the profession should have a standardized concept of the goal of nursing and of nurse-client interaction.

Although diversity is the watchword of western society, at a concrete level there has to be some conformity in practice. Every client deserves to know that, minimally, certain health-related behavioral patterns will be assessed for potential or actual problems relative to the client's own or external norms. The idea is certainly not new. Dorothy Smith (1968) has been prodding the profession for at least 15 years.

Standardization of assessment areas will require thoughtful consideration of related issues and consequences. In addition, proposed formats for standardized assessment will have to be evaluated, both initially and periodically, in all settings and specialties of nursing practice.

It is this author's opinion that the profession must take action to delineate the basic

TABLE 3-6
TYPOLOGY OF ELEVEN FUNCTIONAL HEALTH PATTERNS

Health-perception–health-management pattern   Describes client's perceived pattern of health and well-being and how health is managed

Nutritional-metabolic pattern   Describes pattern of food and fluid consumption relative to metabolic need and pattern indicators of local nutrient supply

Elimination pattern   Describes patterns of excretory function (bowel, bladder, and skin)

Activity-exercise pattern   Describes pattern of exercise, activity, leisure, and recreation

Cognitive-perceptual pattern   Describes sensory-perceptual and cognitive pattern

Sleep-rest pattern   Describes patterns of sleep, rest, and relaxation

Self-perception–self-concept pattern   Describes self-concept pattern and perceptions of self (e.g., body comfort, body image, feeling state)

Role-relationship pattern   Describes pattern of role-engagements and relationships

Sexuality-reproductive pattern   Describes client's patterns of satisfaction and dissatisfaction with sexuality pattern; describes reproductive patterns

Coping-stress-tolerance pattern   Describes general coping pattern and effectiveness of the pattern in terms of stress tolerance

Value-belief pattern   Describes patterns of values, beliefs (including spiritual), or goals that guide choices or decisions

---

areas of assessment applicable to all clients. The result would be that (1) the domain of responsibility and accountability would be clear, (2) the focus for clinical studies would be identified, and (3) the focus for development of expertise in assessment and diagnosis would be clearly delineated for teachers, students, and practitioners.

A typology of assessment categories proposed in the next section is viewed as a step in the direction of unification of *structural areas*. As stated previously, each nurse's *approach* to these areas is dictated by the conceptual framework utilized.

FUNCTIONAL HEALTH PATTERNS TYPOLOGY

The typology[5] of functional patterns in Table 3-6 contains a set of health-related areas quite familiar to nurses. Client reports and nurses' observations provide the data for identifying patterns.

The clinical information collected under the assessment structure shown in Table 3-6 is relevant to all conceptual models because it is *basic* information. The typology represents both traditional and contemporary ideas of nursing practice in a *concise, easily learned set* of category names.

---

[5] The pattern areas were identified by the author about 1974 for purposes of teaching assessment and diagnosis at Boston College School of Nursing. Colleagues have suggested some minor changes in labels and content. Faye E. McCain's (1965) and Dorothy Smith's (1968; Becknell and Smith, 1975) assessment concepts were particularly influential, as were the comments of clinical specialists and students who reviewed and tried out the categories in practice.

The 11 terms are readily committed to memory and thereafter serve as a guideline for assessment and for retrieving from memory the specific items to be assessed in each area (Appendix C). Most importantly, these functional pattern assessment areas lead nurses to nursing diagnoses, not medical diagnoses, thus eliminating a problem that has existed with biomedical systems categories.

In the following sections, general characteristics of patterns will be examined. A description of each of the 11 pattern areas will follow. Finally, arguments will be presented as to why these patterns provide a *structural* framework for the diagnostic process.

A Pattern Focus

The typology presented in Table 3-6 utilizes the term *pattern*, which is defined as a sequence of behavior[6] across time. *Sequences of behavior,* rather than isolated events, are the data used in clinical inference and judgment. For example, a nurse observes that a hospitalized client has an argument with her husband. What does the nurse infer? Nothing, one hopes! Is the quarrel a sign of the client's general pattern of relationships, marital included? Maybe or maybe not. Obviously, information about interactions across time is needed to determine whether relationships are possibly problematic for the client.

Patterns are constructed from clinical data gained in historytaking and examination. Suppose additional information about the couple just mentioned clarifies that the marital relationship is a problematic area. The nurse is still at an elementary level of pattern construction. Other relationships have to be assessed to see whether the problem is generalized or specific. These components of the total relationship pattern may include parent-child, work, social, and other kinds of interactions. When these sorts of data have been collected, the diagnostician can move toward understanding the overall role-relationship pattern and the client's perception of the pattern.

As information is collected, the nurse begins to understand the area being assessed. Gradually, a pattern emerges. It is very important to recognize that what occurs during information collection is the *construction of a pattern* from a client's descriptions and the nurse's observations. Recognizing this (1) prevents superficial data collection that can lead to errors in diagnosis and (2) serves as a constant reminder that patterns are not observable but are constructed by cognitive operations and therefore are always open to challenge by new information.

Understanding may still be elusive until all 11 health areas are assessed. Explanations of one pattern may lie in other pattern areas. As an example of the interaction and interdependence of pattern areas, perception of a threat to the self may be associated with transitory changes in relating to others.

The point to be made is that the "raw data" gathered during assessment are sequences of historical and current behavior across time. These sequences can be conceived as patterns if the observer puts the information together. (Note that lack of pattern in a functional health area is a type of pattern.)

---

[6] Behavior is used as an all-encompassing term. It refers to physiological, psychological, sociological, and any other classifications of behavior.

The second important point is that diagnoses describe dysfunctional or potentially dysfunctional patterns. In assessment and diagnosis the nurse works with *patterns within patterns*. The larger (more inclusive) patterns appear as one proceeds from concrete, observable sequences of behavior (patterns) to clustering and, finally, to a pattern synthesis that can be given a diagnostic label.

Does the process just described sound foreign? Consider that one usually is unable to make a judgment about data, such as heart rate or blood pressure, unless base-line data are available. Even one base-line measure and one current measure describe an elementary pattern across time, if the nurse puts the data together.

As another example, think of a friend's behavior that came to your attention recently. Did you expect or not expect the particular behavior? Why did you even have an expectation? Knowledge of your friend's previous behavioral patterns caused you to notice a difference. To understand the friend's behavior, information about the whole person and the situation (environmental events) was necessary. You have now been led to a synthesis. Many pieces of information have been put together to gain understanding.

The process is not foreign; human beings process information this way every day. When it is important for the life or comfort of another person that the correct synthesis and judgment occur, the process is done consciously and systematically.

The functional typology also helps to identify why a dysfunctional pattern may exist and what strengths, or assets, are within the client-environment situation. This is because the 11 patterns represent a composite of the client's life in the individual environment. Reasons for problems will be found within this composite, as well as the strengths that are needed to solve problems. No one pattern can be understood in isolation; the client and environment function as a whole. An example may clarify this idea: during a home visit a community health nurse collected the following information as part of a data base.

> Husband, 65 years old, has recently retired after selling the grocery store that previously occupied his time from 8 a.m. until 6 p.m. States he has little to do now and gets into arguments with his wife: "She doesn't like me around the house; it interferes with what she wants to do; I just want to spend more time talking to her and doing things together." Wife states she has the house to keep up, meals to cook, and her volunteer activities at the day care center every afternoon. States she can't get things done because "he's in the way" and "he mopes around the house."

The nurse collected two types of data: previous patterns and current patterns. Change was inferred. Even with this minimal information it can be seen that the problem may be in the area of roles and relationships; perhaps family conflict is a tenable diagnostic hypothesis at this point.

Look again at the list of functional health patterns in Table 3–6. In which categories might the etiology of this problem reside? Isn't it probable that data about coping pattern, activity pattern, and value-belief pattern would help the nurse to identify etiological factors and perhaps also to refine the problem? For example, is the husband's activity tolerance low? Is that why he doesn't engage in activities within or outside the home? Are the wife's and husband's values, relative to their relationship, divergent? Is there a lack of resources for retired persons in this community or has a choice been made not to use them? Certainly, questions could be raised regarding the contribution of all other pattern areas to this problem.

This example points out two things. First, the categories provide a structure for analyzing a problem *within* a category, as in the example of husband-wife conflict within family role and relationships. Secondly, a structure is provided to focus the search for causal explanations, usually *outside* the problem category; in the example of the grocer, activities, values, and coping patterns would be explored.

To make information processing even easier, the current list of accepted diagnoses (Appendix A) can be classified into the functional health pattern areas (Appendix B). As will be discussed in another chapter, a nurse can move horizontally from data in a pattern area to problem identification and then vertically through the patterns to identify etiological factors. Diagnosis is facilitated if information is gathered and organized in a way relevant to problem identification.

It will be useful at this time to further define the pattern areas. Keep in mind that these 11 functional health pattern areas are appropriate for nursing assessment of individuals, families, and communities. Also, these patterns form the *basic data base* for nursing assessment in all specialties and across all age groups.

Health-Perception–Health-Management Pattern The goal of nursing is to promote health. Yet it is clients who actually perceive and manage their health. Clients' perceptions of their health status and the practices they use to maintain health can be assessed. This information may indicate a dysfunctional pattern or may influence decisions about interventions for other problems.

Clients may become despondent about changes in their health and believe they have no control over events. "Fate" rather than their own behavior may be viewed as the main determinant of health. Teaching health practices in these situations will be to no avail. Perceptions and beliefs have to be dealt with first.

The objective in assessing the health-perception–health-management pattern is to obtain data about general perceptions, general health management, and preventive practices. Specific details are explored in other relevant pattern areas. For example, if a client says laxatives are taken for constipation, this information is held and noted. The question that follows may be, "Do you find you can solve most of your health problems yourself?"

In this pattern area, cues to potential health hazards in client practices, potential or actual noncompliance, and unrealistic health or illness perception should not be missed.

Individual Assessment When asked, each of us can offer a generalization about our health pattern. Sometimes the reference is to recent years, for example, "I've really felt good these last few years." Other statements may refer to childhood, such as, "I was a sickly child and ever since . . ." or "I never paid much attention to what I did; this illness has really taught me a lesson." Health perceptions can be used as a basis for understanding a client's past practices, including preventive measures, and for predicting future motivation toward health promotion.

Questions about health perceptions and health management may also elicit descriptions of illness. As the client talks about illness, *listen* for health perceptions and health management practices. For example, an adult client says, "After about a month of . . . [symptoms] , I tried to find a doctor that would see me." Listening would cause the nurse to think, "Delay in seeking help? No established resource for health care? Knowledge of community resources? Routine checkups?" Perceptions, meanings, responses, and practices are the *nursing* data.

Examination is generally done after obtaining subjective reports during a history. Observation of an individual's actual practices is difficult. Usually a nurse has to rely on clients' reports unless information is available from home visits or a client in a hospital can be given responsibility for certain treatments.

Family Assessment The family's perception of their health as a group usually is expressed in "we" statements such as "We've always been a healthy family because I see to it that . . . ." Usually one question phrased to obtain the group perception elicits both a perceived health pattern and explanations for the pattern. When individual members' health and health management (as perceived by the family representative speaking) are described, the nurse has to cluster data. A generalization about the family has to be made if each member's pattern and practices are described specifically. Listen to learn who seems to be the influential member in health-related decisions. This information may be useful if health practices need improving.

Community Assessment Listening to residents of a community, one may hear, "The drug problem here is terrible; this used to be a good community to raise children"; "We need a stop sign here for the children's crossing"; "They closed the clinic and now we have to go to the city"; or "Everybody's got the flu and it spreads through the schools; I can't remember a worse winter for sickness." Some of these statements provide cues to how people perceive the community's health pattern. Others provide cues about health management in the community. Sampling key groups can usually elicit historical patterns of "then and now" or "we've always been . . . ." The perceived reasons for patterns and practices usually are stated without prodding. If a problem is identified by a community group, the first step in health promotion is already accomplished. Other groups may have to be helped to gain insight into problems that exist.

Objective data on the health pattern of a community can be obtained from mortality and morbidity statistics, accident rates, and other data of public record. Assessing the use of health facilities and examining health legislation may also provide cues to a community's management pattern. Even more basic, do such services as home care, school health, and care of the aged exist?

Nutritional-Metabolic Pattern Clients' nutritional patterns and underlying dietary habits have always been a concern of nurses because of nurses' recognition that all life functions and well-being depend on adequate intake and the supply of nutrients to tissues. The focus of assessment in the nutritional-metabolic pattern area is food and fluid consumption relative to metabolic need.

The assessment objective is to collect data about the typical pattern of food and fluid consumption. Additionally, gross indicators of metabolic need are assessed, such as growth states (child growth, pregnancy, and tissue healing). Subjective reports are obtained regarding food and fluid consumption, problems perceived by the client or others, the client's explanations of problems, actions taken to solve problems, and the perceived effect of those actions.

Physical examination focuses on the skin, bony prominences, hair, oral mucous membranes, teeth, height and weight relative to age norms, and temperature. These indicators may provide validation of client reports regarding nutrient intake, nutrient supply to tissues, or metabolic need. As a minimum, the nurse screens for patterns indicating nutritional and fluid deficits, excess intake, and skin alterations or breakdown.

Individual Assessment The assessment of individual clients includes a typical daily intake of food, fluids, and nutrient supplements such as vitamins. Changes in nutritional-metabolic patterns may be elicited through interview or observed during examination.

Assessment of the skin provides important data about quality of nutrient intake and supply of nutrients to this tissue. Indicators of nutritional pattern include tissue healing after injuries; skin integrity; and integrity of mucous membranes, hair, and nails. Skin and mucous membranes, in particular, are highly metabolic organs. Cell duplication is rapid and, accordingly, so is utilization of nutrients. Because of high requirements, changes can be observed when problems exist in food or fluid consumption. Also, growth and physical development depend on nutrition and metabolism.

Family Assessment Family or household patterns of food, fluid, and supplement consumption are especially important. Many of our habits, as well as likes and dislikes, are learned in the family setting. The family member who does the shopping and cooking is most important to the assessment (as well as to subsequent intervention): This may be the family member who makes the nutrition-related decisions. Again the aim is to obtain general patterns; if the need arises, a nurse may shift to individual assessment of one or more members.

Community Assessment Groups of people living in a geographic area have nutritional-metabolic patterns. You've heard comments to substantiate this: "All these people are on food stamps, and you should see what they buy"; "Look at the elderly in this place; they're all thin; never enough money for food"; or "Just sitting in the park you see all the pink-cheeked, healthy babies and kids; you know, our schools have thrown out all those junk food machines." By interview, observation of people, and checking community resources a nurse can obtain an overview of qualitative and quantitative aspects of a community's pattern of food and fluid consumption.

Elimination Patterns Regularity and control of elimination patterns are important in most people's lives. Perhaps culturally based toilet training and media commercials about body odor and waste disposal emphasize this functional health pattern. It is an important area in which to assess clients' concerns.

The assessment objective is to collect data about regularity and control of excretory patterns (bowel, bladder, skin, and wastes). Subjective descriptions, problems perceived by the client or others, the client's explanations of problems, remedial actions taken, and the perceived effects of those actions are the data of concern. Examination includes gross screening of specimens, inspection of prostheses (devices such as ostomy bags), and noting any odors. Minimally, the nurse screens for patterns of incontinence and irregularity. Habits in regard to elimination and data from other pattern areas (nutritional, for example) may explain a dysfunctional pattern.

Individual Assessment The individual client's descriptions of regularity, control, quantity, and other characteristics of bowel, bladder, and skin excretory patterns are assessed. If problems are perceived by the client or others, the nurse obtains explanations, finds out what remedial actions have been taken, and asks about the perceived effect of the actions.

The excretory pattern indicators (quantity, regularity, etc.) are applicable even if a client has deviation from the normal route of excretion. There is still a bowel or urinary elimination pattern.

Laypeople have many misconceptions about regularity and control. Dependency on laxatives or enemas may mean that the client has a knowledge deficit regarding bowel regulation. This diagnosis should not be missed. Waste disposal, as discussed below, is also a component of excretory pattern that may be relevant to individual assessment in the home.

Family Assessment   When asking about family excretory patterns, the nurse focuses on waste disposal and related hygienic practices. Thus in a home visit the nurse may inquire whether garbage disposal is a problem. Observation would include sanitary practices related to waste disposal. These components of the excretory pattern would also be pertinent to an individual living alone.

Community Assessment   Communities are aggregates of individuals, households, and industries. Each of these social units has an excretory pattern of waste disposal that can influence the community. In recent years much attention has been given to hazardous waste disposal and air pollution. These topics as well as common sanitation or disposal practices are included in community assessment. Usually data can be collected from community leaders and by observation of statistics about certain infections, diseases, and radiation or pollution levels.

Activity-Exercise Pattern   Movement is one of the most important functional patterns. It permits people to control their immediate physical environment. Assessment of activity patterns can lead to the detection of poor health practices, prevention of major functional losses, or helping clients to compensate for loss.

The objective of assessment is to determine the client's pattern of activities that require energy expenditure. Components reviewed are daily activities, exercise, and leisure activities. Subjective descriptions of these pattern components, problems perceived by the client or others, the client's perceived reasons for any existing problems, actions taken to solve the problems, and perceived effects of those actions are elicited. Observation is an important aspect of assessment in this pattern area.

Individual Assessment   A screening of daily routine activities is done. These include the client's perceived capabilities for movement, self-care (feeding, bathing, dressing, grooming, and toileting) and, if relevant, home management. Each can be classified using the system in Table 3–7. Classifications also exist for assessing activity tolerance of clients with cardiac or pulmonary problems.

Irrespective of the client's mobility level, some degree of either active or passive exercise is needed. During assessment the type, amount, and frequency of exercise should be elicited. People also need leisure activities. Assessment of the activity-exercise pattern includes the type of recreational activities and the amount of time spent pursuing them.

The screening examination of the client may be limited to gait, posture, muscle tone, absence of body part, and prostheses or assistive devices employed. If indicated,

TABLE 3-7
CLASSIFICATION OF FUNCTIONAL ACTIVITY LEVEL

Score	Activity level
0	Total independence
1	Requires use of equipment or assistive device
2	Requires assistance or supervision from another person
3	Requires assistance or supervision from another person and equipment or device
4	Dependent and does not participate in self-care

Source: Adapted from McCourt (1981).

assessment of his or her range of motion in joints, hand grip, and ability to pick up a pencil will provide additional data. Pulse rate and rhythm and respiratory rate and depth may explain subjective reports about activity tolerance.

Minimally, screening assessment should reveal any actual or potential dysfunctional activity patterns. In particular, deficits in mobility, self-care, home management, and diversional activity should not be missed. The potential for joint contractures and in-effective airway clearance are also problems nurses have identified as within their scope of diagnostic judgment. These two conditions can predispose to activity pattern dysfunctions. In general, if a client has a cardiac, neurological, or respiratory disease, in-depth assessment is warranted. Also, developmental problems may be revealed by assessment of specific motor skills in children.

Family Assessment   Families can exhibit activity patterns. Some households run at a hectic level, others seem almost lethargic. Pace of activities is a characteristic of family activity; it may or may not be related to the number of family members.

Other than clichés, such as "The family that plays [leisure pattern] together, stays together," minimal information exists in nursing about family activity patterns. Doing things together and sharing recreational interests would appear to increase family solidarity. No diagnoses have been identified in the area of family activity patterns.

Community Assessment   Communities have rhythmic activity patterns. Some "roll up the sidewalks" at 9 p.m. and others are bustling night and day. In communities, activity can be associated with noise and crowding and may elicit complaints from residents who wish for more peace and quiet. Community activity patterns are also often beneficial, such as scheduled recreation. These resources permit individuals and families to socialize and enjoy leisure. Any community could be described in terms of its diversional activities, both recreational and cultural.

Evidence that generalizations can be made at the community activity level include statements such as, "There is nothing to do in this town" or "I'm so busy since I retired, with all the senior citizen activities going on." Because political, recreational, and cultural activities fulfill the lives of people, community assessment should include this pattern area.

Communities also have mobility patterns—public transportation systems. Information in this area is important for understanding accessibility to facilities for health care, recreation, or socialization.

Cognitive-Perceptual Pattern   To think, hear, see, smell, taste, and touch are human functions taken for granted until deficits arise. Prevention of deficits and helping clients to compensate for losses are important nursing activities.

The objective of assessing the client's cognitive-perceptual pattern is to describe the adequacy of language, cognitive skills, and perception relative to desired or required activities. Subjective descriptions, problems perceived by the client or others, compensations for deficits, and the effectiveness of efforts to compensate for them are elicited during the history.

During examination, observations are made of cognitive and sensory capabilities. Data in this pattern area are critical for future nursing intervention. For example, if judgment capabilities are inadequate, a client may need supervision. If the person is blind, safety may be a problem.

Individual Assessment   Cognitive and perceptual pattern components are assessed. Cognitive functions include language capability, memory, problem solving, and decision making. These are basic functions but should be evaluated relative to the complexity of environment chosen by the client. A mentally retarded person may be functioning quite independently in a sheltered environment. An active business executive in the same type of environment may exhibit symptoms of sensory or cognitive deprivation.

Examination of cognitive patterns occurs during the history. The nurse observes the client's language skills, grasp of ideas and abstractions, attention span, level of consciousness, reality-testing, and any aids required for communication. Some problem the client describes during assessment can be selected to measure problem solving and decision making. In fact, in each pattern area the client's perception of problems, reasons for problems, actions taken, and perceived effectiveness of actions provide a wealth of data on cognitive functions.

The subjective report of the client regarding patterns of vision, hearing, touch, taste, and smell can be supplemented by actual testing. For example, keep some newsprint in your pocket and use it to screen for visual difficulties. Don't miss assessing for prostheses such as glasses or hearing aids.

The ability to feel pain or discomfort is another sensory capability of human beings. If pain is present, especially chronic pain, ask the client how he or she manages it. The answer may reveal deficits in pain management that require intervention. Nurses have many ways of helping people deal with pain.

In assessing cognitive functions and sensory modes, be alert to compensations clients may use that mask basic dysfunctions. Safety of the client may be jeopardized if problems are not detected. Remember that at times we all have memory lapses, make illogical statements, and fail to recognize a familiar object or person. It may be necessary to elicit impressions from family members to differentiate between common, temporary lapses and progressive deficits.

Cues to sensory deficits, sensory deprivation or overload, and pain management problems must not be overlooked. Impaired reasoning, knowledge deficits related to health practices, and memory deficits are additional problems that may exist and may even be the basis for other dysfunctional patterns.

Family Assessment   The cognitive-perceptual pattern of a family is evidenced in how family decisions are made, the concreteness or abstractness of thinking, and whether decisions are oriented to the future or present. Data in these areas may be the basis for understanding other problems such as family disorganization and stress. Nurses have a number of ways of helping families in the cognitive-perceptual area of health functioning.

Community Assessment While assessing a community a nurse can obtain data on decision making, especially regarding health-related matters. Are the school board and parent-teacher association effective? How are community decisions made? Sitting in on meetings of committees dealing with health issues usually provides a wealth of information. Do all groups participate, and are their voices heard regarding health matters? Is future planning done, or are crisis reactions the pattern? These questions can elicit data about the cognitive processes operating in a community.

Sleep-Rest Pattern Preoccupations with sleep arise only when it eludes us; otherwise it is something taken for granted. In today's busy world, rest and relaxation may also elude a lot of people.

The objective in assessing a sleep-rest pattern is to describe the effectiveness of the pattern from the client's perspective. Some are well rested after 4 hours of sleep; others need much more. Rest and relaxation are also assessed in regard to client perceptions. What may be relaxing to some is considered work by others. If problems are perceived by the client or others, explanations, previous actions taken, and perception of their effect are elicited.

Individual Assessment The nurse screens the client's sleep-rest pattern by finding out about the person's general feeling of readiness for daily activities after sleep. If problems are perceived, the dysfunctional pattern is described. Rest and relaxation comprise a second component to be assessed in this pattern.

If problems are present, assessment should include sleep onset, sleep interruption (including dreams), or early awakening patterns. Sleep pattern reversal (day-night reversal) is another problem that should not be overlooked. Use of sleeping aids, both prescription and nonprescription, should be elicited during pattern assessment. As previously stated, the client's perception of a dysfunctional pattern provides valuable cues. Clients who appear to sleep but report sleep deprivation may not be getting sufficient deep sleep.

Family Assessment There may be a general pattern of sleep within a family. Some adhere to "early to bed, early to rise." Rest and relaxation patterns also are frequently built into family patterns. These can be assessed. Sometimes the family pattern is disturbed because of one member's sleep problem. This situation may require a shift to individual assessment.

Community Assessment Communities usually have patterns of sleeping, resting, and relaxation. Some towns are described as "never shut down." Disturbances in the community sleep-rest pattern can be inferred from residents' comments about continuous highway noise or airplanes going over all night. Such disturbance produces health concerns and can increase levels of stress.

Self-Perception–Self-Concept Pattern Many psychologists have tried to describe the consciousness of being, or awareness of existence, that all humans have. This sense of being is commonly referred to as the self. Clients have perceptions and concepts of themselves, such as body image, social self, self-competency, and subjective mood states. Negative evaluations of the self can produce personal discomfort and also can influence other functional patterns. Change, loss, and threat are common factors that may impinge on self-concept.

The objective of assessment in this pattern area is to describe the client's pattern of beliefs and evaluations regarding general self-worth and feeling states. Problems the client or others identify, explanations or reasons they identify for the problems, actions taken to try to solve the problems, and effects of those actions are also described.

Assessment of self-concept and self-perception usually is not effective (accurate and thorough) unless the client has a sense of trust in the nurse. People tend not to share personal feelings unless the nurse has already established an empathic and non-judgmental atmosphere. As Powell reminds us, "But, if I tell you who I am, you may not like who I am, and it is all that I have" (1969, p. 12).

Individual Assessment   A person's self-perception–self-concept pattern may be screened by obtaining data about (1) general feelings of self-worth and personal identity and (2) general emotional pattern. If cues or situations warrant, more in-depth assessment can be done.

Observation during an admission interview can reveal nonverbal cues about self-concept and self-perception. Body posture and movement, eye contact, and voice and speech pattern are important to observe. Cues to identity confusion, altered body image, lowered self-esteem, perceptions of powerlessness, situational depression, and fear should not be missed.

Family Assessment   Families have perceptions and concepts about their image; their status in the community; and their competency, as a unit, to deal with life. Emotional patterns tend to be shared because of the close relationships in a family or household. Situations that affect one member usually produce an effect on the entire family group. To help a family realize its potential, the nurse needs to assess how the family members perceive their family.

Community Assessment   Just as families and individuals have patterns of self-worth and personal identity, so have communities. Image, status, and perceived competency to deal with problems are characteristics that can be assessed.

The image of a community may be reflected in housing conditions, buildings, and cleanliness. Community perception of self-worth may relate to school systems, crime rates, accidents, and whether residents and outsiders consider it "a good place to live." Competency in dealing with social and political issues and community spirit cause self-evaluation to be positive. Knowing the level of community "pride" may assist a nurse in developing innovative health programs. The emotional tone (fear, depression, or a generally positive emotional outlook) can usually be related to findings in other pattern areas. For example, tensions in the community relationship pattern may explain a general feeling of fear in the residents.

Role-Relationship Pattern   Much has been written about relationships, including the human need for others and the influence of relationships on personal and group development. People engage in many levels of relationships. Some are very close, such as family relationships. Others are superficial and without any true sharing, as described in the lyrics of "The Sounds of Silence" by Paul Simon:

> And in the naked night I saw
> Ten thousand people, maybe more,
> People talking without speaking,
> People hearing without listening,
> People writing songs that voices never shared.
> No one dared
> Disturb the sounds of silence.[7]

The objective of role-relationship pattern assessment is to describe a client's pattern of family and social roles. The client's perceptions about his or her relationship patterns (satisfactions and dissatisfactions) are also a component of this pattern area.

Individual Assessment   The major role-taking and relationship patterns in a person's life situation are the components of the role-relationship pattern. Family roles, work or student roles, and social roles are some of the major aspects assessed. Clients' satisfactions and dissatisfactions with role responsibilities and relationships are elicited. If the client perceives problems in this pattern area, perceived reasons for the problems, actions that have been taken to remedy the problems, and effects of those actions are assessed.

Family roles are usually particularly important in the individual's life. Discussion with a client in this area discloses how many are in the family group or household, including both children and adults, and whether there is a nuclear or extended family. Roles and relationships are usually reviewed before the sexuality-reproductive pattern. This sequence permits a natural transition in the discussion.

Loss, change, or threat produce the major problems in the role-relationship pattern. The cues that should not be missed are related to problems such as grieving, conflict, social isolation, impaired verbal communication, and potential for violence.

Working roles and relationships are an important area to assess. Statistics indicate that many people (nurses included) suffer occupational role stress (McLean, 1978). Assessment should include whether the client perceives the work environment to be safe and healthy. Does the work role leave time for rest and leisure? Because work has the potential to contribute to self-fulfillment, the client's satisfaction with work roles and organization of work activities is assessed. Financial concerns, unemployment, and other issues related to work are identified. Assessment of the school-age client or college student should elicit any problems related to roles and relationships in these settings.

Family Assessment   Roles and relationships of a particularly close kind are a fundamental aspect of family life. Relationships can be supportive and growth-producing. At the opposite extreme, violence and abuse can permeate relationships of families under stress.

As with individual assessment, structural aspects of the family are assessed. These include living space, number of members, their ages, and their various roles.

There are a number of ways the dynamics of family relationships can be assessed. One is in terms of interdependence, dependence, and independence. Another approach is based on the ways relationships influence the family's developmental tasks. Family

[7]©1964, 1965 by Paul Simon. Used by permission.

developmental tasks, according to Duvall (1967), include (1) physical maintenance; (2) resource allocation; (3) division of labor; (4) socialization of members; (5) reproduction, recruitment, and release of members; (6) maintenance of order; and (7) maintenance of motivation and morale.

Community Assessment   The basic function of a community lies in its collaborative relationships and allocation of role responsibilities. Nursing assessment is particularly concerned with whether a community structure of roles and relationships permits residents to realize their health-related potentialities. Patterns of crime, racial incidents, and social networks are indexes of human relationships in a community.

Sexuality-Reproductive Pattern   Sexuality is the behavioral expression of sexual identity. It may involve, but is not limited to, sexual relationships with a partner. Just as in other functional patterns, cultural norms regulate expression.

Currently in western society the norms for sexuality are in a state of flux. The distinction between what is masculine and what is feminine is sometimes blurred, and the scope of acceptable sexual expression is widening within some groups. Yet society imposes limits. Sexual abuse of children and incest are not tolerated. When clients choose modes of expression that are marginally acceptable, problems can arise. Individual problems may also arise when discrepancies exist between the expression of sexuality the person has attained and the expression he or she desires.

Reproductive patterns involve reproductive capacity and reproduction itself. The cultural norms that affect reproduction are also undergoing change. The number of children in families is smaller and in many cases pregnancies and births are planned.

The objective of assessment in the sexuality-reproductive pattern is to describe problems or potential problems.

Individual Assessment   A screening assessment of an individual client's expression of sexuality is focused on developmental patterns and perceived satisfactions or dissatisfactions. If problems are perceived, the nurse obtains the client's explanation of the problem, a history of remedial action taken, and the client's opinion about the effectiveness of those actions. It is important not to miss problems related to expression of sexuality in clients of any age.

Assessment of reproductive patterns involves collecting information about the client's stage of reproductive development in relationship to developmental milestones such as menarche or climacteric. Number of pregnancies and live births provide information about a female client's reproductive pattern. Development of reproductive capacities (secondary sex characteristics and genital development) should be assessed in young clients. It is important not to miss problems associated with contraceptives, reproduction, menstruation, or climacteric.

Family Assessment   The information collected in assessment of a family's sexuality pattern includes a couple's level of satisfaction with their sexual relationship, any problems they perceive, how the problems are managed, and the results of actions taken to resolve the problems. When there are children in the household, the nurse would be interested in what information about sexual subjects is taught to children as well as when and how this is communicated. If the adults feel uninformed or uncomfortable in discussing sexual subjects with children, the nurse who is aware of the problem can provide important assistance. Although previously considered a very personal matter, sexual relationships and feelings related to sexual identity have become more openly discussed. This trend toward freer discussion may not affect all clients; thus the nurse obtains information in a sensitive manner.

The reproductive pattern assessment includes any problems the couple perceives, explanations they offer for the problems, actions they have taken to deal with the problems, and the result of the actions. The number and ages of children, number and outcomes of pregnancies, and birth control methods in use are included in the family data base.

Community Assessment Community attitudes toward sexuality are assessed. Do educational programs exist in schools or churches? Does the community desire such programs? If the residents view sex education as a function of the family, are there programs for parents?

Crime in general was assessed in the area of relationships. In the sexuality-reproductive pattern it is useful to note the incidence of sex-related crime or sexual abuse of children in the community. A high incidence may indicate the need for increased community awareness and action.

The reproductive pattern of a community is reflected in birth, miscarriage, and abortion rates. Maternal and fetal mortality rates are also very important indicators. The accessibility of health services as well as availability of childbirth education programs should be assessed. Access to family planning and abortion services is assessed in terms of the community's desire for such services. In areas with high rates of adolescent pregnancies, the availability of programs for continued schooling is assessed.

Compiling such information enables the nurse to evaluate community needs and available services. Problems are identified when needs and health services do not match. The sexuality-reproductive pattern of individuals, families, and communities can be viewed as a component of the role-relationship pattern. It is listed separately so that sexual and reproductive assessment are not neglected. An additional reason for separating the two is that sexuality and reproduction involve a different level of relationships than those established in social or work groups. The assessment interview should flow smoothly from self-concept pattern to relationships with others and then on to sexual relationships.

Coping–Stress-Tolerance Pattern Stress is a part of living for any person at any age. In fact, many say that without stress there would be no growth. For example, learning to walk places stress on bones, a factor necessary for their integrity and development. Separating from the security of home also produces stress but leads to social development.

Stressor, coping, and *stress tolerance* are three terms whose definitions are intertwined. A *stressor* is an event that threatens or challenges the integrity of the human being. It produces a psychophysiological response that can lead to growth and further development or to disorganization manifested as anxiety, fear, depression, and other changes in self-perception or roles and relationships.

People respond to events differently. To know if a particular event is stressful for a person, family, or community the nurse has to ascertain the *client's* perception or definition of the situation. Community disasters, loss of a family member, illness, or hospitalization are usually perceived as a threat to integrity or to the usual pattern of life activities; thus, these are stressors. The meaning of potentially stressful events and the perceived degree of control over the events influence the amount of stress induced.

The way in which people generally respond to events perceived as a threat is their *coping pattern*. Clients' general patterns of coping may or may not be effective in handling stressful situations. Some clients employ problem solving; others respond with denial or other mental mechanisms. All these are learned behaviors for dealing with stress. The more effective the coping pattern, the greater sense of control the client can exert over the threat to integrity.

Stress-tolerance pattern describes the amount of stress the client has handled effectively. This, of course, is related to the amount of stress previously experienced and the effectiveness of coping patterns. A client's stress-tolerance pattern predicts, to some extent, potential for effective coping; however, people can mobilize resources and withstand levels of stress that exceed their previous experience.

The objective of assessment in this pattern area is to describe the stress tolerance and coping pattern of a client. Not to be missed are changes in the effectiveness of a coping pattern, which can occur if a threat to integrity is perceived as beyond personal control (personal coping capacity). This type of situation should lead the nurse to make a more in-depth assessment of support systems available to the client.

Individual Assessment The nurse asks the client to recall stressful life events, briefly tell how they were managed, and evaluate the effectiveness with which he or she coped with those situations. This history provides information about stress tolerance and coping pattern.

Data from other pattern areas may indicate that the client perceives a current or an anticipated threat to integrity. If such a threat is perceived, assessment proceeds to an examination of perceived control; that is, the nurse inquires how the client plans to deal with the situation and has the client evaluate the likelihood that the proposed coping pattern will be effective.

Why the emphasis on the individual's perception of events? This is because, as Selye says, "It is not what happens to you, but the way you take it [that matters]" (1979). Surgical mortality rate may be less than 1 percent, a low probability of death, yet if the client perceives the threat of death as high, surgery will be a stressor. Clients' personal concepts, constructed from the knowledge they have, determine their reactions. In a sense it is irrelevant what reality is; reality "is" whatever the client perceives. This is why subjective data are so important. Intervention begins with the way the client views the situation.

Family Assessment Dimensions of family assessment in this pattern area are similar to those in individual assessment. It is well to remember that family life revolves around a set of interrelationships. These relationships can be the supportive structure of a coping pattern but also can be a source of stress.

Community Assessment Stressors are sometimes experienced by a whole community. These are usually revealed in the data of previous pattern areas and may include such problems as unemployment, racial or ethnic tensions, drug problems, or accident rates. Natural disasters may threaten community integrity and require outside support for coping patterns.

A pattern of coping with community-wide stressors is usually revealed by interviews with community members. Leaders are quick to evaluate the effectiveness of community coping and "what works in our town." A community's stress tolerance depends upon supportive relationships between community groups.

Value-Belief Pattern A pattern of valuing and believing is found at all ages. As people develop, the emerging pattern of values and beliefs becomes more complex and, generally, more conscious. Beliefs and values include opinions about what is correct, proper, meaningful, and good, in a personal sense. Collective value and belief patterns also exist within a society or culture. These group norms may or may not be consistent with the personal pattern of a particular client or health care provider. Conflicts can arise. When important alternatives present themselves, values help determine choices. Choices deal with what is right or wrong for the person. *Right and wrong* relate to action; *good and bad* refer to outcomes or goals (Steele and Harmon, 1979, pp. 1-4).

Belief patterns describe what people hold to be true on the basis of faith or conviction. They are arrived at by inference and form the basis for attitudes or predispositions. Beliefs are the philosophical and theological dimensions of personal knowing. They include explanations at a very abstract level, including explanations of life, existence, and why certain things are valued. Common, day-to-day actions may not require this level of thought and explanation. Illness and other significant events provide the time and motivation to review life, goals, and what is important.

Patterns of valuing describe the importance or worth accorded to goals, actions, people, objects, and other phenomena. The value pattern can influence a client's health-related decisions about personal practices, treatments, health priorities, and even life or death.

The objective in assessing clients' value-belief pattern is to understand the basis for health-related decisions and actions. This understanding increases sensitivity to value-belief conflicts that may arise if preventive action isn't taken.

Individual Assessment Life requires decisions. Thus, as human beings develop they construct a system of beliefs and values, in fact a philosophical system. This system provides guidelines for important decisions and ways of behaving. It may or may not be tied to theological and religious beliefs and values.

The assessment of value-belief patterns focuses on what is important to clients in their lives. Beliefs and values can be regarded as spiritual in the broadest sense of "human spirit." Usually nurses assess more specific areas, such as religious preference or religious practices. This broader view of "what is important" includes, but is not limited to, religious practices.

Understanding a client's personal value-belief pattern can increase sensitivity to potential conflicts and help clients examine ways their belief system can assist them in decision making. Clients' use of philosophical or theological values and beliefs as a predominant coping strategy has not been systematically studied in nursing. The nurse who understands the client's spiritual beliefs (including, but not limited to, religious beliefs) may be able to support coping strategies of this type.

Family Assessment Families have value-belief patterns. Some say the sharing of values and beliefs is one of the important characteristics of a successful marriage.

Dissimilar value-belief patterns within a marital or family relationship usually produce conflicts observed in other pattern areas, such as role-relationships. Conflicts also arise when members, such as teenagers, are in the process of developing a conscious awareness of values and beliefs. Because of the potential for family disorganization, value-belief pattern conflicts should not be missed during assessment.

Community Assessment Communities have health-related values; understanding these is critical in diagnosing conflicts when working with community groups. Value patterns underlie decisions about where tax money should be spent; and whether or not the community should have an abortion clinic, sex education in the schools, senior citizen centers, and special education for the handicapped. These and many other community issues that affect health ultimately rest on the predominant value-belief pattern of a community.

Functional Pattern Characteristics

Patterns have four characteristics that deserve discussion. Two relate to their focus, one to the use of the term *functional*, and one to usability.

Client-Environment Focus Interaction between the client and environment is an essential, common thread throughout all functional patterns. From this interaction, patterns develop. For example, patterns of role-relationships and self-concept are influenced by the environment, particularly people and culture. This influence begins at birth and is more pronounced as language and nonverbal behavior are learned. Taking and giving emotional support is another example of client-environment interaction; in this instance the interaction influences coping patterns.

Crop production, food additives, and environmental temperature all influence a nutritional-metabolic pattern. As another example, much has been said in news reports about human activities that negatively change the natural environment, such as industrial waste elimination patterns. This example illustrates a change in natural environmental patterns produced by human beings that then, in turn, influences human patterns. Client-environment interaction is an integral part of information collection in each pattern area.

Developmental Focus Nurses are concerned with human development of children and adults. Consequently any structure for information collection must include development. What is human development? Could it not be conceived as the development of the functional patterns? Human growth and development are reflected in each pattern area. Elimination patterns change, particularly in the area of control. Maturation toward adult norms occurs in role-relationship, cognitive-perceptual, and other patterns as years go by. The 11 functional patterns are judged, in part, against age norms, or developmental norms. Thus, a developmental focus is built into the functional typology.

Functional Focus Questions may be raised about using the term *functional patterns*. Traditionally, "ways of living," or functional patterns, have been an important focus of nursing's health promotion, assistance, and rehabilitation activities. Yet *functional* is a term used in other professions also. It may be useful to consider differences and similarities. In medicine the word *function* is used to describe physiological function, such as respiratory function, cardiac function, or brain function. The diagnostic focus is on functions of organs and systems, not functions of the whole individual.

Compare information nurses and physicians collect in assessment. Physicians, in the process of identifying medical diagnoses, want to know whether respiratory function is impaired. Clinical data of concern are respiratory depth and frequency, skin color, coughing, dyspnea, fatigue, and so forth.

Nurses, in the process of identifying possible nursing diagnosis, ask other things. Consider the example of a client with impaired respiratory function, a factor influencing activity tolerance. Nurses ask about stairs in the home, meal preparation, shopping, changes in body perception, and relationships. They want information about air pollution and work environment. At other times they try to influence people's effects on the environment. Air pollution that can be detrimental to the activity pattern of a client with respiratory disease is a case in point.

Information collected by nurses is relevant to human patterns, quality of life, and the achievement of human health potential. The information collected is used to identify human patterns that result from human-environment interactions. This is quite a different level from organ or system functions. The distinction is the difference in focus of medicine and nursing.

Both physicians and nurses collect data about functional patterns, but different patterns. Obviously, their interventions are also different. Does this mean that cardiorespiratory or genitourinary functions are not of interest to nurses? Certainly not; an abnormal cardiorespiratory pattern influences function, or "way of living." Nurses need information about cardiorespiratory function to complete their understanding of a client's functional health patterns. Are the same data about health patterns of interest to the cardiologist? Certainly, but they are not *critical data* in the diagnosis of disease (Booth, 1979).

Another question is whether nurses are ever concerned solely with cardiac or neurological assessment. In caring for a client who is unable to monitor his or her own heart rate or pupil dilation, nurses collect information for two purposes. One purpose is to understand or predict functional patterns, as has been discussed. The second reason is that the nurse reports complications and disease progression to a physician when the client lacks the expertise or ability to do this. This is the area of practice where tentative medical diagnoses may be made by nurses for purposes of referral.

Usability in Practice   Appendix C presents a list of pattern indicators that should be included in a basic assessment of functional patterns.[8] This list will provide the nursing data required by most current assessment tools; it also screens for all the problems described by the current nursing diagnoses. Assessment in greater depth is indicated

---

[8] These areas for data collection are derived from the definitions of the 11 functional patterns. These pattern indicators have been tested clinically for usability, reviewed by practicing clinical specialists in all of the nursing specialty areas of practice, and have been used in approximately 250 admission assessments in acute care hospitals.

when this basic assessment suggests a deviation from norms or when other existing health problems (medical or nursing) predict a functional problem. Both situations (deviations from norms and predictions on the basis of coexisting problems) lead the nurse to generate *possible* diagnoses. The possible diagnoses, particularly their defining signs and symptoms, become guidelines for further assessment in these situations.

Consider an example. If a client has a heart condition, theoretical knowledge predicts that his or her activity-exercise pattern may be influenced by the disease. The nurse, sensitive to this possibility, knows an in-depth assessment of the pattern may be required. Look at the Appendix B grouping of problems. Which might be predicted to be present?

Cardiovascular system pathology can be associated with decreased activity tolerance, impaired home maintenance management, and, depending on the severity, perhaps self-care deficits. Diversional activities may be altered if the client's chosen activities require power, speed, and endurance.[9] The signs and symptoms defining these health problems should be used to guide in-depth assessment.

The length of time required to complete an admission assessment varies greatly. The time spent depends partly on the expertise of the nurse to zero in on the pertinent data and partly on the client. The more health problems a client has, the more time is needed to identify them and the underlying dysfunctional patterns.

The issue of an assessment tool's usability relative to the time available in clinical settings is important to nurses. A truism of clinical practice is that nurses never have enough time. This is not necessarily because they do not organize efficiently; sometimes clients' care needs exceed the staff time available.

It is hard to say which functional health patterns are not important to assess when a nurse is "too busy." Value-belief patterns? That one sounds abstract; can it be sacrificed? To do so is risky; later it may be found that all nursing care efforts have been in vain because the client's values or beliefs were ignored.

Is some information needed in all categories? It seems that an administrative problem exists if not every client entering the health care system can have a basic health assessment. If assessment is important, then it has to be done; if valued, then it will be done. Nurses have a difficult time depriving clients of something nurses feel is needed. When assessments are not done, usually it is because of the value-belief system of the nurse; when other valued activities cannot be carried out, the problem is referred to administration.

The practical response to the time dilemma can be problem screening in each pattern area. For example, a new client could be asked, "Most mornings when you wake up, do you feel rested and ready for the day's activities?" This screening question for the sleep-rest pattern may provide sufficient information to make a judgment about whether or not a problem exists. Other health problems, age, or observations can provide cues to help the nurse decide when the risk of screening, as opposed to full health assessment, can be taken.

Screening assessments are indicated when the client is in critical condition. When

---

[9] Alterations in cardiac output and abnormal tissue perfusion, as currently defined, seem to be rewording of the medical diagnoses. In this author's opinion these are diagnoses for the purpose of referral to a physician. More will be said about this type of diagnostic activity in a later section.

the client is unable to respond to questions, the family or others provide a history; or assessment may be done primarily by physical examination. The main objective when the client is critical is to preserve life; the data collection should take this into account. Later, when the client is stabilized, a complete health pattern review can be done.

In summary, functional health patterns provide a basic data base for use with any conceptual framework. They supply the concrete structure for collecting information in a comprehensive, purposeful manner. The structure reveals what to collect; how to go about collecting clinical information is the subject of the next chapter.

WHAT IS A PROBLEM?

The preceding discussion of functional health patterns makes it possible now to specify more clearly what health problems are the focus of nursing diagnosis. Previously we have either referred to the list of diagnoses in Appendix A or said that problems are health-related conditions that respond primarily to nursing care. Clearer guidelines are required during information collection. The nurse making an assessment must know what clinical data to pay attention to.

What one attends to depends primarily on one's purpose. The main purpose of collecting information from a new client is to see whether health problems exist. If so, nursing care is offered.

Clinical information may indicate that *all* patterns are at an optimal functional level. This finding suggests health and a high level of well-being. Another finding may be that *some* patterns are functional. These patterns are strengths in the client's situation that may be used to influence or resolve problems.

Clinical data may indicate an actual or potentially dysfunctional pattern. A dysfunctional pattern is a problem when it (1) generates therapeutic concern on the part of the client, others, or the nurse,[10] and (2) is amenable to nursing treatment. The signs and symptoms of the problem and the etiological factors are given labels. Problem and etiological factors constitute a nursing diagnosis.

A dysfunctional pattern can be viewed as a self-care deficit (Orem, 1980), a maladaptation (Roy, 1980), a behavioral system instability (Grubbs, 1980), or a human need (Yura and Walsh, 1978). Dysfunctional health patterns can be thought of as responses to a stressor (Little and Carnevali, 1976) or to conflicting needs (Soares, 1978). Certainly they are human responses (Campbell, 1978; American Nurses' Association, 1981). Dysfunctional patterns are sufficiently concrete to accommodate various conceptual viewpoints.

Pathology and its treatment can alter functional patterns; these alterations are the secondary functional effects of disease or treatment. Examples are changes in usual coping patterns and stress tolerance with disease, changes in elimination patterns and metabolism with bed rest, and the not uncommon readjustment of value-belief patterns after a life-threatening illness.

Figure 3–1 depicts secondary functional effects of disease. Consider a common case.

---

[10] *Therapeutic concern* is a term used by Taylor (1971) to refer to a client's desire to receive treatment or a nurse's desire to provide it.

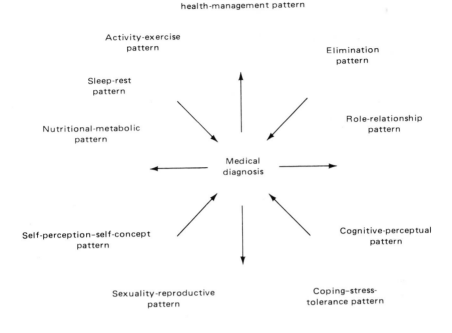

FIGURE 3-1
Effect of disease on functional patterns, and of functional patterns on development of a disease.

A person is hospitalized for weight loss, frequent urination, thirst, and an elevated blood glucose level. Medical tests support a diagnosis of diabetes mellitus. Nurses familiar with the typical newly diagnosed client with diabetes will attest to the fact that secondary effects are widespread. The pathology, its treatment, the personal response of the client and family, and the long-term management of the condition influence all functional patterns, as illustrated by the arrows in Figure 3–1 proceeding from medical diagnosis outward to pattern areas.

In addition to disturbances in functional patterns secondary to disease, dysfunctional patterns can occur when no evidence of disease is present. A client may be designated healthy from a medical perspective but still require nursing care. This phenomenon is also illustrated in Figure 3-1. Arrows proceeding from functional patterns to medical diagnosis represent the idea that unresolved dysfunctional patterns can increase susceptibility to various diseases, stressors, and microorganisms.

Few escape the media messages that life patterns can predispose to illness. One is told to walk or jog (exercise-activity pattern); cut down on saturated fats (nutritional-metabolic pattern); stop smoking, lose weight, and get regular checkups (health management pattern), learn to handle stress (role-relationship pattern), set priorities and ignore inconsequential annoyances (value-belief pattern), and remember "number one" (self-perception–self-concept pattern). This list is just to prevent cardiovascular disease.

Many people need help to work out productive health patterns. Nurses have always assumed responsibility for health promotion and health maintenance. Systematic, early identification and treatment of actual and potential problems (dysfunctional patterns) would probably have demonstrable effects on the health of the population.

Thus far it has been argued here (1) that from a nursing perspective health problems are defined as dysfunctional patterns, (2) that potential or actual dysfunctional patterns are labeled as nursing diagnoses, and (3) that nursing's major contribution to health care is in prevention and treatment of dysfunctional health patterns. This conceptual background provides a beginning answer to the earlier question, What is a problem? But to make a judgment that a dysfunctional pattern exists requires more concrete guidelines than this provides.

Types of Health Problems

To obtain more specific guidelines for diagnosing a dysfunctional pattern, let us consider those that most frequently generate therapeutic concern. They include (1) dysfunctional changes from base line and (2) stabilized dysfunctional patterns.

First of all, patterns may change from the client's individual base line. When historical and current data indicate two different patterns, change obviously has occurred. For example, a client may report that he has had to "slow down lately." Walking two city blocks and climbing a flight of stairs to his apartment causes shortness of breath; greater fatigue is present than previously. He may say he's been wondering lately whether his job is "too much for him," since his heart "can't be improved." Clearly these cues point toward a change in this patient's activity-exercise pattern.

A second type of health problem is a stabilized dysfunctional pattern. No recent change has occurred but the pattern is unhealthful. Historical and current data provide support for this judgment. For example, a geriatric clinical specialist found that her clients, residents of an inner city housing complex for the elderly, considerably restricted their activity-exercise patterns. Many confined themselves to their own building, except for arranged bus trips, because of a high incidence of violent crime in their neighborhood. The pattern was judged unhealthy for the clients, although adaptive in their environment. Ways had to be found to protect them from violence.

A stabilized pattern can also be unhealthful if developmental potential has not been realized. An example would be provided by a child who has not developed self-care activities appropriate to his developmental level. There are a number of theories and milestones (norms) of development across the life-span that can be used to make judgments about functional patterns, such as when tying shoelaces or dressing independently can be expected. Underdeveloped potential can exist in individuals, families, and even regions of the world. Nurses are concerned when underdevelopment results from, or leads to, health problems.

The purpose of discussing the various types of dysfunctional patterns is not to make diagnosis more complex. Rather, it is to provide some concrete guidelines. When clients describe functional health patterns (what is eaten, how they cope with stress, perceptions of health, and so forth), watch for or probe for:

1 Changes from an optimal to a dysfunctional pattern. Is there a change? Is it unhealthful?

2 Stabilized dysfunctional pattern. Is there a long-term history of continuing unhealthful behavior?

3 Stabilized dysfunctional developmental pattern. Is development delayed or interrupted?

Keeping these questions in mind increases sensitivity to cues when information is being collected.

Etiological Factors

Information collection permits the nurse to construct a description of each of the client's 11 functional patterns. When a problem is identified in a pattern area, the next question is why. Etiological factors are explanations—answers to that question. The probable explanation, or cause, usually lies in *one or more of the remaining patterns*. This assumption is based on the interdependence and interaction of functional patterns and on the belief that the client responds as a whole person-situation configuration.

Consider an example. A change in self-perception, such as anxiety, can influence all other patterns, including nutritional patterns, sleep-rest patterns, and, in severe cases, activity patterns. As another example, consider the 11 functional patterns in Table 3-6. Suppose a client developed a dysfunctional perceptual pattern, such as uncompensated visual deficit. In which patterns would you expect problems to occur? To some degree in all, depending on the meaning of the dysfunction in the client's life.

Each pattern is an expression of the whole and in turn influences the whole. In identifying the etiology of a problem, look for another dysfunctional pattern that may be a probable cause. If a nurse can determine the underlying dysfunctional pattern, intervention should be effective in resolving the problem. Identifying the etiology is not always easy to do, because cause and effect relationships are usually complex and contain an element of uncertainty. Diagnoses are formulated at the most complete level possible within the time, resources, and data available. Both the problem and the etiology are always open to revision.

Causality is important in everyday thinking. Most adults have some intuitive notion of the concept. Simply, it means that a cause-and-effect relationship exists between certain things. A finger used to flick a light switch "causes" a light bulb to light. This level of explanation usually suffices, except when the light does not go on. Then it is necessary to seek other levels of explanation, such as flow of electrical current and the workings of a light bulb.

Even deeper levels of causation have to be sought when people in adjacent homes are unable to turn on their lights by flipping their switches. Cause and effect are not so simply explained when a whole area of the country experiences a blackout. Hypotheses about the relationship between power production and electricity distribution have to be formulated. It becomes clear that there are many levels of explanation and a chain of cause-and-effect relationships.

We experience every day the fact that our actions do indeed change things. By inductive reasoning from experience, we attribute cause to action. This observed link between action and outcome produces one notion of cause and effect. The other, also arrived at by induction, is the concept of natural cause. From the sidelines it is observed that A has caused B or that A is causing B. Combining the two notions of causality in clinical practice, it is reasoned, If A is causing B and the nurse intervenes in the A conditions, then a change in B should result.

The first question to be raised is, What is the rationale for saying A is the cause of B? Stated differently, What is the basis for judging that a particular phenomenon is the etiology of a particular problem? What level of causal explanation is sought in nursing practice? What level in nursing science? A major issue is, What level of certainty should be reached before saying *this* is the etiology, or cause? The questions are of major importance because precious human resources will be used to intervene (or teach the client to intervene) in causal factors.

Determining the etiology of a dysfunctional pattern is very important before the nursing process is further implemented. Nursing intervention is based on the factors that cause or maintain a problem as well as on the health problem itself. For example, suppose a communication deficit is caused by an uncompensated speech impairment. Written communication or sign language may be appropriate. But if the communication impairment is caused by psychological withdrawal, these interventions would be inappropriate and ineffective. Thus determining etiology is important from the practical perspective of nursing intervention.

Concept of Cause The accepted rules for stating that A causes B have been debated by philosophers for centuries. Numerous schools of thought still exist (Cook and Campbell, 1979, pp. 9-36). The use of the idea and word *etiology* in diagnosis requires a consideration of some debated issues: sequence of cause and effect, logical justification, sufficient and necessary cause, and probable cause.

Sequence of Etiology and Problem To say a factor, A, is the cause of another phenomenon, B, requires that A precede or occur with B. In the natural sciences, this chronology is a requirement for a causal relation. In the human sciences and health professions, an additional idea is accepted: that future goals, potentialities, or intentions can cause present human behavior.

When motives or intentions are cited as causes, one is invoking future-directed cause for a present problem. Consider an example. Perceived invulnerability to a health condition that might develop in the future may cause noncompliance with a preventive care regimen. Establishing an acceptable causal relation requires that the stated etiology can be demonstrated (1) to *precede* the health problem or (2) to be a future-directed motive or intention.

Logical Justification A second issue in discussions of causality is logical justification of the proposal that A causes B. The rules of logic require that one avoid juxtaposition such as is seen in young children's "explanations" that use the words *because* or *therefore*. In their thinking, events are just stuck together with no better reason than that one thing varies with another (Piaget, 1969). An example of justaposition of events or ideas is provided by a little boy who believes that trees in the park act as fans to cause the wind (Chesterton, 1922). If event A, a change in the trees, is accompanied by event B, a change in air flow, then the child claims that A causes B. Lacking the ability to think logically, the child cannot generate explanations except those of direct association (Piaget, 1969). This juxtaposition usually leads to the construction of invalid inferential conclusions about relationships between events.

Sufficient and Necessary Cause The above example also demonstrates that it may be difficult to prove that any one factor *is* the cause and that others are not. For example, can the little boy be proved wrong? It is impossible to remove all the trees from the world in order to see whether wind occurs independently of them. This complexity is equally present in health care situations. How can it be known with certainty that a particular etiology is both *necessary* and *sufficient* to cause a problem?

It is unlikely that any one single factor is both a sufficient and a necessary cause for a client's problem. *Sufficient* means that *all* the conditions that contribute to the problem are present; *necessary* means that the problem cannot occur without the factor. In diagnosis, the nurse attempts to identify a set, or chain, of factors that logically could be sufficient conditions for causing a problem (dysfunctional pattern) to develop (Gough, 1971).

The relationship between knowledge deficit and noncompliance provides an example for discussion of necessary and sufficient cause. Is knowledge of a prescribed treatment regimen *necessary* for compliance? Yes—a person who is ignorant of the treatment regimen cannot follow it. Thus, a knowledge deficit is a *cause* of noncompliance because knowledge is *necessary* for compliance.

Is knowledge of a prescribed treatment regimen a *sufficient* condition to produce compliance in all cases? No—experience and research demonstrate that clients with full knowledge of the treatment regimen are noncompliant.

Knowledge deficit is not a *sufficient* explanation of noncompliance in all cases. Therefore, it can be said that knowledge is a necessary but not a sufficient condition for compliance with a treatment regimen. The sufficient conditions for development of noncompliance usually include multiple, interacting factors.

Multifactor etiology is a more likely explanation than single-factor etiology. Thus one has to go beyond knowledge deficit as a reason for noncompliance to identify other personal and situational causes. This identification of the several contributing causal factors will approximate the *conditions sufficient* for problem development.

Probable Cause Identified etiological factors may seem sufficient to cause a problem. Yet there is still the consideration of whether they represent the *true causes* in a particular case. In the human sciences, one has to accept that causal factors do not *always* produce the same problem in the same person or in different persons. The causal relationships derived from research and used in practice are probabilistic (Cook and Campbell, 1979, p. 31). In probabilistic relationships it cannot be said with absolute certainty that A causes B. Causal relationships in the health professions are recognized as plausible, not ultimate, necessary, or sufficient causes (Taylor, 1971). Thus a third consideration in practice is that etiological factors are thought of as *probable causes*.

What are the implications of the three issues in causality discussed above? The major implication is that etiological factors are probable causes. They are treated as hypotheses, not facts. The second is that error can be reduced by one's being conscious of the deductive reasoning behind a proposed relationship between a health problem and a cause. For example, *why* should a knowledge deficit cause noncompliance? Third, etiology preceeds or occurs with a problem. The exception is a client's goals or intentions that are future-directed but could be an etiological factor of a current problem.

Intervention is based on both the problem and its etiology. Predicted outcomes of intervention may not occur; one reason may be that the causal hypothesis (the supposed etiology) was incorrect. A later chapter will discuss how to identify etiological factors and state them in a way that guides care planning.

What is a Potential Problem?

Since modern nursing began, health promotion and preventive intervention have been an integral part of clinical practice. Thus the identification of potential problems is equally important as diagnosing actual problems. Potential problems can occur without a client's having a medical diagnosis or can occur secondary to an acute or chronic disease.

A *potential problem* is a potentially dysfunctional health pattern. Prediction of a potential dysfunction is made when sufficient risk factors are present. A *developmental risk* or a *risk of change* toward a less functional health pattern are two types of risk states.

To say that a client is susceptible to (or at risk for) a health problem requires the presence of risk factors. Usually the historical or current data include a combination of signs in one or more patterns. For example, the Surgeon General's report on health promotion and disease prevention (U.S. Department of Health, Education, and Welfare, 1979) states that 40 percent of American children ages 11 to 14 are estimated to have one or more risk factors associated with heart disease: overweight, high blood pressure, high blood cholesterol, cigarette smoking, lack of exercise, or diabetes. If children in a particular community are found to be similar to these national figures, this finding represents a set of potential problems, or potential dysfunctional patterns, requiring parent and child health education.

Potential for injury is another example of a risk state. Forty percent of hospital admissions for burns are due to scalding from excessively hot water in showers or bathtubs; 56 percent of fatal residential fires are cigarette-related, many due to smoking in bed, according to the Surgeon General's report (U.S. Department of Health, Education, and Welfare, 1979). An example of a potential problem secondary to disease and its treatment is potential noncompliance. Multiple prescriptions and other factors increase the risk that a client may not follow the treatment regime even when desire and intention were initially present.

The diagnosis of potential problems can be limited to individuals who have a greater number of risk factors than the population as a whole. For example, everyone has a potential for injury while crossing a city street, cutting vegetables in the kitchen, or shaving. Most clients are not at any more risk than the rest of the so-called normal population doing everyday activities. But those in the particular subpopulations with sensory-perceptual problems, a mobility deficit, or a bleeding tendency may be substantially at risk while performing these everyday activities.

Perhaps comparing two groups within a population of clients on a surgical service will clarify this idea. A client who is of normal body weight, doesn't smoke, has no chronic lung disease, and has been reasonably active is going to have surgery to remove the gallbladder. Compare this client to another, scheduled for the same operation, who smokes heavily, has chronic bronchitis, is 60 pounds overweight, and has relatively poor muscle tone because of a sedentary activity pattern. Which client has a potential for, or is at risk for, atelectasis postoperatively? Stated differently, which client should have intensive nursing treatment to prevent this pulmonary complication after surgery? Clearly, the second client is at high risk for atelectasis. (Postoperatively the risk increases if neither of these clients carry out deep breathing and coughing exercises due to incisional pain.)

This comparison illustrates the idea of population at risk. The first person represents the normal population having a cholecystectomy (gallbladder removal). The second client having this surgery comes from a different population whose characteristics of heavy smoking, chronic bronchitis, and weak muscle tone greatly predispose to atelectasis after surgery.

One may ask *why* a particular client has a potential for atelectasis. The form of the question implies a search for etiological factors; the answer has to be in the form of a *because, due to,* or *related to* statement. The client in the example is at risk for atelectasis *because* of heavy smoking, obesity, weak muscle tone, chronic bronchitis, and upper abdominal surgery. This is a restatement of the risk factors, which are also the signs of the potential problem.

In clinical settings where diagnosis is just beginning to be used, clinicians may wish to call attention to the risk factors. This can be done by recording the diagnosis as *potential for atelectasis* and stating, in parentheses, *see risk factors.* This statement is more concise and less repetitive when risk factors have already been recorded. Ultimately, when risk factor specification is standardized, all nurses will have learned the signs of potential- or high-risk states.

To conclude this discussion, it may be said that a problem, from a nursing perspective, is a dysfunctional health pattern. A problem represents a dysfunctional change in a pattern or an unhealthful pattern that has stabilized. Developmental problems exist when development is stabilized at a dysfunctional level relative to the client's potential.

A potential problem is a risk state. It indicates the presence of factors that predispose a client to a dysfunctional health pattern. Potential fluid volume deficit, potential alterations in parenting, and potential noncompliance are examples that describe dysfunctional nutritional-metabolic, role-relationship, and health-perception-health-management patterns, respectively.

Both the problem and the etiological factors are named in a nursing diagnosis. An exploration of the issues related to causality suggested etiological factors (1) are *probable* causes, (2) are *logically* related to the problem, and (3) precede or occur with a problem. Identification of etiological factors is a prerequisite for care planning. Intervention is directed toward the causal factors that can be changed and are predicted to have an impact on the problem.

Risk factors, the signs indicating a potential problem, are in a sense the cause. A potential state is a predicted state, not an actual state with an actual cause; thus, etiology is not specified. Intervention in this case is directed toward reducing risk factors.

SUMMARY

This chapter contains important ideas for using nursing diagnosis and the diagnostic process. There is an ethical responsibility in diagnosis. One aspect of that responsibility is to have a consciously defined purpose and a systematic approach. Clients should not be subjected to an unorganized set of questions, and the reasons for collecting information should be clear. Hence a conceptual framework is necessary for using the diagnostic process.

A few current conceptual frameworks were described in order to demonstrate that they provide a nursing focus for diagnosis. Particular attention was given to concepts of the client and of nursing's goal. These concepts are particularly relevant to the focus of information collection for diagnosis. No unified framework for nursing, accepted by all, exists or can be predicted to exist in the near future. At a *basic level*, all frameworks require similar assessment data.

A typology of 11 functional health patterns was provided to organize the collection of this basic assessment information. The pattern areas are:

Health-perception–health-management   Sleep-rest pattern
    pattern   Self-perception–self-concept pattern
Nutritional-metabolic pattern   Role-relationship pattern
Elimination pattern   Sexuality-reproductive pattern
Activity-exercise pattern   Coping–stress-tolerance pattern
Cognitive-perceptual pattern   Value-belief pattern

To combine these patterns with conceptual frameworks, the patterns are thought of as areas of self-care agency (Orem, 1980), adaptation (Roy, 1980), behavioral systems (Grubbs, 1980; and Johnson, 1980), manifestations of the life pattern (Rogers, 1970), or areas of human need (Yura and Walsh, 1978).

The pattern areas represent a standardized assessment format. The advantage of this is that a common basic data base is collected from each client, irrespective of age, level of care, or medical disease. The standardized assessment procedure based on the pattern areas has the additional advantages of (1) not needing to be continually relearned (it is expanded as clinical knowledge accumulates), (2) leading directly to nursing diagnoses (Appendix B), and (3) encompassing a holistic approach to human functional assessment.

Each pattern area is a biopsychosocial expression of the whole person. Human development occurs in these patterns; thus they also provide for developmental assessment of client-environment interaction.

Change in one pattern area is reflected in other areas because the patterns are interdependent. When a problem is diagnosed in one area, the etiological factors usually are found in one or more of the other pattern areas.

People of any age can develop problems in functional patterns. Dysfunctional or potentially dysfunctional patterns are the health problems described by nursing diagnoses. A diagnosis also describes the etiological factors contributing to the problem. This chapter includes a discussion of current issues underlying the idea of causality. It was suggested that etiological factors are only *probable* causes of a problem because clincial diagnostic situations always contain some degree of uncertainty; both health problems and etiological factors have to be open to revision when new data or new insights are obtained.

BIBLIOGRAPHY

American Nurses' Association. *Standards for nursing practice*. Kansas City, Mo.: American Nurses' Association, 1973.

American Nurses' Association. *Scope of nursing practice: A social policy statement*. Kansas City, Mo.: American Nurses' Association, 1981.

Becknell, E., & Smith, D. *System of nursing practice*. New York: Davis, 1975.

Booth, G. Psychobiological aspects of "spontaneous" regressions of cancer. In C. Garfield (Ed.), *Stress and survival: The emotional realities of life-threatening illness*. St. Louis: Mosby, 1979.

Campbell, C. *Nursing diagnosis and intervention in nursing practice*. New York: Wiley, 1978.

Chesterton, G. *Tremendous trifles*. New York: Dodd, Mead, 1922.

Cook, T. D., & Campbell, D. T. *Quasi-experimentation: Design and analysis issues for field testing*. Chicago: Rand McNally College Press, 1979.

Dunn, H. What high-level wellness means. *Canadian Journal of Public Health*, November 1959, *50*, 447–457.

Duvall, E. *Family development* (3d ed.). Philadelphia: Lippincott, 1967.

Gough, H. Some reflections on the meaning of psychodiagnosis. *American Psychologist*, February 1971, *26*, 160–167.

Grubbs, J. The Johnson behavioral system model. In J. P. Riehl & C. Roy (Eds.), *Conceptual models for nursing practice* (2d ed.). New York: Appleton-Century-Crofts, 1980.

Hall, L. E. Quality of nursing care. Address at meeting of Department of Baccalaureate and Higher Degree Programs of the New Jersey League for Nursing, Newark, N.J., February 7, 1955. Published in *Public Health News*, New Jersey State Department of Health, June 1955. [Cited in H. Yura & M. B. Walsh, *The nursing process: Assessing, planning, implementing, evaluating* (3d ed.). New York: Appleton-Century-Crofts, 1978.]

Helson, H. *Adaptation level theory*. New York: Harper & Row, 1964.

Johnson, D. *One conceptual model of nursing*. Unpublished paper presented April 25, 1968, at Vanderbilt University, Nashville, Tennessee.

Johnson, D. The behavioral systems model. In J. P. Riehl & C. Roy (Eds.), *Conceptual models for nursing practice* (2d ed.). New York: Appleton-Century-Crofts, 1980.

King, I. M. *Towards a theory for nursing: General concepts of human behavior*. New York: Wiley, 1971.

Levine, M. E. *Introduction to clinical nursing* (2d ed.). Philadelphia: Davis, 1973.

Little, D., & Carnevali, D. *Nursing care planning* (2d ed.). Philadelphia: Lippincott, 1976.

Lonergan, B. J. *Insight: A study of human understanding* (3d ed.). New York: Philosophical Library, 1970.

McCain, F. Nursing by assessment—not intuition. *American Journal of Nursing*, April 1965, *65*, 82–84.

McCourt, A. Measurement of functional deficit in quality assurance. *Quality Assurance Update*, Kansas City, Mo.: American Nurses' Association, May 1981, pp. 1–3.

McLean, A. (Ed.). *Reducing occupational stress: Proceedings of a conference, Westchester Division, New York Hospital–Cornell Medical Center, May 10–12, 1977*. Washington, D.C.: U.S. Department of Health, Education, and Welfare, 1978.

Miller, J. G. *Living systems*. New York: McGraw-Hill, 1978.

National League for Nursing, Department of Baccalaureate and Higher Degree Programs. *Criteria for appraisal of baccalaureate and higher degree programs in nursing.* New York: National League for Nursing, 1977.

Neuman, B. The Betty Neuman health-care systems model: A total person approach to patient problems. In J. P. Riehl & C. Roy (Eds.), *Conceptual models for nursing practice* (2d ed.). New York: Appleton-Century-Crofts, 1980.

Orem, D. *Nursing: Concepts of practice.* New York: McGraw-Hill, 1980.

Orlando, I. J. *The dynamic nurse-patient relationship: Function, process and principles.* New York: Putnam, 1961.

Patterson, J. G., & Zderad, L. *Humanistic nursing.* New York: Wiley, 1976.

Piaget, J. *Judgment and reasoning in the child.* Totowa, N.J.: Adams, 1969.

Powell, J. *Why am I afraid to tell you who I am?* Chicago: Argus Communications, 1969.

Putt, A. M. *General systems theory applied to nursing.* Boston: Little, Brown, 1978.

Riehl, J. P., & Roy, C. A unified model of nursing. In J. P. Riehl & C. Roy (Eds.), *Conceptual models for nursing practice* (2d ed.). New York: Appleton-Century-Crofts, 1980.

Riehl, J. P., & Roy, C. Discussion of a unified nursing model. In J. P. Riehl & C. Roy (Eds.), Conceptual models for nursing practice. New York: Appleton-Century-Crofts, 1974.

Rogers, M. *An introduction to the theoretical basis of nursing.* Philadelphia: Davis, 1970.

Roy, C. *Introduction to nursing: An adaptation model.* Englewood Cliffs, N.J.: Prentice-Hall, 1976.

Roy, C., & Roberts, S. L. *Theory construction in nursing: An adaptation model.* Englewood Cliffs, N.J.: Prentice-Hall, 1981.

Selye, H. Stress without distress. In C. A. Garfield (Ed.), *Stress and survival.* St. Louis: Mosby, 1979.

Smith, D. M. A clinical nursing tool. *American Journal of Nursing,* November 1968, *68,* 2384–2388.

Soares, C. A. Nursing and medical diagnoses: Comparison of variant and essential features. In N. L. Chaska (Ed.), *The nursing profession: Views through the mist.* New York: McGraw-Hill, 1978.

Steele, S. M., & Harmon, V. M. *Values clarification in nursing.* New York: Appleton-Century-Crofts, 1979.

Taylor, F. K. A logical analysis of the medico-psychologic concept of disease (Part I). *Psychological Medicine,* 1971, *1,* 356–364.

U.S. Department of Health, Education, and Welfare. *Healthy people: The Surgeon General's report on health promotion and disease prevention.* Washington, D.C.: U.S. Government Printing Office, DHEW (PHS) Publication No. 79–55071, 1979.

Yura, H., & Walsh, M. *Human needs and the nursing process.* New York: Appleton-Century-Crofts, 1978.

Zderad, L. *Future directions in nursing theory.* Taped seminar paper presented at Nurse Educator Conference, New York, December 4–7, 1978. (Cassette available from Nursing Resources, Inc., Wakefield, Mass.)

CHAPTER 4

THE COLLECTION OF CLINICAL INFORMATION

The diagnostic process was defined previously as including four activities: information collection, information interpretation, information clustering, and naming the cluster. Chapter 3 began the discussion of information collection. Frameworks for making decisions about *what* information to collect were the focus. This chapter continues the discussion, but the focus is on *how* information is collected.

Three basic factors must be taken into consideration in any discussion of how to collect clinical information about a client's health status. One is the *situational context* in which the information is collected. Both physical and interpersonal characteristics of a situation are influential. A second factor is the *nature of the information* available. Certain characteristics of clinical information influence both how it is collected and how it is used. The third influential factor is the *diagnostician* who collects the information. The cognitive and perceptual capabilities of the diagnostician are tools employed to collect health status information.

All three factors operate simultaneously in every clinical situation where information is being collected. For example, in a hospital room (situational context), a nurse anticipating that a client may be having pain looks closely (diagnostician) for facial grimacing related to pain (nonverbal nature of the information). How is information collected? By knowing the nature of the information desired, setting up the ideal situation for its collection, and finely tuning the senses required for perceptual recognition.

In the first section of this chapter the reader will find an overview of *assessment*, the term used in nursing to describe information collection. Also included will be a discussion of what is "good" information. Following this we will consider how to structure the assessment situation, the nature of clinical information, and the perceptual capabilities of the diagnostician.

ASSESSMENT

According to common usage, the term *assessment* means evaluation. In an analysis of its use in nursing, Bloch (1974) comments on the great variation in what the word means. Some authors use the term to refer to the four activities of the diagnostic process. Others define assessment to include *two* separate processes—data collection[1] and problem definition.

The different cognitive and interpersonal processes can be studied when assessment is separated into problem definition and data collection. *Problem definition* is a cognitive operation that uses data. It may or may not involve interaction with the client. *Data collection* and its validation always require a nurse-client interaction. Separation of the two processes involved in assessment is useful when focusing on the different operations involved, but in actual practice tentative problem identification occurs *during* data collection.

When talking about process, as opposed to structure, separation of components of the diagnostic process is artificial. Therefore, this is how the terms will be used in this book:

> *Assessment* refers to data collection. *Diagnosis* refers to information interpretation, clustering, and labeling. Assessment and diagnosis *overlap*, and together they constitute the diagnostic process.

It is important to realize that data collection continues during all nurse-client interactions. The same can be said of the overall diagnostic process; fewer problems are missed if a diagnostic approach is taken to all information seeking, beginning with the initial encounter at admission. In this and all data gathering situations, it is important to obtain a good data base for clinical judgments. In the next section we will explore what that means.

Good Assessment Data

Good clinical judgments are based on good information. This raises the question of what "good" information is and the related question of how to structure an assessment situation to obtain this kind of data. *Valid* data are valued as "good." The content of information is valid if it represents the properties of what is being judged. A description of food and fluid intake represents one property of a nutritional pattern; thus it is one piece of valid information for making a judgment about this pattern. Is the client's description of what his wife prepares for each meal valid information about his dietary intake pattern? No; unaccompanied by other data it does not provide direct information about food and fluid intake and leads to risky judgments based on assumptions.

There are degrees of validity. Highly valid clinical data *directly represent* critical properties of a pattern. Information of lower validity requires assumptions that may

---

[1] *Data* is synonymous with the term *information.*

or may not be true. The clearer the definition of functional health patterns, the easier it is to seek valid data with which to make judgments about patterns. Thus definitions of the critical properties of a pattern have to be continually improved as new knowledge accumulates.

Reliable information is also valued as "good." Information is reliable if it is an accurate measure of a property. There are degrees of reliability. For example, which measure of food and fluid intake is most accurate and, therefore, most reliable: (1) a client's description of daily food and fluid intake, (2) a nurse's daily observation of the client's food and fluid intake, or (3) the wife's description of the meals prepared for the client?

To make a judgment about a food and fluid intake pattern, most would prefer to use the second option, the nurse's observations. This preference is based on the idea that an outside observer (and a professional) is free of bias and more accurate. It may be that the client is just as accurate as the nurse, but we do not know this. The wife's description of meals she prepares has lowest reliability; we do not know whether the client eats the meals.

The above example has further implications. The cost of obtaining information through observation is high. If there is no reason to suspect the client is unreliable, his verbal report may be accepted. In some situations observation is impossible; client reports are then accepted as the most reliable information obtainable. In other situations judgments are so important that, irrespective of time and costs, direct measurements are performed by the diagnostician. Situations have to be judged individually. Accuracy of measurement, and thus reliability, is an important concern during information collection. This is why good lighting for observations, careful listening to verbal cues, well-formulated questions, and a situation of acceptance, interest, and caring are stressed.

In summary, valid information obtained by reliable measures provides a base for valid and reliable judgments about functional health patterns. Each of the previously mentioned factors—structuring the assessment situation, the nature of information, and the diagnostician—influences the validity and reliability of information. In the next section we will consider how the assessment situation can be structured to obtain valid and reliable data.

STRUCTURING THE ASSESSMENT SITUATION

Structure is provided in the admission assessment by a systematic history and examination format. The way the format is implemented contributes to the goal of obtaining valid and reliable information. Psychological, or motivational, set (attitudes and expectations) of the clinician and client are also influential; this, as will be seen, contributes to the establishment of a therapeutic relationship. Characteristics of various assessment situations are discussed in this section; it is important to note the different focus of each type of assessment situation. As the greatest emphasis will be placed on the admission assessment, readers unfamiliar with this may find it helpful to scan the examples in Appendix G.

Initial Nursing History and Examination

Whenever a client is added to a nurse's caseload, an initial assessment is made of the 11 previously described functional health patterns. This establishes the nursing data base. Initial assessments are referred to as a data base because (1) basic historical and current information about all health patterns is collected and (2) the information is used as base-line criteria against which any future changes are evaluated.

An admission assessment consists of a *nursing history* of functional health patterns and an *examination* of indicators of patterns. The former is done by interviewing the client or others; the latter, by observation and other examination techniques. Generally, a comprehensive assessment is necessary. If a client's condition is critical (physiological or psychological instability exists), only screening assessment of patterns may be warranted.

Nursing History Information collection in the admission nursing history permits a systematic description of the 11 functional health patterns and the client's perception and explanation of any problems. Explanations clients provide for particular behaviors or situations are important. They can be diagnostic of knowledge deficits and health management deficits, among other things.

In primary care (ambulatory care) settings, a functional health pattern assessment and a biomedical systems assessment can be integrated. In these settings the history and examination are designed to detect dysfunctional health patterns *and* diseases. Tentative diagnoses of disease are referred to a physician or treated under protocols.

In home care a complete assessment is done when a family is initially visited. Similarly, community nurses responsible for program planning do a community assessment to reveal environmental and other problems influencing health patterns of groups. For example, in community assessment the *history* may include general dietary patterns of an elderly population; hazardous waste elimination patterns within a geographic area; the community's self-image pattern; and its level of activity as indicated by patterns of participation in work, political, or recreational activities. *Examination* of the community may include observations of people on busy streets or buses and observations of resources and facilities. (The local barber or bartender has a wealth of community information.)

Two important differences exist between history taking by interview and by having the client fill out a questionnaire. If the client fills out a form, the responses are taken at face value. No interpersonal interaction occurs as the questions are answered. In an interview, as Froelich and Bishop state (1977, p. 3), meaning is derived from what the client says. This requires interpersonal interaction. The purpose of an interview is to clarify, permit elaboration, and thus arrive at an understanding of responses. History-taking by interview is most common in nursing practice.

A successful interview is guided, not dominated, by the nurse. Actually, the client should be talking about 80 percent of the time and the nurse, 20 percent. The nurse guides the interview by opening a topic (pattern area), assisting with the narrative, focusing, and closing a topic (Froelich and Bishop, 1977, p. 89). The first decision is how to begin; the last involves termination.

Beginning an Assessment An initial assessment begins with the nursing history.

Introductions are important because people consider names personal. Address the client by name, introduce yourself, and state your title, for example, student nurse, registered nurse or clinical specialist. Explain your purpose. All of the following introductions have been observed in clinical settings; which one begins to establish a professional relationship?

1 Mr. Jones? I'm Ms. Arnold, a student nurse at the university. I'd like to talk to you about your health and how you're managing.

2 Hi, Mr. Jones. I'm Ms. Arnold, a student. I have to do a nursing assessment on you.

3 Mr. Jones? I'm Joan, but most of my friends call me Jo. I'd like to see if you have any problems.

4 Bill Jones? I'm Ms. Arnold; before I go off duty I have to do your nursing care plan.

The over-friendly approach of numbers 2, 3, and 4 is not appropriate in initiating an admission assessment. Examples 2 and 3, with the "have to do" phrase, may communicate that other activities would be preferred. In number 4, especially, the client is made to feel that he is delaying the nurse from going off duty; this situation generates the expectation of a rushed job. Rather than focus on a task to be done, focus on the client's needs as in number 1, which is the preferred introduction. The idea of how to begin health pattern assessment will be expanded further in later chapters on diagnostic strategies.

Helping the Client to Describe Health Patterns As each pattern is assessed, try to relate the next pattern area to a previous statement. Use a transition statement; otherwise the nursing history appears to be an interrogation. Insert an appropriate transitional comment, then follow with a question.

Some examples of transition may be helpful. A number of problems may be verbalized while the client reports data about his or her health-perception–health-management pattern. The transition to nutritional pattern can be made by saying, "Let's jot down those problems; we will want to talk further about them. I seem to need more specific information about some things. You mentioned that planning meals was difficult. What kinds of foods have you been eating at breakfast, lunch, dinner, and for snacks? Let's begin with breakfast." This leads into the nutritional pattern.

Attempt to construct a comfortable transition, especially in areas usually considered personal. For example, after inquiring about family structure and relationships, move on to sexuality patterns: "You mentioned that you've been married nearly 10 years; do you both find sexual relationships satisfactory?" or, less direct, "Do any marital problems arise now and then?" or "Has this illness been associated with any problems in sexual relationships?" Creating transitional statements will take practice. The main idea to keep in mind is to personalize the interview. Pick up on something that has been said and relate it to the next topic for discussion.

There are various types of questions and remarks that facilitate history taking. One is the *open-ended question*. The topic for discussion is specified in a general question and usually elicits descriptions and current concerns. An example would be "What's it like for you when all the children are at home for the day?" This is in contrast to the *direct, leading question*, which requires a specific yes or no answer.

An example is, "Do you get upset when all the children are home for the day?" After a client has responded to an open-ended question, direct questions may provide particular cues. These are needed when a specific diagnostic possibility is being tested.

Probing questions are frequently needed to obtain clarification. These are questions that permit the client to elaborate. They are commonly used when a client employs abstract terms or offers judgments such as *nervous, depressed,* or *ulcer.* Beware of accepting such words at face value: the client may define them totally differently than you do. Probe with a follow-up inquiry such as, "What feelings do you notice when you're nervous?" Sometimes it will be discovered that cardiac rhythm irregularities are occurring. Similarly, *ulcer* may mean a skin abrasion.

It is also not uncommon for clients to circumvent an area that is emotionally charged, such as death. They may not be sure the nurse can accept their beliefs or feelings. The nurse who suspects this must probe with care and at the same time be accepting and supporting.

Support, reassurance, empathy, and silence are communications that assist the client in describing health patterns. Support demonstrates interest, concern, and understanding. It can enhance description or close it off, depending on when understanding is communicated. Reassurance communicates that the client has worth and self-reliance. Empathy accepts or clarifies feelings or behavior. Supportive silence permits the client to continue a response when description is difficult. Examples of these communications follow:

Support

Client: I have a terrible time trying to get to sleep at night.
Nurse: That must be difficult. What seems to be . . . ?

Reassurance

Client: I have a terrible time trying to get to sleep at night.
Nurse: I think we can come up with some things you can do. What seems to be . . . ?

Empathy

Client; I have a terrible time trying to get to sleep at night.
Nurse: That can cause you a lot of worry and concern. What seems to be . . . ?

Silence can communicate interest or withdrawal. For example, when the client uses the words *terrible time*, the nurse could shift forward very slightly, holding eye contact. This movement indicates interest and concern. Shifting away from the client and from eye contact indicates withdrawal from the problem, irrespective of what the nurse says or the silence that intervenes. The client may be sensitive to this body language and may not elaborate, thinking the nurse is uncomfortable or not interested.

Questions and remarks can be reflective or confronting. A *reflection* echoes a portion of what the client just said. For example, a child may say, "I get upset in school"; the nurse then says, with a gentle, supportive, questioning tone of a voice, "Upset?"

Confrontation focuses attention on feelings or behavior. It is used to probe more deeply. A client may describe some change. Three or four sentences later it is evident that this change began 2 months after a divorce. The nurse, feeling attention should be focused on the time sequence, may say, "Do you think that was related to your feelings after your divorce?" Confrontations can be based on the need to validate an inference or an observation during the diagnostic process; confrontation during an intervention may have other objectives, such as insight development.

During the assessment of emotionally charged areas, a client may begin to cry. Accept this demonstration of feeling without feeling guilty. Feelings of guilt are a sign to the nurse that his or her focus has turned inward toward self rather than outward toward the client. Crying is a cue to depth of feelings, such as frustration or sadness. Empathy, reassurance, or silence combined with touch usually is helpful. After the client gains some composure the nurse can ask whether he or she can help in any way. This is better than suggesting that the interview stop; the only recourse then would be to leave, since presence indicates waiting to continue.

Early indications of fatigue or increasing anxiety need to be observed. Try to validate these impressions with the client. Both fatigue and anxiety during the interview should be treated as data. Fatigue is a cue to activity tolerance. It should be noted and a decision made about shifting from a detailed assessment to a few screening questions. Judgment has to be used regarding the signs of increasing anxiety. Either the topic or the discussion of the topic with a not-yet-trusted nurse may be producing a perceived threat to the self. The client can be asked whether he or she wishes to talk further about the topic or to continue later. There are many good books about interviewing and assessment that deal with situations such as these and prepare the beginner for handling this type of situation if it arises.

Examination Following the nursing history an examination is done. Observations are made of physical characteristics such as gait and mobility, skin integrity, heart rate, and range of joint movement. Cues obtained during history taking provide impressions of speech (tone, rate, and quality) and possibly interactions if another person is present (parent-child or client-other relationships).[2] Assessment occurring in the home provides opportunities to observe living conditions, safety hazards, and the client's neighborhood.

Five sensory modalities (vision, hearing, cutaneous touch, smell, and kinesthesia) provide a means for obtaining clinical data during examination. (Taste, the other sensory modality, is rarely used.) The nurse is a sensitive measuring device for listening, interpersonal interaction, observation, inspection, and examination (auscultation, palpation, and percussion). An amazing amount of information can be collected through the use of the five sensory modalities and these four methods of data collection. As educational programs incorporate additional physical examination skills into clinical courses, the areas listed under examination in Appendix C can be expanded.

---

[2] Interaction in the full sense of the word cannot be accomplished when a patient is unconscious, extremely hyperactive, or markedly out of contact with reality. In these instances information is acquired from a knowledgeable person or by examination.

(Many excellent books about the methods of clinical data collection are available; some are listed in the bibliography at the end of this chapter.)

All of the above observational and examination methods provide information about functional health patterns. For example, a pattern of exercise-activity described in the history can be understood in the context of an observed gait impairment. A school child's poor hygiene may be understood after examination of living facilities.

Deeper understanding of functional patterns is acquired *only* if physical assessment findings *are collected for this purpose.* Seems obvious? Apparently it is not, because sometimes physical examination data are separated from nursing history data by using a biomedical systems format (gastrointestinal, cardiovascular, and similar categories). If functional health patterns are a reasonable focus for nursing assessment and diagnosis, think about *all* clinical data as indicators of these patterns. What is observed during examination may be the outcome of existing or emerging functional patterns the client described during the history. Or the observational data may explain why certain patterns exist, have changed, or are emerging developmentally.

Examination of the client and situation verifies or expands understanding gained during history taking. Generally, dysfunctional patterns are elicited during the history; examination of the client provides further data, not surprises.

Terminating the Admission Assessment After information is collected about each functional health pattern by history taking and examination, termination of the initial assessment begins. There are three objectives at this time: (1) to offer the opportunity for the client to add further information or express additional concerns, (2) to summarize, and (3) to make plans.

As one's experience increases in diagnosis, it becomes possible in most cases to structure diagnostic hypotheses simultaneously with history taking and examination. After asking whether the client has further information or concerns, the nurse summarizes and makes plans in the context of ongoing events. The following is an example of terminating an initial assessment of a 60-year-old female client admitted one day before gallbladder surgery; the diagnoses are moderate anticipatory anxiety related to postoperative dependency, exogenous obesity related to caloric intake–energy expenditure imbalance, high risk for atelectasis, and alteration in socialization related to stress incontinence:

Interaction	Purpose
Nurse: You've mentioned a few things that we can help you with while you're in the hospital. Is there anything we haven't talked about that is of concern to you?	Give cues that summarization is forthcoming.
Client: No, I can't think of anything; the worst thing is not being able to control my urine when I can't find a bathroom quickly.	

Interaction	Purpose
Nurse: That can be troublesome; there are ways to manage that and we'll also have to see what ideas the doctor may have. Is that something that will be troublesome now?	Summarization and plans for the concerns that have been expressed. (Notice that in summarization the actual diagnostic labels need not be used.)
Client: Oh, no, the bathroom is right here and I have a bedpan in my table.	
Nurse: You mentioned wanting to lose weight; that's another thing we can work on after your surgery. It seems that your diet and fluid intake have been good. Also, you mentioned bowels have been regular the past week. All these things are important for healing after surgery. Your concern about the surgery is something we'll want to talk about after lunch. I've got some ideas that might help you control what happens. This afternoon we'll go over how you can manage things like discomfort and prevent other problems with particular exercises. Read the little booklet; if your daughter comes in this afternoon, should we include her?	Summarization and plans for expressed concerns. (Notice that for some diagnoses the nursing care will not be started until after surgery). Leave client with feeling of ability to cope with problems or concerns identified.

Preoperative preparation plans and plans to further discuss anxiety response. |
| *Client:* Oh, yes, she would like to know all about it, too. | |
| *Nurse:* Good. See you around two-thirty. Enjoy your lunch. | |

Summarization and planning with the client at the time the assessment ends may not always be possible, especially when the nurse is in the early stages of learning diagnosis. Secondly, even the experienced diagnostician may not be able to formulate diagnoses "on the spot" because of complexity of the health problem or because of missing data. The nurse should not feel pressured to diagnose, summarize, and plan at the end of the assessment; it is better to discuss concerns at the symptom level than to share early judgments that may be incorrect. For example, a nurse could say, "We've talked about a number of things; while you're thinking about anything we've missed, I'll just look over what we talked about. . . ." Or, when data are missing or time is needed to formulate a problem, an expression of interest and concern may be sufficient. This could be stated as, "You've mentioned a number of things; I think you can work out some solutions if we talk about these some more" or "Let's both think about what could be causing the family to react this way, and tomorrow we can talk about that."

The idea to be gained from the above examples is that after assessment clients should (1) perceive that something will be done with the information that has been shared and (2) have a feeling of future competency for handling any identified problems with (or without) assistance from the nurse. Basically, what is being described is a sharing of interest, concern, and understanding—the caring response even before the actual care plan has been designed.

Psychological Set in Assessment A psychological *set* is an inclination or disposition to take certain actions or to hold certain attitudes. Disposition influences attention and overall motivation. During history and examination activities the set, or motivation, is to describe and evaluate functional health patterns and subsequently to offer the client help or guidance as necessary. This fact should be kept in mind, because it is not the common, everyday social set. Most interpersonal interactions are not descriptive-evaluative, nor are they purposefully diagnostic. Neither are they necessarily or deliberately therapeutic.

The nurse's motivation in the interaction complements the client's role set. Although sometimes disguised, the client's objective generally is to obtain help in health evaluation, problem solving, or physical activities. The first step in providing help is to describe and explain current health pattterns. Then professional decisions can be made regarding the need for help and the goals of helping.

The most productive motivation of a professional health care provider doing assessment is to *explain* impressions and other data. It has been suggested that a diagnostician approaches clinical observations with a descriptive-explanatory set related to the question, Why? This set should predominate over a concern (1) about personal self-maintenance (What is the client in relation to me? or Can the client help me meet my needs?), (2) about personal role (Who is the client in relation to me? or What role shall I play?), or (3) about acceptable and unacceptable behavior of the client (How well does the client meet my expectations of a client?). Sets to perceive and interpret greatly influence the way client behaviors are categorized (Sarbin, Taft, and Bailey, 1960, pp. 144-159).

Imagine what would ensue if one's primary set in a psychiatric setting was self-maintenance. Clients' behavior might be instantly interpreted as potential violence. Or a nurse with a set to evaluate how a client "stayed in line" with the patient role might be quick to see too much independence and "taking over" during assessment. Far too often care providers slip into nonproductive sets during interactions with clients.

Part of socialization into professional nursing is to learn role behavior, for example, that the motivation predominating in assessment is the descriptive-explanatory, or *why*, set. This is not to say that the other sets are never used. An experienced nurse may reflect on how sensitive the client is to another's (the nurse's) needs. Are social cues to roles (the nurse's role) received? How well does the client assume various role expectations? The nurse-client interaction is used as the object of observation. The nurse pays attention to her or his own affective reactions and impressions generated by the client's behavior. These personal reactions are used as hypotheses about how others react to the client and may provide data about health problems in the role-relationship pattern area. These techniques are particularly useful in specialty areas such as psychiatric nursing assessment.

Assessment from the Client's Viewpoint   Assessment is accomplished more successfully when one is aware of one's own perspective and takes account of the motivation and perspective of the client. According to one school of social psychology, behavior is greatly influenced by the way a person "defines the situation" (Cardwell, 1971).

Extending this idea to assessment would suggest a number of things. Initially, both client and nurse bring past experience, expectations, and values to the situation. Individually, both synthesize these predefinitions with current perceptions. Unspoken questions may arise: What is happening? What role shall I play? How shall I behave? Personal definition of the assessment situation is one factor that influences behavior in interpersonal interaction. This idea provides food for thought. How does the nurse help the client to define and understand the "situation" of assessment and health care? Before discussing approaches, let us extend this idea further.

Diagnosis is also a "definition of situation"; it is a way of defining the health situation. A client usually has some idea of the health problems when assessment begins. This idea includes notions, expectations, and feelings, and they may be realistic or unrealistic. By telling his or her health history and thinking about the questions asked, a client may even be disposed to define the situation a new way. Simultaneously, the nurse gains information to define the situation diagnostically.

Prior to assessment, the individual, family, friends, or society must define the situation as requiring health consultation or care. Otherwise, no action is taken. The client's predefinition of the problem, the data collection process, and the health care system need to be taken into account.

Herzlich and Graham (1973) identified the meanings people attributed to the terms *health* and *illness*. Of interest to our discussion are the findings about when and why people consult health care providers. In these researchers' middle class, urban sample and in other studies (Koss, 1960; Mechanic and Volkart, 1961; Zola, 1979) it was found that perception of symptoms was not sufficient to initiate health consultation. Passage from a perceived state of health to perceived sickness occurred when symptoms interfered with work or social activity. People then defined themselves as needing to know "what is the matter."

Symptoms were viewed as ambiguous; they could either mean nothing or be important. This produced uncertainty. Most importantly, symptoms interfered with activity. These were the reasons consultation was sought. The expectation was that the health care provider would define the situation and give it meaning. Routine health examinations were sought even in the absence of symptoms, for the same reasons; the care provider would reassure that absence of symptoms meant health (Herzlich and Graham, 1973, pp. 78–87).

Interference with functional activities involved in daily living was the main concern that initiated health consultation. Therefore, diagnosing disease is an insufficient response to the client. Diagnosis should also focus on management of functional activities and on the associated capabilities required. This is the province of nursing diagnosis, although it is not a diagnostic area that has been offered to the consumer in a systematic, organized way by nurses.

Most clients will view consultation or entrance into the health care delivery system as focusing on medical diagnosis, medical treatment, and the prognosis of physical or mental *disease*. This is how they have been socialized. The details of health management are usually left for them to work out as best they can. As the literature reveals, one result is a high incidence of noncompliance with therapeutic recommendations (Haynes, Taylor, and Sackett, 1979).

Two reactions from clients are common when nurses begin to assess things other than the physical aspects of a disease. One is amazement that the nurse would be concerned. The second is the "something else is the matter with me" reaction. (The latter also occurs when three or four doctors plus a medical student see a patient.)

Consumers have to become accustomed to defining the health care system as offering both nursing and medical consultation and as oriented to both health and disease. Purposeful communication to inform people about this distinction and about nursing's role in health care is needed. The communication can be incorporated into nursing assessment of the functional health patterns described in Chapter 3.

Consider some examples of initiating an assessment so as to help the client define the situation. The nurse could say, being purposefully vague, "Ms. Klein, I'd like to see if I can help you. Let's talk about some things regarding your care. . . ." The more direct approach is, "Ms. Klein, I'd like to do a nursing assessment. There may be things you would like help with, so we'll talk about the way you plan your diet and . . ." (mentions a few relevant things). The latter clearly implies a strategy for educating the consumer about nursing. It familiarizes the client with vocabulary (*nursing assessment*), definitions, and what benefits may be derived. When the situation is perceived clearly, the client is in a better position to respond to assessment questions. Over and over again this has been demonstrated in psychological studies of cognition (Bruner, Goodnow, and Austin, 1956). Responses are more appropriate when a person knows what is expected, and involvement increases when the benefits are clear. These are points sometimes neglected in clinical practice.

Building on the idea in Chapter 3 of a framework that answers the question of *what* to assess, this section began the examination of *how* information is collected. Various terms are used to refer to this activity, including *assessment, data collection,* or the *admission nursing history and examination.* A history is obtained by interview; examination requires observation and other techniques. These techniques were described briefly and will be further discussed in other chapters. The reader is encouraged to consult the many good books written on interviewing and examination; these provide suggestions for handling most situations that occur during assessment.

Both clients and nurses have expectations for assessment. The nurse seeks information to describe and explain functional health patterns. Clients expect to learn the meaning of symptoms or to be reassured about their health and health practices. As well as the care provider's physiological interpretations of symptoms, clients wish to know the meaning of symptoms relative to the human functions they engage in day by day. These functions are the focus of nursing, and assessment begins the process of nursing. The client may need to be told why nurses wish information so that interview purposes are clear.

ASSESSMENT SITUATIONS IN CLINICAL PRACTICE

Assessment has been described above as information collection occurring at admission of a client to a nurse's caseload. It was also stated that assessment is continuous. To clarify, let us look at various clinical situations where information is required. All involve assessment of the client but differ in the probability of health problems, scope of data gathered, situational context, and immediate purpose. The initial assessment previously described will be included to complete the listing.

Take particular note of differences among the various situations regarding the probability that a problem exists. The diagnostician's preencounter hypotheses (or educated guesses) directly influence assessment in two ways. One is the major question posed; this guides the search for information. The second is the difficulty inherent in conducting the search. Clearly, if one knows what one is looking for (problem-focused assessment), the search is easier than if one does not (universe of possibilities). Before seeing a new client the nurse has no information about the person; thus the total universe of health problems is open. As will be seen in a later chapter, nurses have strategies for quickly narrowing the possibilities.

Initial Assessment

The purpose of initial assessment is to evaluate health status and identify any problematic functional patterns. A complete nursing history and examination are required and usually are completed at admission. Nursing assessment cannot be problem-focused at the start; no current clinical data are available. *The hypothesis of no dysfunctional pattern is as probable as the hypothesis that dysfunctional patterns exist.* The question is: *Does a health problem exist?* The universe of possibilities is open as assessment begins. On the basis of initial cues, likely possibilities are generated by inference and tested by gathering information.

The situation in which initial diagnoses are established is important. Generally, the person or family does not know the nurse. Therefore, consideration has to be given to establishing trust and rapport during assessment. Interpersonal factors are critical for obtaining valid information and for a future helping relationship.

The setting is also critical to the initial assessment. When people are asked to share information about personal "ways of living," privacy must be ensured. The clinician and client, trying to structure a relationship characterized by confidence and rapport, need a comfortable setting free from interruption and distraction.

Problem-Focused Assessment

The objective in this second type of assessment situation is to make a clinical judgment about the status of a previously identified nursing diagnosis. One might assume that diagnoses are made, care is planned and carried out, problems are resolved, and outcomes are measured. This sequence, proceeding so neatly through time, is the "textbook picture" of clinical practice. In reality, people change, events occur, and diagnoses get added, deleted, or revised.

In problem-focused assessment a problematic pattern is assumed to exist. Assessment is based on previously stated diagnoses. *The hypothesis of a dysfunctional pattern is more likely than the hypothesis that no dysfunctional pattern exists.* The question pursued is, *Does the problem exist today and, if so, what is the status of the problem?* This assessment task is relatively structured; the nurse assesses signs and symptoms known to indicate the problem. The scope of the clinical data gathered is narrower than in an initial assessment of a new client and, naturally, time required for assessment is less. Yet the anticipation of new problems and alertness to discover missed problems or misdiagnoses accompanies the problem-focused assessment.

The situational context differs from that of an initial assessment. Change has occurred in the interpersonal dimension; now the nurse and client are not strangers to each other. Whereas in the first encounter trust, confidence, and rapport had to be built, successive encounters focus on extending and maintaining these. Secondly, in the admission or intake assessment, the setting was designed to promote sharing of information in a relaxed atmosphere. In the problem-focused assessment the nurse most likely interweaves assessment and care. The care may include teaching, bathing, or treatments. If so, judgment has to be exercised regarding needs for privacy and absence of distraction.

Emergency Assessment

A life-threatening emergency is always expressed, however subtly, in *all* functional patterns. Yet to determine that an emergency exists, only a few pattern indicators need to be assessed. The purpose of assessment is (1) to identify the situation as either an emergency or a nonemergency, (2) to determine the *nature* of the emergency quickly, and (3) to intervene quickly. Obviously, in an emergency admission *the hypothesis of an acute dysfunctional change in a pattern is more likely than the hypothesis that no acute change has occurred.* The question is, What is the nature of the dysfunction?

Although probably without much conscious recognition, a nurse scans for certain overt, perceptible cues *every time* a nurse-client interaction occurs. This takes approximately 2 to 7 seconds and is done in a particular order. For example, a primary scan of three indicators of change in metabolic and activity patterns (skin color, posture, and facial expression) provides a wealth of information on the heart-lung-brain complex in less than a second. Additional information, if indicated, includes the radial or apical pulse and feeling for passage of air at the mouth. This information dictates whether further emergency assessment is done.

The preliminary scan of skin, posture, and face is usually done simultaneously with a question addressed to the person. Verbal or even nonverbal response would indicate changes in the cognitive-perceptual pattern. Environmental factors are often the major importance to the assessment. For example, if a person in a restaurant develops inability to breathe, panic, and bluish cast to the skin, a "cafe coronary" may be suspected (acute strangulation occurring from aspiration of incompletely chewed food).

Certain crises occurring in the life of a person, group, or community also require emergency assessment. For example, psychotic breakdown and potential for suicide or violence are crises requiring immediate assessment, diagnosis, and intervention.

Indicators of critical changes in self-concept (which may lead to suicide) or relationship patterns (which can result in violence) are cues to whether or not a crisis exists. In community health practice, emergency assessment may be required on the rare occasion of impending mob violence, riot, epidemics, or natural disasters.

Emergency assessment differs from other types of assessment. The time factor between observation and action, and the purpose of intervention, are different. In emergency assessment the life-threatening "diagnosis" is usually identified as a cluster of signs and symptoms. Immediate action and thoughts about cause are simultaneous. The purpose is to preserve life. Consequently, emergency assessment may not impose as high a *cognitive* demand as other types of assessment. Yet emotional and situational demands can be high. Also, time and risk factors contribute to the nurse's overall cognitive-affective state. Human life is valued. This value contributes to the heightened emotional state of care providers when a life-threatening emergency occurs.

Time-Lapse Reassessment

The basic objective in time-lapse reassessment is to evaluate changes in functional patterns. The time lapse since a previous history and examination may be considerable. Three, six, twelve, or more months may have elapsed since the last clinic visit or the last health status review of a client in a residential center. Functional patterns and the client's situation may have changed. Natural growth, health management practices, or long-term care can have demonstrable effects over time. Equally possible, non-productive patterns may have emerged because of health practices or situational factors.

This type of assessment has similarities to the initial and problem-focused assessment. It requires review of the current status of previous problems. It also requires the anticipation that new patterns may have emerged and require examination; accordingly, a total screening of all patterns is done. Only if unexpected changes or problems are perceived is it necessary to probe the history since the last evaluation. *The hypothesis either that a dysfunctional change has occurred or that none has occurred is influenced by previous knowledge of the client.* The question is, *Has change occurred over time and, if so, what is its direction?*

Time-lapse reassessment is common in follow-up of clients in ambulatory care settings and in periodic assessment in residential facilities, long-term care facilities, long-term home care, and school and industrial nursing. Situational factors play a similar role in this type of assessment and in the other types of assessment discussed above. The information load and cognitive strain vary with the occurrence of changes in the client's health status over time.

As is evident in this discussion, the structure of the assessment situation differs in accordance with the possibility that problems are present and the questions directing assessment. The differences among the four types of assessment are shown in Table 4-1. The summary in this table suggests that it is important to know the purpose of assessment so that assessment procedures can be structured to obtain valid and reliable data. The next section should further expand the notion of just how valid and reliable data can be. Additionally, it will become evident that the nature of the information influences *how* it is collected.

TABLE 4-1

COMPARISON OF THE FOUR ASSESSMENT SITUATIONS
AND THEIR STRUCTURAL INFLUENCES

Assessment situation	Preencounter probabilities	Questions directing the assessment	Structure of the environment
Initial (admission) assessment	The hypothesis of no dysfunctional pattern is as probable as the hypothesis that dysfunctional patterns exist	Does a problem (dysfunctional pattern) exist?	Establish a setting for obtaining accurate data (lighting, quiet, etc.) Establish an interpersonal atmosphere conducive to sharing thoughts, feelings, beliefs
Problem-focused assessment	The hypothesis of a dysfunctional pattern is more likely than the hypothesis that no dysfunctional pattern exists	Does a problem exist today? If so, what is the status of the problem?	Extend and maintain an interpersonal atmosphere conducive to sharing thoughts, feelings, beliefs
Emergency assessment, (client classified by instantaneous perception of life-threatening cues)	The hypothesis of an acute, dysfunctional change in a pattern is more likely than the hypothesis that no acute change has occurred	What is the nature of the dysfunction?	Establish a setting for obtaining data quickly and for immediate life-sustaining action
Time-lapse reassessment	The hypothesis that no dysfunctional change has occurred or that dysfunctional change has occurred is influenced by previous knowledge of the client	Has change occurred over time? If so, what is its direction?	Establish a setting for obtaining accurate data (lighting, quiet, etc.) Reestablish interpersonal atmosphere conducive to sharing thoughts, feelings, beliefs

THE NATURE OF CLINICAL INFORMATION

The term *data base* was used previously to describe information collected in the nursing history and examination. In this section discussion will focus on the general nature of the data. The nature of clinical data influences information collection and utilization. Ultimately, it influences diagnostic judgments.

Many difficulties in collecting and processing information can be avoided if one understands the nature of clinical cues. They are the "building blocks" (Cutler, 1979) or "raw data" from which a client's functional health patterns and, subsequently, diagnoses are constructed.

Clinical Cues

Clinical data collected during a purposeful assessment are cues to the health status of a client. A *cue* is defined as information which influences decisions. The nurse's decision may be to collect more information; or the cue may be used directly in diagnostic judgments regarding a particular condition.

Cues can take on different values. For example, marital status has five values: single, married, divorced, separated, and widowed. Some cues can be represented by numerical values, for example, heart rate. Quantification allows more precise measurement. Yet many of the cues to a client's health status are subjective impressions of quality or quantity, such as estimates of depth of respirations, moistness of skin, or severity of discomfort. As much as possible, data should be scaled (and scales carefully defined) or quantified numerically. This quantification increases reliability of measures and subsequently, the reliability of judgments and communications.

Cue Evaluation   Evaluating health pattern data involves comparing the *observed value* with the *expected value*. Population values (norms) from research, individual base lines, or (in some instances) the clinician's past clinical experiences provide the expected values. These are the criteria with which clinical data are compared. The importance of this evaluation must not be underestimated. It is the basis for subsequent diagnostic judgments.

Caution must be exercised in selecting the expected values to be used for evaluating clinical data. *Population norms* specify a range of normal limits for particular groups, frequently age groups. These norms are used as guidelines when evaluating physical attributes such as visual acuity, blood pressure, or protein intake. For evaluating data such as values, beliefs, self-perceptions, or role relationships, general population norms may be inadequate. Cultural, ethnic, racial, national, and religious patterns, as well as personal ones, need to be considered. For example, evaluation of data on toilet-training practices may be in error if specific cultural norms are ignored.

Secondly, when a social norm is in flux, it may not be useful as a criterion for evaluation. Sexuality patterns are an example; evaluation may have to be based partly or entirely on the client's perception of whether a problem exists.

Individual base lines, if available, are important in evaluating data. *Base-line data* provide individualized criteria that permit evaluation on the basis of the client's own functional health patterns. The difficulty arises in obtaining base-line measures. A human characteristic can be influenced by the context of the assessment situation, *including the nurse doing the base-line assessment*. Previous records may be helpful and should be consulted. If true base lines are not available, data obtained in the admission history and examination are used as base-line criteria for evaluating change in subsequent assessments.

The critical need for base-line data is the reason many hospitals require a nursing assessment within 24 hours of admission. Ideally, the assessment should be made as soon as a client enters a hospital, clinic, nursing home, or other health care service and has an opportunity to relax and obtain orienting information. The importance of this assessment in establishing base lines is the rationale for (1) having the history and examination done by a professional nurse; (2) doing the assessment in an environment conducive to relaxation; (3) establishing an interpersonal situation that facilitates development of rapport, trust, and confidence; and (4) ensuring privacy, quiet, and adequate lighting to facilitate conversation and examination.

Types of Cues The information gathered during assessment can be classified on the basis of a number of characteristics. Two important characteristics of cues have just been considered, validity and reliability. These characteristics and the ones discussed below influence the way information is collected and utilized.

Relevant and Irrelevant Cues The terms *relevant* and *irrelevant* are used frequently to pertain to validity. The relevance of a cue depends on the purpose for collecting information. Overall evaluation of functional health patterns is one purpose of an initial assessment. More specifically, the purpose is to obtain data to evaluate health-perception–health-management, nutritional-metabolic, role-relationship, and the other functional health patterns. Specific information about the essential properties of each pattern is considered *relevant* data. This information is what makes the data base informative.

The second purpose of asesssment is to identify dysfunctional patterns if they are present. Early data may suggest a tentative diagnostic hypothesis. The cue search then becomes focused on the signs and symptoms that define the diagnostic category under consideration. These defining signs and symptoms are the *relevant* cues that support or negate a hypothesis. But caution must be exercised in discounting what appears irrelevant in regard to one diagnosis. When investigated it may prove to be an indicator of another problem.

Irrelevant information can produce interference. Large amounts cause cognitive processes to become overloaded with noncontributory or redundant information, the "chaff" as opposed to the "wheat." For example, before completing the assessment of a client's nutritional pattern, one should have sufficient data to determine whether any type of nutritional deficit or excess is present and how the client manages this functional pattern. This necessary information is the wheat. It may be interesting to know also that the client's mother was a good cook, but this information in isolation is probably irrelevant.

The advantage of focusing on relevant data is that less time is needed for the assessment. For example, one could ask five questions about a client's sleep pattern. Suppose instead the client is asked, "Most mornings when you get up, do you feel rested and ready for the day?" If the response to this question is yes, is it relevant in a screening assessment to know the hours of sleep and other particulars? These details would be relevant only if a problem was present. *Each piece of clinical data collected should provide additional information relevant to judgment about a functional health pattern.*

Subjective and Objective Cues Frequently in practice a subjective-objective classification of cues is used. This is probably a false distinction. All observations have some subjectivity because the stimulus has been processed through the observer's mind.

Common usage defines *objective data* as characteristics perceived by some outside observer, whereas *subjective data* refers to characteristics perceived by the client and not the observer. The latter includes subjective perceptions and feelings, such as self-concept or pain. In contrast are the so-called objective data the nurse observes, such as skin color, heart rate, or parent-child interaction. Clinical data are commonly categorized as subjective or objective within the format of the problem-oriented recording system in many health care agencies.[3]

The objective-subjective designation has relevance to the processing of information. The trained observer credits himself or herself with more objectivity than the client. Thus objective data are considered to be free from personal biases, emotions, and the like that can influence information processing. This supposition, of course, is not always true; many times people, nurses included, see what they are ready to see. Yet the clinician *tries* to put aside biases or predispositions and to be objective when analyzing clinical data. Some nurses are more successful than others.

It is well to recognize that there are two primary value systems that relate to subjective and objective data. In the diagnosis of disease or disease complications, objective data are valued for their diagnostic significance. Thus when a nurse transmits data to a physician, the emphasis is usually on objective data. Objective and subjective data are of *equal* diagnostic significance to nurses. Some examples will clarify these two sets of values.

In the process of diagnosing disease, the physician considers subjective reports to be tentative until verification can be obtained by objective measures. In the extreme case, physical symptoms may be categorized as hypochondria if objective measurement does not support subjective reports. A somewhat paradoxical situation exists: if a lesion is observed on x-ray, the situation is reversed; support for the presence of the lesion is sought in subjective data from the client. For example, if lung pathology is found by objective x-ray examination, the patient is asked whether pain, dyspnea, or other subjective symptoms have been experienced. A conflict between the two types of data is resolved either by greater reliance on objective measurements or, in some cases, a "wait and see" attitude.

In psychiatric diagnosis subjective data are essential but are complemented by objective examination to rule out organ pathology. For example, signs of a behavioral disorder would not be given a psychiatric label without ruling out organic problems, such as a brain tumor.

Nurses are concerned equally with both objective and subjective data. They shuttle back and forth between their own observations (the so-called objective data) and the subjective reports of the client. Many manage to arrive at a synthesis. For example, a nurse may objectively measure a pressure sore. Yet there is *equal* diagnostic concern about the individual's coping response to this condition and personal and environmental factors that brought it about.

Subjective client reports have diagnostic value because they help the nurse understand the client's perspective. These subjective data are valued because nurses' *primary* emphasis is on people and their total situation, including, but not limited to, the

---

[3]The problem-oriented recording system is a charting format that requires the separation of objective observations and subjective reports. Its use with nursing diagnoses will be discussed in a later chapter.

disease. Medical care providers of course do not totally ignore the person's ideas, actions, feelings, values, or beliefs, but these are not diagnostic of disease.

When a nurse acts within a nursing framework, the concerns, the data, and the diagnoses are different from those of physicians. When a nurse operates within a bio-medical framework and transmits data to a physician, objective data are valued more than subjective reports. Both frameworks are used in nursing practice.

A related typology of clinical cues is the *sign and symptom classification*. The term *symptom* designates an experience related by a client. Information about symptoms is subjective. It includes the client's perceptions of body temperature, skin sensations, palpitations, feelings of competency or esteem, beliefs, attitudes, and values.

In contrast, a *sign* is an objective indicator of a health problem. A symptom can be a sign, and a client can perceive a sign but may not interpret it. If this is thoroughly confusing, the reader will appreciate why the terms *sign* and *symptom* are frequently used interchangeably. For the reader who wishes to pursue the distinction further, King's (1968) treatise on the subject will be of interest.

Historical and Current Cues   Another useful way of thinking about the clinical data collected for purposes of nursing diagnosis is from a *time perspective*. An understanding of a client's functional patterns is constructed from historical and current cues. This way of classifying clinical data permits one to examine the cues used in nursing diagnoses. Are they based on historical information, current information, or both? Secondly, are diagnoses based only on cues to the client's state or also on cues about the situational or environmental context?

To appreciate the distinction between historical and current information, keep in mind that current data come from "the here and now." Historical data may pertain to last night, 2 days ago, or 10 years ago.

Historical measures of client characteristics provide *historical state cues*. These are previous values of characteristics, such as blood pressure, appetite, family roles, and body perception. In community assessment, traffic fatalities or cardiovascular death rates in previous years may be historical cues.

The data described above provide an individualized base line. One common example is blood pressure. What does a current value of 95/78 mean? If the value for the past 2 years has been 150/90, the interpretation is different than if blood pressure has been consistently in the 90–100/70–80 range. As another example, knowing the past number of hours of sleep helps the nurse interpret and evaluate the present value of this characteristic. Historical state data provide base-line cues for interpreting the current state of a client within the context of the client's own functional pattern.

A nursing diagnosis should never be made exclusively from historical cues. Can you think why this is so and how it could ever occur? Inferences about a particular client's behavior can be derived deductively by combining some information (in this case, historical data) and generalizations from memory. For example, a nurse may infer that because the emotional state of a patient was "angry and complaining about the staff" on the day of admission, this is the current state. In a sense the client is never allowed to escape the history. Using *only* historical cues predisposes to diagnostic error. Clearly, the current state of the client must be assessed. Also, it must be recognized that an inference is created in the mind of the clinician and may or may not stand up to the test of reality. This paragraph contains ideas so important in avoiding diagnostic errors that it may be worthwhile to reread it.

Current data about attributes of the client are *current state cues*. These are the current values for blood pressure, comfort level, activity level, caloric intake, age, laboratory test values, emotional state, and other client characteristics. This type of information, in combination with historical base lines, is used to identify health patterns and detect changes.

Current state cues should always be sought before making diagnoses. The etiology of a self-care deficit, or any other problem, is determined by current or historical cues. To determine whether a change in pattern has been abrupt or gradual, historical data are used.

In addition to collecting information about the state of the person, the nurse measures characteristics of the client's situation. These describe the context within which functional patterns arise. Attention is focused on both historical and current situational cues.

Previous values of unchangeable characteristics of the person (birthdate, for example) or situation are *historical contextual cues*. Events that have already occurred are part of one's life history. Not only are they history, but they are the context (not the state) out of which current functional patterns may have evolved. It is worthwhile to consider a few examples, since this type of cue is very useful in diagnosis.

First consider a rather obvious relationship. During assessment, the nurse elicits the information that the client avoids high-roughage foods. For example, no bran, leafy vegetables, nuts, or other foods with bulk are reported in the diet. This has been the pattern for a decade or more. (Note the historical and current *state* information.) The nurse thinks that the client is missing a good source of vitamins and is susceptible to constipation because of the lack of bulk in the diet.

There are two options: one is to plunge ahead and try to correct this behavior; the other is to wonder why the client avoids roughage. Choosing the latter option, the nurse can ask questions to determine whether there is any explanation in past history. The nurse learns that about 15 years ago the client was diagnosed as having diverticulosis[4] and was told to avoid high-roughage foods. This contextual event (being diagnosed and instructed) happened in the past but is the reported reason for the current dietary pattern.

Historical contextual cues (situational cues) not only are helpful in understanding functional patterns but also play an important role in prediction. There is an indication from research (Gordon, 1972, 1980) that nurses use situational cues to predict the most likely health problems. In an admission assessment, prediction is necessary because the universe of possibilities is open. To fully investigate every conceivable functional health problem is impossible. Therefore predictions (inferences, or hypotheses) are made about the likelihood of various problems. Problems estimated to be of high likelihood are investigated.

Predictions are made on the basis of historical contextual cues and conceptual

---

[4] Diverticulosis is a condition in which there are small outpouches and weak points in the wall of the colon. Older methods of treatment included the avoidance of high-roughage foods.

relationships stored in the nurse's memory. For example, a recent historical event in the life of a person, such as a first heart attack, is information that can be used to predict the likelihood of certain functional problems the nurse knows are often associated with heart attack.

Historical information about the environmental context also helps one understand the background from which functional health patterns arise and develop. This information includes prior living environments, economic conditions, the health and welfare resource systems, and the interpersonal and sociocultural environment. In addition to contributing to the nurse's understanding of health patterns, this information may be useful in the prediction of problems. The reader may be wondering, Why bother to think about possibilities? Why not just collect the assessment data?

The perceptually sensitive observer anticipates. An inference is made from relationships stored in the observer's memory. This inference then forms the basis for a set of probing questions and the search for further cues. Predictive inference *is* anticipation, and it largely depends on contextual cues.

Assumptions or inferences drawn on the basis of the person's history are useful but must be used with caution if incorporated, without validation, into diagnosis. Although the historical event of having an amputation or breast removal is highly correlated with an alteration in body image, amputation is insufficient rationale for diagnosis of body image disturbance. A tentative diagnostic hypothesis (alteration in body image) should be generated to guide cue search. Diagnosis based on only historical cues about the situation can result in an error of historical stereotyping.

A final type of clinical cue is the *current contextual cue*. This is derived from assessment of the current situation. For example, assessment usually includes the structure of the interpersonal environment. Is the person a hermit or part of a large, closely structured family network? What are the neighborhood and community like? What health services are available? What are the current events in a client's life, such as an episode of physical illness, a divorce in process, or a husband dying at home? The current context of the client's life, when combined with the historical context, permits the nurse to construct the client's situational or environmental pattern.

This discussion has separated out for definition, analysis, and attention types of client and environmental cues. In actual practice these cues are not collected in separate packages but are obtained within the assessment sequence. What usually happens is that a piece of information is collected and attended to, and then a question arises: What kind of information is necessary to derive meaning from this cue? One may branch to *historical* information about the client and past environment. This information is usually obtained by questions posed to the client or others possessing the historical data.

Branching may also point toward the need for more *current* data. This is obtained by questions to elicit subjective reports about the client's state. The nurse may also need to examine the current situational context, such as home environment. Obviously, if one knows what type of information is needed (historical or current), assessment proceeds more rapidly.

Why bother with a clinical cue classification? Mainly because cognitive operations need some checks and balances. Habits can arise that affect efficiency and accuracy.

Feedback is not always available after student days are over. One can fall into a pattern of diagnosing only on the basis of here and now, which is probably cognitively inefficient, as will be seen in the discussion of diagnostic strategies. Another habit pattern is diagnosing only on the basis of historical information; this is close to stereotyping and is very risky. Examining the cues one habitually uses provides checks and balances on the needed mixture of historical and current information.

Probabilistic Nature of Clinical Cues   The word *probability* means the same as *chance*. The diagnostic task is a probabilistic one. This means that nursing diagnoses are made at some level of probability, not absolute certainty. In contrast, there are other types of categorizations in which information permits one to infer with certainty. These situations are not too common in the everyday world or in clinical practice.

In the previous discussion of validity and reliability of data, the impression may have been given that reliability and validity can be totally controlled. In this section it will be seen that (because of the nature of cues about people) the degree of control over validity and reliability of data and of clinical judgments varies. Much information is probabilistic. Nurses have to learn to deal with uncertainty when it cannot be totally eliminated by assessment methods.

From the time one first notices things in the surrounding world, one learns about probabilities. They involve whether or not trains are apt to come on time, the possibility of a good grade or pay raise, and the chance that a driver will stop at a stop sign. From childhood on, each person works on learning the *likelihood of events* and *what predicts what*. For example, if an object looks like a book, it probably has printed pages.

In nursing, interest centers on the probability, or likelihood, that a problem exists, given a set of cues, or signs and symptoms. Even the critical, defining cues for a diagnosis may not allow certainty in diagnostic judgments. The probabilistic nature of nursing practice has been described by Hammond. He argues that client conditions produce different cues, and the same cue can be produced by different conditions (1966, p. 34). In other words, the cues available for diagnosing a health problem are not always completely valid and reliable.

Consider an example: *A smile is a cue to friendliness.* Let us say that 80 percent of the time when people are friendly, they smile. On the other hand, smiling may be present 20 percent of the time when people are really hostile and angry. Smiling does not predict friendliness with 100 percent certainty. It is a *probabilistic cue*. If these figures are correct, this cue is associated with only 80 percent predictive validity. That is, inferring friendliness when a person smiles will be a valid inference in 80 out of 100 cases.

The ideal situation would be to find cues that are *certain*. Then clinicians could be "sure" of their diagnoses. Yet human behavior is variable and the ideal probably can never be reached. At least at this point in scientific development one cannot actually "stand in the shoes" of another person and know what the other knows, feels, or believes.

Anxiety is a good example for further demonstration. Consider first of all two people. In reality, they both feel anxious. Yet they manifest different signs or cues;

that is, they express anxiety differently. Now consider one person who is anxious. This person will not necessarily demonstrate the same signs of anxiety in two different social environments or at two different times. Thus a set of cues may be unreliable in terms of various *individuals* and also in terms of one individual in different *situations* and through *time.*

Hammond (1966) describes clinicians as hard pressed to point to one set of cues that *always* indicates a diagnosis. Most textbooks reflect this lack of predictability. Look at the way authors describe the signs and symptoms of nursing or medical diagnoses. They use words such as *"usually* presents the symptoms of . . . ," *"nearly always* associated with these signs . . . ," or *"frequently* demonstrates an elevated . . . ." This "hedging" reminds one of the kind of language used in another probabilistic, uncertain situation—weather forecasting; it has the same built-in uncertainty.

Clinicians generally consider *physical cues* to be more reliable and valid indicators of a diagnosis than *social cues.* For example, redness and blanching over bony prominences of the back are highly reliable and valid signs of potential skin breakdown in white- or yellow-skinned persons. Signs of altered body image are more variable from one individual to another; thus they are less reliable predictors of the diagnosis. This difference in the reliability of signs results in a greater feeling of uncertainty in making the latter diagnosis than in making the former.

To identify subjective states (feeling states) or self-perceptions of clients, it is critical to obtain verbal reports of the person. Subjective data increase the clinician's confidence in the diagnosis, as well as validity and reliability of the diagnosis. In the case of objective phenomena, such as potential skin breakdown, it is not critical that the client confirm the clinician's observation (that the skin is red or blanching).

The cues gleaned from interview and examination have a wide range of predictive accuracy. Additionally, many times judgments have to be made with limited information and time.

Handling Uncertainty There is a way of dealing with uncertain information in situations where errors have to be controlled. The method of approach is to use the cues with the highest validity. Every time a cue that is a valid indicator of a diagnosis (critical defining characteristic) is present, there is a high probability that the health problem is present. Such a cue is, in addition, a reliable indicator across clients.[5]

Highly reliable, highly valid cues are referred to as the *critical defining characteristics* of a diagnostic category. They increase confidence in diagnostic judgments. If one or more cues point to the possibility of a health problem, the remaining critical defining cues should be assessed before the diagnosis is made. (As discussed previously, not all currently identified diagnostic categories have critical signs and symptoms specified.)

Clinical inferences about subjective states, such as pain, body image, or conflict, are plagued with uncertainty unless a combination of observations and verbal reports is used. Subjective feeling states are not observable; only the client's response to the feelings can be assessed. For example, consider the signs of restlessness and facial grimacing, combined with a history of abdominal surgery 24 hours previously. A

---

[5] If a cue is a valid indicator of a health problem then it is also a reliable indicator. This statement is based on the assumption that assessment of the cue has been accurate.

possibility is that the client is having incisional pain. How confident would you be about making this inductive inference from the data?

The more knowledge you have about postsurgical care, the *less* confident you will be! These cues are highly uncertain predictors of pain; they do not discriminate among three or four other conditions that are manifested by restlessness and facial grimacing. Suppose the postoperative client says, "I've tried turning and taking the medicine; nothing helps the pain." Does this cue increase confidence in the diagnosis of pain management deficit? Yes; now the other cues become supporting cues. When the cluster is put together, confidence is sufficient to make the diagnostic judgment.

Can doubt always be erased by more information? No, not unless the cue is a more valid and reliable indicator than the information already secured. A verbal report of pain increases validity in the above example because pain, by definition, is a subjective state really known only by the client. It also must be noted that a verbal report *alone* is not always sufficient data. An adequate level of confidence to infer pain and give a narcotic usually requires both verbal report and observational data; this is because, although feeling pain is a valid indicator, our methods of *measuring* feelings (assessing the client's subjective report) are not always reliable. Verbal reports are used to measure feelings and may be biased by conscious or unconscious motives of the person reporting.

In judging the *validity* of a cue or cluster of cues, consider whether the cues indicate a critical property of the diagnosis being considered (i.e., whether they are valid indicators). Second, consider the degree to which this property is present when the diagnosis is present and absent when the diagnosis is not present (degree of validity).

In judging the *reliability* of a cue or cue cluster used in a diagnostic judgment, consider the degree to which it is a dependable cue (always present or only sometimes present when the diagnosis is present). Consider also the degree to which its measurement is dependable (direct versus indirect measure of the property).

The above considerations are important. Good diagnostic judgments are made on the basis of the most valid and reliable cues that can be acquired in a particular situation. The more valid and reliable the cues, the less uncertainty and the higher confidence the nurse will have in his or her judgments. Of course, the better the diagnostic judgments are, the higher is the probability that the care plan devised for the client will be effective.

It may be an interesting exercise to determine which of the following cues and inferences from data are highly valid and reliable. Evaluate each independently. The task is to select information that is absolutely necessary for accurate diagnosis of an intermittent constipation pattern. For the moment, disregard the etiology. These are the cues:

1 Decreased activity level
2 Hard, formed stool today
3 Palpable mass in abdomen
4 Reports feeling of pressure or fullness in rectum
5 Reports history of frequent straining at stool
6 Appetite impairment
7 Headache

8 Reports two or three episodes per month (history) of hard, formed stool following period of no bowel movement

What needs to be determined are the necessary and sufficient criteria for diagnosing an intermittent constipation pattern. The first inference, number 1, decreased activity level, is obviously insufficient for making the diagnosis; it may be either a factor contributing to severity or an etiological (causative) factor in this diagnosis. Hard, formed stool, item number 2, indicates the possibility of the presence of constipation. It does not provide data about an intermittent pattern. A cue such as this should be investigated in terms of the frequency and precipitating factors.

The third cue, palpable mass in the abdomen, is not definitive. It does not differentiate between stool and a tumor. The fourth cue is similar; a rectal tumor could cause the same sensation but usually would also be associated with other symptoms. Number 5 is history of frequent straining at stool; this indeed does provide a valid cue. Is it sufficient information? No, but it is a key piece of information which we will hold for the moment.

The sixth cue, appetite impairment, is interesting; it may be secondary to constipation but deserves investigation to ensure that it is not a cue to another condition. It could be a predisposing or causative factor of constipation if sufficient fluids and bulky foods are not being ingested. Headache, cue number 7, is not unusual with constipation but is not diagnostic. It does deserve explanation even in isolation. Thus far we have one cue; the rest of the information could be signs or symptoms of other conditions. Therefore the cues represent unreliable and nondifferentiating evidence for the diagnosis under consideration. They could be supporting cues for the presence of a *current* state of constipation. but not an intermittent pattern.

The eighth cue, a history of hard, formed stool two or three times per month following a period of no bowel movement, is a highly valid predictor of the diagnosis being entertained. It is a verbal report; unless the reliability of the client is questionable, it does provide sufficient confidence for the diagnosis. Is this one cue sufficient to identify the health problem? Is it a necessary or critical cue, without which the validity of the diagnosis would be questionable? Is it a conclusive sign? The answer to these questions is yes. Cue number 5, frequent straining, is redundant; it really does not provide any further information but only supports that the stool, as described in cue number 8, is probably hard to evacuate.

Redundant cues serve a function. They provide a check or support for a diagnostic judgment and can increase confidence level when information is uncertain. Up to a point, redundant cues are probably psychologically necessary. In excess, they provide quantity, not quality, in a data base.

The etiology of this health problem still has to be identified. A number of options are open. If the eight pieces of data were actually collected in a real situation, questions would arise. Should etiological factors be investigated immediately? Or should the problem be referred to a physician for differential medical diagnosis?

The cues appetite impairment and palpable mass, in conjunction with the problem of intermittent constipation, suggest the need for differential medical diagnosis. Could a tumor be present? It is highly advisable to refer the problem to a physician if the nurse is not competent to discriminate among the etiological factors of intermittent constipation, especially a tumor. A second option is to discuss with a physician the findings and the possibility of administering an enema. The palpable mass may be stool accumulated in the colon; if so, it would disappear when the enema was expelled. In the absence of abdominal tumor, the client's constipation problem may be amenable to nursing therapy. Etiological factors to be investigated by nursing include dietary patterns, abdominal muscle tone, bowel habits, anxiety, and decreased activity.

This example illustrates the need to examine the data collected, predict alternative explanations, and test possibilities. It also demonstrates the uncertain nature of clinical data. Essentially, two main factors should influence judgment. These are the validity and reliability of information available *and* theoretical knowledge one can bring to bear in interpretation.

The Important Cues   Cues or clusters of cues that are important for diagnosis are of four types. The first type is the cue that signifies change in a client's usual patterns that is unexplained by expected norms for growth and development. Change can be positive and health-supporting or it may be negative and potentially dysfunctional. An example of the latter would be change in the role-relationship pattern so that the client becomes socially isolated.

The second type of cue that requires attention is deviation from an appropriate population norm. For example, a person may have *no change* in frequency of elimination but depend on laxatives and enemas to maintain regularity. This represents a deviation from "normality."

In another situation a client may be within the norms of his or her ethnic group but deviant in terms of the general or dominant social norms. This situation can produce problems for the person within one or many functional pattern areas, a possibility that would need to be validated with the client.

The third type of cue or cluster of cues that can be diagnostic is behavior that is nonproductive in the whole-person context. This determination requires consideration of interaction among functional health pattern areas. For example, a person may have no change in nutritional pattern. This does not mean that the pattern is productive for the person. It may be causing an elimination problem, or a nutritional deficit may be present if requirements have increased. These problems are detected only by evaluating information relative to the whole.

The fourth type of cue or cue cluster important for nursing diagnosis is that which indicates pattern development. Each of the functional health patterns is continually evolving as the person grows older. For example, it is expected that a young child's activity-exercise pattern will evolve as neurological development permits more coordinated movement. Similarly, value-belief patterns change with life experiences, including experience with dying. Cues to development of functional health patterns are important. They may signify developmental lags or evolving patterns that are dysfunctional for the client.

Describing signs and symptoms only from the viewpoint of the nurse can lead to errors of omission. The way a client "defines the situation" must be taken into account. For example, it may be "apparent" that a particular mother and father are very concerned, caring, and capable. But if their child says, "Mommy doesn't love me," this statement is a cue. It should not be brushed aside with some superficial reassurance. If that is how the child defines the situation, that is how it is for her. Similarly, if a person says there is no other recourse than suicide, in reality as that person perceives it there may not be another way. When a person newly diagnosed as diabetic says, "I can't manage," the response "Of course you can" may cut off critically important cues.

Clients' descriptions of their problems, their ideas about the causes of the problems, and their responses to the problems provide data about health perceptions and actions; these data are extremely relevant to nursing diagnosis. When a person reports having noted a decrease in social contacts for the past year, important cues can be obtained by asking questions. "Why do you think this has occurred?" explores the client's ideas about causal relationships. "How have you managed that?" provides information about action that has been taken in response to the problem. "Did that seem to help?" asks the client to evaluate the effectiveness of the action taken. Questions similar to these provide cues to health perception, health management, coping patterns, and the client's perception of his or her own competency.

Dismissing cues with superficial reassurance may decrease the nurse's anxiety and the time spent in assessment. Yet the underlying problem will not go away. It will probably come back to haunt the staff in a different guise because the original communication was not attended to. "Uncooperative" behavior (from the nurse's or doctor's perspective), frequent calls for staff, and repeated visits to an emergency room are common ways clients express unresolved problems.

Clients' explanations, actions, and evaluations may be extremely insightful or totally erroneous. In some instances the causes of a problem can be traced to the client's definition of the situation and actions based on this definition. These findings are important cues to knowledge deficits or health management deficits. Some clients provide information voluntarily. Others are reluctant to describe their ideas and actions for fear of being incorrect. Try to encourage expression; avoid communicating "You should have known better," either verbally or by facial expression.

Any discussion of important cues must consider the cues that define currently accepted nursing diagnoses. These are health problems within the scope of nursing practice, and cues to their presence must not be missed. For example, if dietary pattern, body weight, and other characteristics are not assessed, a nutritional deficit may be missed.

A dilemma exists. Most diagnoses are not well defined. Therefore, what are the "important" cues? At this stage of development the list of accepted diagnoses (Appendix A) and their defining criteria (with their deficiencies) are the best available in the nursing literature (Kim and Moritz, 1981).[6] The following brief discussion, about what needs to be done to ensure that critical criteria for using diagnostic labels are available, is relevant to the subject of important cues.

Diagnostic Cues The *defining characteristics* of a diagnostic category are signs and symptoms specified by convention. They are official, formal definitions usually published in a taxonomy manual for use by diagnosticians within the particular pro-

---

[6] Accepted diagnoses and their signs and symptoms are also listed in the manual that accompanies this book.

fession. For clarity in communication, all members of the profession are expected to use the diagnostic labels only when the critical defining signs and symptoms are present.[7] When the signs and symptoms used to make a diagnosis are not the accepted critical defining signs and symptoms, communication with diagnostic labels becomes impossible. Two clinicians might use the same label to refer to two totally different problems requiring totally different therapy.

One major problem with the current list of nursing diagnoses is the lack of critical defining signs and symptoms for each diagnostic label. Either the signs and symptoms listed for the accepted diagnoses are too lengthy or critical ones are not identified. Review and clinical validation are necessary; this work has been started, but until it is completed the probability that the same label is applied consistently to the same set of cues may be low.

A second factor that presents difficulty in identifying the critical criteria for using many of the current diagnostic labels is the breadth of the category label. Terms such as *alteration in parenting* or *sensory perceptual alteration* encompass broad problem areas. Studies of specific problems are needed. For example, in one study five client characteristics are listed as reliable predictors for the diagnosis of potential skin breakdown[8] (Norton, Exton-Smith, and McLaren, 1962, p. 225). When the five cues are present, the diagnosis can be made and the label applied. This kind of specificity is what needs to be available for each nursing diagnosis.

Standardization of diagnoses (official, formal definition) cannot be done until defining characteristics of categories are refined. At the present time nursing has a set of generally ill-defined diagnoses. Yet this situation is better than 10 years ago. To borrow a quote from another profession: "Inadequate as it is, it remains the best classification available and summarizes a vast amount of experience" (Engle and Davis, 1963, p. 519).

It is hoped that students and clinicians bothered by the lack of precise definition will be motivated to assist in the work being done. *Ignoring the list because of its lack of specificity will only perpetuate the problem.* As will be seen in the following section, dealing with ambiguity and uncertainty is the hallmark of clinical practice! Another hallmark is that nurses attempt to decrease uncertainty and thereby increase reliability of their clinical judgments.

This section has provided an introduction to the nature of clinical information used in nursing diagnosis. Four important types of clinical cues to the health status of the client were identified. These were cues indicating change in a functional pattern, deviation from pattern norms, dysfunctional patterns, or pattern development.

The uncertain, or probabilistic, nature of clinical data was described. Because of the human capacity for variability in behavioral expression, signs and symptoms predict with less than perfect certainty. Nurses have to learn to deal with this uncertain environment. It was suggested that highly valid and reliable information has to be used.

---

[7] As with every rule, there are exceptions. Critical cues predict with very high probability, not absolute certainty. If one criterion is not present, clinical judgment about applying the diagnostic label has to be exercised. Other critical cues may provide sufficient support for the diagnosis.

[8] The characteristics are physical condition, mental condition, activity level, mobility level, and bladder control. The values of each determine the level of risk.

Additionally, the nurse must recognize that judgments based on uncertain data are subject to error. A continual openness to new contradictory or supporting information has to be maintained.

Clinical data can be relevant or irrelevant to the purpose of assessment or to a particular diagnostic hypothesis. Knowing what data are needed prevents cognitive processes from being overwhelmed with irrelevant information. Information that does not increase the reliability or validity of judgment is irrelevant. The focus in data collection has to be on the cues that "pay off" in terms of health status evaluation.

The distinction between subjective and objective data was discussed. It was suggested that when a nursing framework is being used, both types of data provide important cues. Nurses are equally concerned with so-called objective observation of the client and the client's situation and with the person's subjective perceptions, responses, beliefs, and attitudes. The client's perspective on his or her situation is considered as important in assessment as the nurse's perspective on it. Rather than discount clients' subjective, personal biases and feelings, nurses use these data in diagnosis.

Historical and current client and contextual data were related to functional health pattern assessment. For understanding a pattern, both types of data are necessary; this is why assessment consists of both history-taking and examination. The errors and decreased efficiency resulting from an overemphasis on either historical or current data were pointed out. The section may be summarized by saying *important cues* are relevant; they may be historical or current, subjective or objective, and related to the client's state or situational context. Lastly, important cues are those that represent the most reliable and valid data available.

DIAGNOSTICIANS' BASIC TOOLS

This section will focus on the diagnostician, who can be thought of as both a measuring device and an information processor. Thinking of oneself as a sensitive measuring device permits some objectivity. It is possible to stand aside and examine the way a nurse's cognitive and perceptual processes can influence information collection.

Cognitive and perceptual abilities are the basic "tools" used in information collection. Nurses have been developing these capabilities since birth. They include *perception, memory, inference*, and the use of *abstractions*. In fact, a complex skill used in nursing diagnosis began to develop during infancy. Learning that a toy ball did not cease to exist after rolling behind the chair ushered in the development of inference. Diagnosis requires sharpening cognitive and perceptual abilities and one important additional ingredient, clinical knowledge. The discussion will begin with this factor because, as will be clear later, people perceive on the basis of previously acquired knowledge.

Clinical Knowledge

Knowledge is a necessary, but not a sufficient, condition for expertise in nursing diagnosis. What is an adequate knowledge base? It is difficult to say. Minimally, knowledge of the functional pattern areas described in Chapter 3 is needed for health status evaluation and diagnosis. Specifically, the following are necessary areas of knowledge for nursing diagnosis (other areas would be required for nursing intervention):

1 Range of norms for the 11 functional health patterns (age norms)
2 Natural development of functional patterns during the life-span
3 Variations in patterns related to culture, environment, disease, and other influences
4 Common dysfunctional patterns (nursing diagnoses)
5 Indicators of dysfunctional patterns

The practical approach is to gain a working knowledge of the functional patterns and of high-incidence nursing diagnoses. It is most important to use the patterns consistently in assessment. From this practice and from further study one learns what patterns clients exhibit, what factors are associated with the patterns, what nursing treatment is successful, and what outcomes result. Knowledge develops with experience, but the clinician has a responsibility *to see that experience contributes to knowledge.* Fulfilling that responsibility takes analysis and reflection; it does not happen automatically. The cognitive and perceptual abilities discussed in the following sections and in Chapter 5 are the means used to learn about clients; they are also the means used to continually increase clinical knowledge.

Perceptual Recognition of Cues

In clinical situations vast amounts of information impinge on the nurse's sense organs at any given moment. This information enters what is called sensory memory. Information decays quickly in sensory memory unless it is *recognized* and *transferred* to short-term memory. Recognition involves an inference about identity. Coding a sensory experience makes it possible to categorize it—to say, for example, *this* is a textbook and *that* is a novel.

Recognition is the mental operation of establishing the correspondence between sensory data and a category conceived and stored in memory. Sensation can occur without recognition, that is, without identity classification. Studies of clients with a certain brain pathology (aphasia) support the belief that recognition occurs in two phases. For example, these clients can discriminate writing on a blackboard but have no idea what it means; they lack recognition.

Holt (1961, p. 378) identifies various causes of failures in recognition: (1) lack of categories in memory (for example, lack of clinical knowledge); (2) lack of training in discrimination (for example, in discrimination of skin color changes); (3) blocks in memory scanning (that is, in retrieving identity categories) because of fatigue or emotional upset; (4) demanding too exact a degree of correspondence between sensory data and categories in memory or accepting too gross a correspondence (insufficient data for identification); and (5) lack of precise criteria for recognition (category stored in memory has not been, or cannot be, precisely defined). Everyone has experienced failures caused by these reasons. In clinical practice, steps have to be taken to reduce the causes of failure to a minimum.

Attaching a word symbol or category name to a sensory event is an act of perceptual recognition and categorization. The process of recognition and categorization is evident in statements such as "the new patient is a *female*" or "her skin is *warm.*" *Female* and *warm* are examples of concrete perceptual inferences and concrete identity categorizations. In a particular clinical situation these kinds of perceptions may be cues to a diagnosis if the nurse uses them to go beyond mere recognition of identity. Before discussing this idea, let us consider what contributes to being a sensitive observer.

Sensitivity to Cues   There are three major requirements for becoming a sensitive observer. One is to have knowledge categories available for coding relevant sensory data so that the identity and meaning of what one observes can be determined. A second factor in becoming a sensitive observer of health-related cues is to anticipate, or look for, cues on the basis of knowledge that certain client behaviors are likely in particular situations. Third, observers have to focus their attention so that sensory data are not missed. These three factors influence perceptual sensitivity to cues and subsequently influence diagnostic judgments.

Ways of representing the perceptual world of nursing practice are learned primarily from others. Descriptions, names for things, and meanings are provided in nursing's "cultural heritage." During learning, images are constructed and stored in memory. Think for a minute; conjure up an image of a thermometer. Describe it. Presumably the reader does not have one handy; thus some mental image from past learning has to be scanned. Images are also referred to as cognitive categories.[9] They are representations in memory from past interactions with the world. In fact, categories and their interrelations are each individual's own personal descriptions of the world. If, when verbalized, they are not reasonably congruent with others' descriptions, the discrepancy is called madness or creativity!

Categorization helps one learn to respond to things judged as comparable or equivalent (things in the same category). When skin is categorized as *mottled*, nurses derive certain meanings from this perception. A different meaning is derived when sensory data are put into another category, *sallow* skin.

Categories may be detailed discriminations or global representations. This varying specificity is determined by the interests and needs of the person and, basically, by past interactions with the environment. For example, English teachers pay close attention to grammar and sentence structure. They have categories available for coding auditory or visual data about grammatical errors, such as dangling participles. Compared to nurses, English teachers may fare poorly in perceiving and categorizing heart rhythms or nonverbal messages. They lack discriminating categories and category systems in these areas.

Many sophisticated discriminations are required in nursing. For example, nurses learn to discriminate among at least nine changes in skin color: jaundice, mottling, flushing, bronzing, sallowness, ashenness, glossiness, pallor, and cyanosis.

Much of nursing education involves categorization. The nurse learns (1) to isolate important details from the environment, (2) to categorize observations, (3) to work with the descriptive labels used in health care, (4) to recognize relationships among categories, and (5) to make general responses to categorized situations. Most importantly, learning to categorize permits the nurse to order and relate one thing to another, such as one cue to another, clusters of cues to a diagnosis, and then diagnosis

---

[9] Earlier in the book, nursing diagnoses were described as *conceptual categories*. In this section the focus is on *perceptual categories* that are the cues, or building blocks, used in attaining a diagnosis.

to general therapy. It also permits anticipation of things not immediately observable (Rosch and Lloyd, 1978, p. 1).

Anticipation   *Sensitivity* is a term used frequently in nursing. Clients use it in the context "such a sensitive nurse." Supervisors, clinical specialists, and nursing instructors may use the term similarly *or* in the negative: "She's just not sensitive to clients." One can surmise that sensitivity is highly valued in a nurse because people rarely confront each other directly with accusations of insensitivity to people. Sensitive observers see not only the very obvious and apparent things but also the not-so-apparent. They anticipate and predict.

Perceptual sensitivity to client behavior depends in part on anticipation of behavior. If something is anticipated, or expected, less information is needed for recognizing and coding sensory input. This is because categories for recognizing the input are more accessible in memory. To become aware of relationships among cues and to know the meaning of cues, one must learn the appropriate categories for coding clinical data and must know the relationships among categories.[10] Knowing the likelihood of events permits anticipation and perceptual readiness. Perception is accurate as long as what is expected corresponds with the events that actually take place.

An example may further clarify how anticipation increases perceptual sensitivity. Suppose a nurse knows that 3 days of bed rest can produce muscle weakness. When a client begins to get out of bed after confinement, a slight buckling of one knee may be sufficient to identify the possibility of muscle weakness. Lacking background knowledge of the expected likelihood of muscle weakness, another nurse might miss the relatively subtle cue of knee buckling and the client might not be supervised as ambulation begins. An impressive cue, such as falling, might be necessary before recognition could occur.

Neisser argues that anticipation plays an active role in all perception (1978, pp. 95–96). To illustrate, he uses the example of someone intently reading in a room with the door open. A visitor arrives and the person looks up, because he either heard him or saw him "out of the corner of his eye." Stored information directed perceptual exploration; the man who was reading anticipated where the door was and looked in that direction. Having turned his head to the door, he scanned the visitor's face with repeated shifting eye movements. Each activity was a *consequence* of the information already picked up; therefore, it is difficult to say perception occurred at any one moment. The example continues, illustrating the anticipatory, or inferential, nature of the perceptual process:

Even without the contribution of peripheral vision, my visitor would not find me perceptually unprepared. After all, he must appear in the doorway. If I am working in my office, I already know where the doorway is, and what lies beyond it, just as I know the location of other familiar objects. This means that I can anticipate the distances and possible motions of any arriving guest. Information about his location and movements fits into a preexisting spatial schema. A visitor who entered through

---

[10]Categories and relationships could be constructed, but the disposition, curiosity, and time to do this are not constantly present. Thus a tendency exists to ignore information that cannot be coded.

the wall, or materialized in the middle of the room, would be more like a ghost than a person. His ghostliness would be the first thing I noticed about him, and would color everything I saw afterward. (Neisser, 1978, p. 96)

Neisser (1978, pp. 92-94) suggests that perception, rather than being something discrete and within the mind, more likely involves the observer and the environment. Figure 4-1 depicts his assumptions. Guided by stored past experience, the observer explores the environment in order to sample available information. Neisser uses the term *schema* (plural, *schemata*), as seen in Figure 4-1, to refer to past experiences in memory that guide perception (1978, p. 97). A schema permits a person to anticipate (infer) what may be observed, even before observation occurs. Anticipations lead to actions; for example, the observer's glance was toward the door because past experience "says" a person will enter a room through a door.

As depicted in Figure 4-1, moment-to-moment exploration brings information back to the mental schema. This new information may modify the schema. A similar event occurs when an incorrect clinical observation is called to one's attention. In these ways perception is self-corrective in the long run; we learn from our mistakes.

In summary, cue perception (hearing, feeling, or seeing) depends on (1) schemata, or categories, constructed from past learning and experience; (2) perceptual exploration; and (3) information available in the environment. Cue perception is guided by what is already known, yet it influences knowing by providing new information to guide subsequent perceptual activity. The corrective effect of cumulative experience explains the generally accurate perception experienced by adults. This theory of perception suggests that information collection in clinical situations is facilitated by *knowledge of what to expect.*

Attention In addition to having categories for coding sensory inputs and knowing the likelihood of events, sensitive observers focus their attention. People have the capacity to direct their attention selectively to particular aspects of their environment. The functional advantage of focused attention is that one is more apt to "see" what is

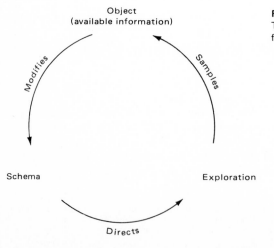

FIGURE 4-1
The perceptual cycle. (Adapted from Neisser, 1976, p. 21.)

important relative to the goal of the moment; distraction by extraneous stimuli is reduced. This selectivity can be lifesaving when one is crossing a busy street and advantageous when looking for a friend in a crowd.

During client health assessment, focusing of attention increases sensitivity to relevant information. For example, the functional health patterns previously discussed focus one's attention on 11 areas of health-related behavior relevant to nursing. This focus increases readiness to perceive cues to these patterns.

In summary, unless appropriate categories and category systems are available for coding sensory events, perception can be delayed or inaccurate. Inability to place sensory input into an appropriate category, when one is motivated to do so, results in a "long, close look." This prolonged observation is common in the child or adult who pauses to stare at something of interest that cannot be immediately categorized. Learning, asking questions, and curiosity increase availability of categories. In contrast, ignoring observations or events that one cannot classify or understand inhibits learning and may lead to diagnostic error.

If perception depends on stored representations of the world and retrieval from memory when sensory input occurs, a question arises: How does one store the clinical information required for thinking and perception?

Short-Term Storage and Retrieval

Humans retain information for long and short intervals. For example, nurses observe and retain information about a pulse rhythm for a minute (the usual observation period); they remember a telephone number until dialing is complete; and they recall the type of surgery a person had last year. The concepts of short- and long-term memory storage are used to explain remembering and forgetting. They are important ideas in assessment, because lost information can lead to error.

Images, thoughts, and information of which one is currently aware are the contents of *short-term memory stores*. Information can be held for seconds or a minute or more. According to a current theory of memory, a perceptual configuration of the environment (for example, the features of a blister) is held for scanning until *long-term memory store* (knowledge) can be retrieved, placed in the short-term store, and scanned (Atkinson and Shiffrin, 1971). This is the way identification occurs. The person finds the best fit and labels the perceived configuration. In this example, features of the lesion under observation would conform to *blister* features stored in memory, and the label stored in memory (*blister*) would be applied.

Atkinson and Shiffrin (1971, p. 83) refer to short-term storage as "working memory" and as consciousness. It is within this short-term memory that perceptual inference, conceptual thinking, problem solving, and decision making go on. Miller (1956, pp. 81–97) suggests that the human mind can hold only about five to nine separate pieces of information in the short-term store. To overcome this limited capacity, "chunking" is used. Pieces of information are put into broader categories, or "chunks," by abstraction. For example, in listening to a client relate a typical dietary pattern, one could use the four basic food groups to "hold" information as the person recites all the foods eaten in a typical day. Diagnostic concepts are also a form of chunking clusters of signs and symptoms into broad categories.

Chunking prevents overload. Without chunking, loss of pertinent pieces of information can occur. In clinical situations the nurse must hold information in short-term memory storage until it can be recorded, processed in decision making, or understood by retrieval of other past experiences from long-term memory.

If short-term memory images are lost within a number of seconds, how does a nurse remember a pulse rate or rhythm? Indeed, how does one remember the last numbers of a 7- to 10-digit telephone number after dialing the first few? *Rehearsal* of information, such as repetition of a telephone number, decreases the rate of loss of the digits and sequence. Yet if similar information, such as other numbers, enters the short-term store, forgetting occurs (Atkinson and Shiffrin, 1971, p. 88). This is a common event everyone has experienced.

Transfer of information to long-term memory storage explains humans' ability to remember after long time lapses. Long-term recall is partially dependent on intentional rehearsal of information to be remembered. (What is thought to occur in rehearsal is that neurons maintain reverberating circuits or undergo some type of structural or functional change.) In addition to intentional rehearsal, constant thinking or rumination about an event can firmly establish memory.

New information can cause loss of information if rehearsal is interrupted. It is well to remember this when collecting all the nursing history and examination data. Inventions to compensate for the limited human capacity to hold information in consciousness include the pencil and paper.

Some nurses do not take notes during a history and examination. This could give the client the impression that the information provided is not important enough to write down. In addition, research findings suggest that it is highly unlikely that continuous information over a period of even 20 minutes can be retained (Atkinson and Shiffrin, 1971). Five to ten minutes are necessary for minimal consolidation in long-term memory and an hour or more for maximum consolidation (Guyton, 1976, p. 752).

Another important point relevant to assessment is that remembering and forgetting seem to be influenced by information coding. Experiments have demonstrated that ability to remember (to recall memories from long-term storage) depends on (1) the way in which information was rehearsed and stored and (2) the retrieval probe that is used (Atkinson and Shiffrin, 1971, p. 89).

Have you noticed that some nurses have to retrieve nursing knowledge by using a disease category probe? This is because their clinical knowledge was originally learned and stored in this way. This cognitive organization around disease categories facilitates practice if nursing is only disease-related. Person-focused nursing requires that knowledge be organized within categories that describe any human being, with or without disease. The 11 functional pattern areas are an example. In long-term memory these areas are then "cross-referenced" with the likelihood of alterations in patterns associated with disease. This method of categorization enables the nurse to organize nursing knowledge *and* medical knowledge and to integrate the two classes of information. A retrieval probe can retrieve all three bodies of knowledge (nursing, medical, and integrated) if the situation warrants. If the client is seen only for health promotion, a disease-oriented probe is not necessary to retrieve clinical knowledge of functional patterns.

The idea of memory probes and long-term memory retrieval can also be applied to assessment. Suppose one wished to get rid of those pages and pages of an assessment tool that defy memorization. Assessment items could be coded in memory under the 11 functional pattern areas. For example, a nurse would learn, that is, place in long-term storage, the items to be assessed in the nutritional-metabolic area (Appendix C). The specific items of data in each area could be retrieved and used to guide questions and observations during history taking and examination. A small sheet with items listed could be devised until learning was complete.

Advanced Organizers   A set of categories, such as the functional health patterns, serve as advanced organizers for storing specifics. *Advanced organizers* are "ideational scaffolding" for the retention of details (Ausubel, 1968, pp. 148-152). The payoff in this type of cognitive organization lies in ease of retrieval; the succinct list of patterns can be used as quick probes for the data to be collected in each area. The key to any retrieval is an appropriate "search set." The key to learning is to organize and categorize details in meaningful ways—meaningful for clinical practice.

SUMMARY

In this chapter the most critical component of the diagnostic process has been explored, information collection. Unless valid and reliable information is used as a base, health problems may be ideas constructed by the diagnostician rather than descriptions of the client's real signs or symptoms. To avoid having imagination take over, diagnoses must be firmly based in clinical data.

In the first section of this chapter assessment was defined as collection of information (collection of data). It was emphasized that this component of the diagnostic process is continuous during all nurse-client interactions. Four types of assessment situations were identified. These included the *initial assessment* at admission, which includes both history and examination. The purpose of the initial assessment is to establish diagnoses (if health problems are present) that can direct care planning.

The *problem-focused assessment* has as its purpose the daily or periodic evaluation of the status of a diagnosis. In some situations, such as residential or long-term care, the time lapse between health status assessments (*time-lapse reassessment*) may be long. A complete history and examination are recommended; yet problem-focused assessment and time-lapse reassessment are designed as follow-ups to previous assessment data. An *emergency assessment* differs from the three other types of assessment in the level of problem formulation and the immediacy of intervention. The differences in scope of data, context, and purpose of these four types of assessment were discussed.

The admission assessment was examined rather closely. Both the client and the nurse have a psychological set toward the interaction; their sets are complementary in most instances. The client wishes to resolve ambiguities and seek help; the nurse has a descriptive-evaluative set and wishes to offer help. Ideas were explored in regard to beginning the assessment, assisting the client to describe his or her health patterns, and terminating the assessment. Assessment was considered in the context of establishing a therapeutic relationship.

After this overview of information collection, discussion turned to other factors that influence a nursing data base. The situational context that permits a client to share information was discussed.

Two other influential factors were examined. One factor is the *nature* of clinical information and its influence on data collection. The probabilistic, or uncertain, nature of clinical data influences subjective confidence in diagnoses. In an uncertain situation, collecting more and more data is not the answer; rather, the most valid and reliable predictors have to be sought. Important cues were described as those that contribute to evaluative judgments. These cues may be of various types: subjective, objective, historical, and current. Important cues are relevant to health status evaluation and permit reliable and valid judgments.

The last section of this chapter focused on the diagnostician's influence on what data are collected. The diagnostician was viewed as a sensitive measuring device. An examination of perceptual recognition and perceptual sensitivity to cues emphasized the importance of clinical knowledge. It is on the basis of knowing what to expect that sensory input is coded, cues are anticipated, and attention is directed. Examination of short- and long-term memory storage resulted in suggestions for collecting information and for organizing clinical knowledge necessary for assessment.

At this point the reader should have a beginning grasp of nursing diagnosis. The process of arriving at a diagnosis has been outlined in a broad sense. This chapter and the one preceeding it have emphasized one component of the process, information collection. Information is continually collected throughout all nurse-client interactions. At certain points, when the data indicate, diagnoses are formulated. One particular point is when health problems are evident following an admission assessment. If diagnoses are present they are used as a focus for the initial nursing care plan.

Information collection is not a random process. Professionals know why information is needed—the long-range goal for which it is collected. Stated differently, they have a conceptual framework from which they view the client, their goal, and the ways that may be used to reach the goal. A framework for professional practice focuses attention on *what* information is important.

It has been suggested that people of all ages, at all levels of health, and with any type of disease have certain functional patterns. Behavior within these pattern areas may be viewed as adaptations, as self-care, or from other perspectives. Irrespective of the conceptual framework applied, the behavior exists and constitutes the basic data of concern to nurses.

After preceding chapters established that a framework is necessary for determining *what* data to collect, the present chapter focused on factors influencing *how* data are collected. Yet nurses do not just collect data; they also make evaluative judgments. If health problems are present these judgments are referred to as diagnostic judgments, or nursing diagnoses.

The reader is being led through the diagnostic process. The question at this point is what to do when a cue or cluster of cues seems to indicate a dysfunctional health pattern. The answer is to generate the likely possibilities and collect data to test each one. The next chapter will expand on this answer by considering diagnostic strategies.

BIBLIOGRAPHY

Atkinson, R. C., & Schiffrin, R. M. The control of short-term memory. *Scientific American,* 1971, *225,* 82–90.

Ausubel, D. *Educational psychology: A cognitive view.* New York: Holt, Rinehart & Winston, 1968.

Bartlett, R. C. *Remembering.* Cambridge, Eng.: Cambridge University Press, 1932.

Bloch, D. Some crucial terms in nursing: What do they really mean? *Nursing Outlook,* November 1974, *22,* 689–694.

Bruner, J. S., Goodnow, J. J., & Austin, G. A. *A study of thinking.* New York: Wiley, 1956.

Cardwell, J. D. *Social psychology.* Philadelphia: Davis, 1971.

Cutler, P. *Problem solving in clinical medicine: From data to diagnosis.* Baltimore: Williams & Wilkins, 1979.

Engle, R. L., & Davis, B. J. Medical diagnosis: Present, past, and future. I. Present concepts of the meaning and limitations of medical diagnosis. *Archives of Internal Medicine,* October 1963, *112,* 512–517.

Froelich, R. E. & Bishop, V. M. *Clinical interviewing skills* (3d ed.). St. Louis: Mosby, 1977.

Gordon, M. Predictive strategies in diagnostic tasks. *Nursing Research,* January–February 1980, *29,* 39–45.

Gordon, M. *Probabilistic concept attainment: A study of nursing diagnosis.* Unpublished doctoral dissertation, Boston College, 1972.

Guyton, A. *Textbook of medical physiology* (5th ed.). Philadelphia: Saunders, 1976.

Hammond, K. Clinical inference in nursing: A psychologist's viewpoint. *Nursing Research,* 1966, *15,* 27–38.

Haynes, R. B., Taylor, D. W., & Sackett, D. L. *Compliance in health care.* Baltimore: Johns Hopkins University Press, 1979.

Herzlich, C., & Graham, D. *Health and illness: A social psychological analysis.* New York: Academic Press, 1973.

Holt, R. Clinical judgment as a disciplined inquiry. *Journal of Nervous and Mental Disease,* November 1961, *133,* 369–382.

Kim, M. J., & Moritz, D. A. *Classification of nursing diagnoses: Proceedings of the third and fourth national conferences.* New York: McGraw-Hill, 1981.

King, L. S. Signs and symptoms. *Journal of the American Medical Association,* October 28, 1968, *206,* 1063–1065.

Koos, E. L. Illness in regionville. In D. Apple (Ed.), *Sociological studies of health and sickness.* New York: McGraw-Hill, 1960.

Mechanic, D., & Volkart, E. H. Stress, illness behavior and the sick role. *American Sociological Review,* 1961, *26,* 51–58.

Miller, G. A. The magical number seven, plus or minus two: Some comments on our capacity for processing information. *Psychological Review,* 1956, *63,* 81–97.

Neisser, U. Cognition and reality. San Francisco: W. H. Freeman, 1976.

Neisser, U. Perceiving, anticipating, imagining. In C. W. Savage (Ed.), *Perception and cognition: Issues in the foundations of psychology, Minnesota studies in the philosophy of science* (Vol. 9). Minneapolis: University of Minnesota Press, 1978.

Norton, D., Exton-Smith, A. N., & McLaren, R. *An investigation of geriatric nursing problems in hospitals.* (Part 1, Section 9, Study of factors concerned in the production of pressure sores and their prevention.) London: National Corporation for the Care of Old People, May, 1962.

Piaget, J. *Play, dreams and imitations in children.* New York: Norton, 1951.

Rosch, E., & Lloyd, B. *Cognition and categorization.* Hillsdale, N.J.: Lawrence Erlbaum Associates, 1978. (Distributed by Halsted Press Division, New York: Wiley, 1978.

Sarbin, T. R., Taft, R., & Bailey, D. E. *Clinical inference and cognitive theory.* New York: Holt, Rinehart & Winston, 1960.

Zola, I. K. Culture and symptoms: An analysis of patients' presenting complaints. In R. E. Spector (Ed.), *Cultural diversity in health and illness.* New York: Appleton-Century-Crofts, 1979.

CHAPTER 5

DIAGNOSTIC STRATEGIES: NARROWING THE POSSIBILITIES

In previous discussions information collection has been treated independently of the overall diagnostic process. This separation permitted an emphasis on important topics but neglected the fact that information is interpreted and clustered while it is being collected. It may be recalled from Chapter 1 that the following four activities occur not as steps but as continuous actions during the diagnostic process:

1 Collecting information
2 Interpreting information
3 Clustering information
4 Naming the cluster

The focus of this chapter is on diagnostic strategies for interpreting information and for narrowing the universe of possible problems. This chapter will also deal with tentative diagnostic labels for cue clusters. *Naming* in the full sense of problem formulation, or diagnosing for purposes of treatment, is discussed in Chapter 6.

After a brief overview the reader will be led through various *levels* at which the diagnostic process can be understood. At the observable level nurses are seen to ask questions and examine a client. Then, after a period of time, they verbalize and record a diagnosis. How do we explain this behavior, especially when it seems their diagnoses are valid and reliable? The first level of explanation that will be discussed is that they have a strategy. The selection of information, the sequence of collection, and the way they use the information are a sequence of decisions, which by definition is a strategy.

Strategies permit attainment of objectives. Three interrelated objectives are important. One is accuracy in diagnosis. The second is efficiency. The third objective is to prevent overload of cognitive capacities; otherwise accuracy may be jeopardized.

Learning how to make a diagnosis requires probing more deeply. Exactly what is going on when a diagnostic strategy is employed? Rather, what do we think is going on? From studies of diagnosticians and others, it appears that decisions about information collection and utilization are based on diagnostic hypotheses generated from data obtained early in the assessment process. In fact, over and above the standard assessment questions and examination guidelines, data gathering is directed by hypotheses.

The richness of information gathered by a human being, as opposed to a questionnaire or computer, results from hypothesis generation. The diagnostician thinks of alternative diagnoses and proceeds to investigate these. Some may be discarded, some held, and others revised; also, new diagnostic hypotheses may be generated.[1]

How do nurses know what questions to ask and what to examine if these things are not specified by the predetermined assessment tool? Where do hypotheses come from? Answers to these questions are at a deeper level of explanation: clinical reasoning and inference.

The section of the chapter that is devoted to clinical reasoning will discuss how cues and clinical knowledge are combined to yield inferences. There the reader will find the basic explanation for the previously discussed hypothesis-directed cue search, hypothesis-testing strategies, and nurse behavior observed during history taking and examinations.

As will be seen, abilities underlying diagnostic strategies have been developing since childhood. To practice nursing, one must further refine these abilities, since judgments that result from information interpretation and clustering can have an impact on the client's comfort or life.

STRATEGIES, HYPOTHESES, AND DECISIONS

Actions are behaviors that can be observed. Strategies, hypotheses, and decisions are not observable. They are *theoretical constructs*, that is, they are ideas used to explain the behavior of people who are attempting to identify or categorize something from multiple cues. Let us see what goes on during assessment that is explained by these constructs.

Each client admitted to a nurse's caseload is assessed. Certain data *must* be collected to describe a client's functional health patterns, such as those identified in Appendix C. Nurses cannot rely solely on the items listed on an assessment tool or guideline. Just filling out a form usually results in insufficient and unreliable data.

Whether or not cues suggest that there is a health problem, clarification and verification of information are necessary. To clarify and verify data, one must go beyond the basic assessment guidelines. *Clarification* refers to clearer understanding. Whenever clients use abstract terms or global statements, data have to be clarified. For example, what are the feelings the client is classifying as "anxious"? What does "I eat a good diet" mean? Do specific fears underlie a statement such as "I'm afraid of dying"? What does "I feel weak" mean?

Verification of data means double checking. This is necessary when (1) there is

---

[1] The terms *hypothesis* and *hypothesis testing* are employed in order to be consistent with literature in cognitive psychology, which the reader may wish to pursue at some point. The terms are not used as they would be in a research context, but as a model for explaining information processing.

doubt about the client's or nurse's perception, (2) there is conflict among cues, or (3) the information has been created by inference.

Certain information *must* be obtained to describe functional health patterns; these requirements can be predetermined by a standardized assessment tool. Yet two factors must be recognized. One is the uncertain nature of the data. Further questions or observations to clarify or verify clients' reports are usually required. The second factor is the appearance of cues possibly signifying a health problem in a pattern area. Investigation of health problems requires a diagnostic strategy.

An assessment tool that provides for clarification, verification, and pursuit of all diagnostic cues would be too heavy to carry. That is why there is a need to learn strategies for collecting and processing information. Clinical knowledge plus diagnostic strategies permit a nurse to deal with the variety and complexity of client situations encountered in practice.

During the diagnostic process one must make a series of decisions about acquiring, retaining, and utilizing information. The sequential set of decisions is a *strategy*; decisions include what information to collect, in what sequence to collect it, and how to use the information (Bruner, Goodnow, and Austin, 1956, p. 51).

Consider an example. During information collection there is an interrelated sequence of questions and observations. This sequence reflects decisions about data collection and utilization. A client describes some behavior or event and a clinician asks a related question. Following the client's response another inquiry or observation is made. The information brings the clinician closer to an understanding and description of the client's functional health status.

Research indicates that decisions are directed by hypotheses generated from cues or clusters of cues. A *hypothesis* is an idea—a hunch—a person "formulates, remembers, tests, and revised in light of incoming information" (Bourne, Dominowski, and Loftus, 1979, p. 172). Diagnostic hypotheses are possible problems or possible etiologies that direct the search for cues to confirm, reject, or revise the hypotheses.

In past years, students were told not to consider possible problems until the entire assessment was completed. Recent studies have suggested that experienced as well as inexperienced diagnosticians generate hypotheses on the basis of early cues. In fact, instructions *not* to generate hypotheses early cannot prevent the behavior (Elstein, Schulman, and Sprafka, 1978).

Every clinician has a way of doing assessment and diagnosis; that is, each has a hypothesis-testing strategy. The strategy may or may not control memory and inferential strain. Additionally, it may or may not ensure that maximum information is obtained. In some instances the strategy employed may lead to a high risk of error.

Objectives of a Hypothesis-Testing Strategy

Objectives are predetermined outcomes to be reached, for example, to arrive safely in Milwaukee on Saturday. The broad objectives of an ideal diagnostic strategy are to attain a concept of the state of a client (1) efficiently and (2) accurately.

According to Bruner and his colleagues, a successful strategy has to balance information intake, cognitive strain, and risk of failure. Strategies can be evaluated according to their effectiveness in attaining the following objectives; the first two objectives are related to efficiency of a strategy and the third focuses on accuracy:

1 Ensures that maximum information is obtained from each observation and question

2 Keeps cognitive (inferential and memory) strain within manageable limits, especially within limits imposed by one's cognitive capacity

3 Regulates the risk of failing to attain a concept of the state of a client within limits imposed by the situation. (Bruner et al., 1956, p. 234)

The reader already may have made the inferential leap that these objectives are important if one is to avoid certain pitfalls. Briefly, they are: insufficient or irrelevant information for a health assessment, forgetting, incorrect inferences, omissions, and incorrect diagnoses.

Bruner and his coauthors comment, "What is most creative about concept attainment behavior is that the patterning of decisions does indeed reflect the demands of the situation in which the person finds himself" (1956, p. 55). A diagnostic strategy changes in response to situational demands and cognitive capabilities. People gamble when things are going well. They become conservative risk takers when the going gets rough.

A recipe for use in all situations by all clinicians would be useless. What can be offered are objectives and a description of different hypothesis-testing procedures from which a strategy can be constructed. Being aware of the costs and benefits of various procedures prevents one from becoming locked into one strategy when the situation dictates flexibility.

HYPOTHESIS-TESTING DIAGNOSTIC STRATEGIES

In discussing diagnostic strategies we shall consider the diagnostic situation that begins with no information. Any health problem within the universe of all nursing diagnoses is possible. In fact, the hypothesis or possibility that no health problem is present (the client is in optimal health) is as likely as the hypothesis that one or more problems are present. This is the situation at the start of an admission assessment, from a cognitive perspective potentially the most complex diagnostic task.

In addition to meeting the objectives of a general strategy outlined in the previous section, a diagnostic strategy should:

1 Narrow the universe of possible health problems quickly
2 Focus on high-probability diagnostic hypotheses
3 Ensure that the most valid and reliable data are collected
4 Ensure accuracy and confidence in judgment within the limits of certainty that can be obtained

Knowing how to *narrow the universe of possibilities* makes the diagnostic process manageable. It is unlikely that a client would have all known health problems or even all the currently identified nursing diagnoses. The focus should be on those with the highest predicted likelihood for a particular client-situation. Predicting likely possibilities involves clinical reasoning. Accordingly, we will need to consider this level in order to explain how nurses know what data will lead to likely hypotheses.

Diagnostic hypotheses have to be tested. To investigate a possible diagnosis, information is needed. Decisions about what information to collect will also require consideration of the basic level, that of clinical reasoning. How can a sequence of questions and observations (1) be used to test hypotheses, (2) ensure valid and reliable data, and (3) ensure accuracy and confidence in judgments about holding, discarding, or revising diagnostic hypotheses? This question will focus the discussion of the remaining three objectives of a diagnostic strategy in the next chapter.

Narrowing the Universe of Possibilities

Experienced clinicians say certain cues are "automatically" associated with certain diagnostic hypotheses. This "explanation" does not help the beginner. When just starting to acquire clinical knowledge or just beginning to focus consciously on identifying dysfunctional patterns, the nurse needs specific guidelines for narrowing the universe of possibilities.

The universe of possible states of the client can be divided into two sets (subparts). One is optimal functional patterns and the other is actually and potentially dysfunctional patterns. The subset of dysfunctional patterns contains many possibilities. First let us consider the client who has optimal health patterns. Then we will deal with how the subset of health problems can be narrowed.

It is certainly possible that the admission assessment will show that no dysfunctional pattern is present. Functional patterns may be judged to be optimal. In this case ask yourself, What is the cause? If a functional pattern is *optimal*, there may be two reasons. One, the client may have health-related knowledge and apply it in everyday living. Point this out to the client after you complete your data analysis. Feedback is important.

A second reason for an optimal pattern is *chance*. This is why the diagnostician is encouraged to pursue reasons for behavior. Clients may not realize the positive health action they take, its importance to their living, and why habit patterns should be maintained. A chancy situation exists if there is no firm foundation for the client's healthful practices. Nursing interventions directed toward consciousness raising and health education would be indicated.

Assessment can be approached as a process of ruling out health problems. The approach would be: Assume dysfunctional patterns unless the data support optimal patterns. Advocates of this position would take a diagnostic approach to all assessment. They may be biased toward *overdiagnosis* but usually are *not* biased toward errors of omission.

A second approach in assessment is: Assume optimal health unless the data indicate a dysfunctional pattern. Advocates of this approach would reject ruling out problems and a diagnostic approach to assessment. A bias may exist toward *underdiagnosis* and *errors of omission* with this assumption.

Neither of these alternatives, the diagnostic approach nor the health-focused approach, has been studied relative to diagnostic errors. This author favors the diagnostic approach with built-in safeguards against a bias toward overdiagnosing. This preference will be evident in suggestions to use situational information and pattern areas to increase sensitivity to cues and to generate likely diagnostic hypotheses.

Use of Preencounter Information   The diagnostic process begins with the first information obtained. In fact, with *no* information about a client, general expectations about possible nursing diagnoses can arise from the setting in which the nurse practices. For example, it is reasonable to assume that a client admitted to a hospital, long-term care facility, or rehabilitation center has problems that require nursing care. Otherwise the person could receive health care in the community. It is equally true that a client who comes to a clinic or private practitioner's office, or a family that requests a home visit, probably perceives some health problem.

The clinician's expectations about a client's probable diagnoses can be still more specific in specialty practice, such as a cardiac surgical unit. Before seeing a new client, the nurse in such a setting can predict a cardiac problem and surgery. This ability to predict in advance leads to sensitivity to cues. For example, is there a problem coping with fear or anxiety about surgery? Is there a knowledge deficit regarding what will happen or how to do breathing exercises postoperatively? Is the family coping effectively? These are the kinds of hypotheses cardiac surgical nurses generate from knowledge and past experience even before seeing a client.

In addition to the practice setting, the nurse may draw upon information from other sources to generate hypotheses before seeing the client. A medical diagnosis of the present illness, a previous record of hospitalizations, or records of clinic visits may create expectations because nurses have learned that particular pathologies are associated with changes in functional health patterns.

Also, comments by medical or nursing colleagues may generate diagnostic hypotheses. A physician calls and says: "I'm sending in a patient, she's been having a hard time with her husband over the surgery." Or another nurse may say: "I just saw him come in on the stretcher, he doesn't look good." Expectancies start to form.

An initial impression begins with the first piece of information and can be formed before any interaction with the client. Impressions or predictions may prove true or may be totally inaccurate. Hold them, but not firmly. Wait for the assessment data and make sure hypotheses are rejected if not supported by those data.

These few words are designed to dispel the notion that before interaction with a client there is no information. Expectancies arise because of the setting, medical diagnoses on the admitting sheet, previously recorded history, or colleagues' comments. They are used to generate tentative diagnostic hypotheses and to guide the search for cues. Beware; they can also bias toward a particular diagnosis. This danger can be avoided if diagnoses are based on actual clinical data, not the nurse's inferences or beliefs.

Use of Pattern Assessment Sequence   Beginning the history taking with the client's health-perception–health-management pattern appears to facilitate hypothesis generation and to increase sensitivity to cues. This pattern provides a context: clients' perceptions of their overall health pattern, and their health management practices, may suggest hypotheses to be investigated. Review of this pattern area may also elicit health management (or disease management) practices that relate to other pattern areas.

Logically, of all the pattern areas, health-perception–health-management provides the broadest information related to health. It gives an overview; thus it can be used to predict where problems may exist in other patterns and which other patterns require in-depth assessment. This predictive feature of health-perception–health-management data was not recognized immediately. The logic of the sequence became apparent as a result of the attempt to understand why many graduate students placed this pattern area first in their client histories and examinations.

In addition to suggesting possible diagnostic hypotheses, assessing the health-perception–health-management pattern is a good starting point from the client's perspective. It is relevant, irrespective of the level of care or setting. As the reader may recall, defining the situation and learning how to manage are uppermost in the client's mind when seeking health care.

There has been no research about the relationship between the sequence in which patterns are assessed in the nursing history and the nurse's cognitive processing of the information obtained. Therefore it is not known whether or not nurses' utilization of information is facilitated by any certain sequence. As the pattern areas are used in the nursing specialties, a useful sequence may evolve.

There are a few ways of deciding what assessment sequence to use after the health-perception–health-management pattern has been assessed.[2] For one thing, there should be a logical sequence from one content area to the next. For example, it seems logical to assess self-perception-self-concept, then role-relationships, and then the sexuality-reproductive pattern. One flows from the other. Similarly, the nutritional-metabolic and elimination patterns seem logically related.

From a psychological perspective, the value-belief pattern (including spirituality) and the sexuality-reproductive pattern may be considered highly personal areas. Most nurses would not assess these areas until rapport had been established and the client was at ease. Hence these patterns would be placed later in the sequence.

The sequence of pattern assessment can be related to individual situations. In a psychiatric setting, perhaps self-perception–self-concept or role-relationship patterns would be assessed early. In a medical or surgical setting, the nutritional-metabolic pattern might be the second area assessed, followed by the elimination pattern. With experience the clinician can develop an order that considers the client and situation and facilitates information processing in the history. For the first few nursing histories, try this sequence:

1 Health-perception–health-management pattern
2 Nutritional-metabolic pattern
3 Elimination pattern
4 Activity-exercise pattern
5 Sleep-rest pattern
6 Cognitive-perceptual pattern
7 Self-perception–self-concept pattern

[2] It may be useful to scan the definitions of the pattern areas on page 81.

8 Role-relationship pattern
9 Sexuality-reproductive pattern
10 Coping–stress-tolerance pattern
11 Value-belief pattern

Defining and Using a Problem Space Concepts for identifying and describing the world of experience are stored in long-term memory. Among these are diagnostic concepts, or nursing diagnoses. Embedded in a network of nursing knowledge, these previously learned health problems, possible causes, and defining signs and symptoms are the source of diagnostic hypotheses. For example, a clinician may have learned diagnostic concepts for describing various nutritional problems. By a process of inference, present cues are seen as equivalent to previously learned cues *and* the health problem categories they define. Additionally, stored knowledge may include information about the frequency of occurrence of these problems in various age groups or particular situations. Recall of this stored knowledge is used to generate hypotheses during assessment.

Recall must be selective. The universe of nursing diagnoses is large and it would be impractical to think that every diagnosis would be relevant to every client-situation. Thus the domain of possibilities has to be narrowed.

Newell and Simon (1972), cognitive theorists, propose that the universe of possibilities is narrowed to a limited *problem space* by early information. A problem space can be thought of as an area of clinical knowledge, such as nutritional problems. Hypotheses about the particular client and situation can be formulated by retrieving diagnostic concepts from this defined problem space.

Restle (1962) provides a similar but more colorful notion. His conception also supports the idea of a universe of available diagnostic concepts. Initial cues give rise to a *specific pool of hypotheses*. Within this pool, some hypotheses are relevant to the client and situation; others are not. During information collection the pool is gradually decreased by a process of elimination. The result is that the diagnostician begins to close in on the most reasonable diagnostic hypotheses.

Differences can be expected between novice and expert diagnosticians. Two observable differences are the speed with which the correct problem space is defined and the speed with which a relevant pool of diagnostic hypotheses is retrieved from memory. Selecting the right problem space and retrieving probable hypotheses depends on past learning and experience.

The novice may not have learned sufficient concepts for describing the range of problems encountered in practice. Or a network of relationships between predictive cues and likely possibilities may not have been established. The ability to anticipate or predict, as was discussed in Chapter 4, depends on having diagnostic concepts accessible for retrieval.

Pattern Areas as a Problem Space Initial hypotheses are usually formulations of *broad* problems. These first hypotheses would be inadequate for planning treatment. Their advantage is that they enable the nurse to focus in on a problem space so that retrieval from a pool of more specific hypotheses is facilitated.

Each pattern area describes a domain of functional and dysfunctional patterns. The pattern area can be used as a broad diagnostic hypothesis to direct the search for cues. Thus the 11 pattern areas narrow the universe to 11 *tentative hypotheses* at the start. As a way of testing these 11 hypotheses, the nurse tacitly poses 11 questions, as follows:

1 Does this client have a health-perception–health-management problem?
2 A nutritional-metabolic problem?
3 An elimination problem?
4 An activity-exercise problem?
5 A sleep-rest problem?
6 A cognitive-perceptual problem?
7 A self-perception–self-concept problem?
8 A role-relationship problem?
9 A sexuality-reproductive problem?
10 A coping–stress-tolerance problem?
11 A value-belief problem?

Use of Diagnostic Concepts as Specific Hypotheses   As assessment in each pattern area proceeds, information accumulates. Specific nursing diagnoses, currently available in memory, are used to cluster cues indicating a dysfunctional pattern.[3]

As an example, at the beginning of the assessment of the nutritional pattern of a child, adult, or family, initial cues may indicate an actually or potentially dysfunctional pattern. One or more specific hypotheses may be generated from the following diagnostic categories:

1 Total nutritional deficit
2 Potential nutritional deficit
3 Protein deficit
4 Vitamin or mineral deficit (specify)
5 Exogenous obesity
6 Potential nutritional excess
7 Fluid volume deficit (level I)
8 Potential fluid volume deficit

These diagnostic possibilities (hypotheses suggested by the early assessment data) guide further cue search. Lists could be made for each pattern area similar to those in the index of a diagnostic manual or in Appendix B.

The nurse will at times encounter data that *cannot* be organized and clustered under any currently identified nursing diagnosis. This fact is a good working assumption. It prevents forcing data into categories. One word of caution: Before generating new categories, one must be sure about having adequate knowledge of those currently identified and their defining signs and symptoms.

Having discussed ways hypotheses can be retrieved, let us examine some data. The

---

[3] If you are in the process of learning specific nursing diagnoses, during assessment use the concepts *you have available* in memory as hypotheses. Later, consult a diagnostic manual (Gordon, 1982) or book (Kim and Moritz, 1981) for currently identified terminology.

following small collection of clinical data provides an example of hypothesis generation and sequential decisions about information collection. Try to determine the hypotheses that arose and how these may have controlled the cue search. Breaks in the nurse's recordings will be made for comments.

Mr. D is a healthy-appearing, single, 60-year-old salesman with well-controlled high blood pressure.

Health-perception–health-management pattern. Views self as healthy and enjoying life. Takes medications as prescribed.

Nutritional-metabolic pattern. In reviewing dietary pattern he states that he avoids meats except hamburger, doesn't like eggs or fish, and rarely eats raw vegetables or fruits. He comments that everything has to be cooked well.

The initial impression, "healthy appearing," indicates that body weight, facial expression, speech, skin, and mobility do not *globally* appear problematic. This tentative impression provides a background for the rest of the assessment.

When the nutritional-metabolic pattern was assessed, the nurse began by raising the question (broad hypothesis), Does this client have a nutritional problem? The first component reviewed (consistent with the broad hypothesis) was dietary intake pattern. Note the client's response. It supports the broad hypothesis and indicates the possibility of problems. He is eating only soft foods. This kind of diet can be associated with an inadequate nutritional pattern. The report of a soft diet initiated a search for cues guided by less broad hypotheses: Does the client have a nutrient, caloric, fluid, vitamin, or mineral deficit? Inferences from the medical diagnosis, essential hypertension, and initial impression suggested a 50:50 chance that any dysfunctional pattern existed. This is typical in the admission assessment, in which there is an equal probability that a problem does or does not exist. Now data are collected to test the hypotheses generated.

Detailed review of typical daily intake reveals less than minimum requirements for protein and vitamin intake. Other nutrient intake is sufficient. When asked if this dietary pattern represents a change, Mr. D replied, "Well . . . yes, I guess in the last year or so."

The nurse's hypothesis, nutritional problem, led to a search for details of the daily intake, comparison to standard requirements, and an evaluative judgment of the data. Note how some of the original hypotheses are discarded and the problem narrows to protein and vitamin deficit. The next question to the client established that there has been a pattern change that evidently occurred over a year. At this point the decision should be to raise the question of *why change occurred* and pursue some causal hypotheses. A broad question about the reason for change did not elicit useful information; questions became more specific.

No indigestion or "stomach trouble" was reported. A question in regard to chewing difficulty produced the report that Mr. D had had a lot of back teeth pulled as a teenager. Examination revealed many missing back teeth, multiple dental caries, and broken teeth.

Three cue-search decisions are evident. One was to elicit cues in the area of gastrointestinal tolerance for food. The second decision was to seek cues to chewing difficulties. This cue-search led to a third decision, to examine the client's teeth as a possible reason for the soft diet. Two questions were asked, one in the area of gastrointestinal tolerance for food and the other in regard to chewing. The hypothesis of chewing difficulty directed the search for cues by examination.

The nurse's inquiry about indigestion was probably based on the proposition that *if* symptoms or concerns exist about a gastrointestinal problem, *then* soft foods are eaten. Based on this proposition, the hypothesis that the problem was *gastrointestinal* was tested. The client reported no indigestion or "stomach trouble." This, plus the absence of any pathology noted on medical examination, was sufficient information for discarding this causal hypothesis.

A second causal hypothesis, chewing difficulty and dental problems, was raised. It probably rested on the proposition that discomfort in chewing could produce a change to soft foods. The age of the client and his verbal report were supporting data. A decision was made to examine the client's teeth, and the data provided support for the hypothesis of dental problems.

The example illustrates hypothesis generation and hypothesis-directed decisions. More information is needed before stating a diagnosis. This would include the client's perception of the dental problem, actions he has taken to deal with the problem, and factors in other pattern areas that may be interacting to produce this problem. The possibility that Mr. D. has a knowledge deficit about minimum daily dietary requirements would also need to be investigated.

In this example multiple hypotheses were tested simultaneously by asking about dietary pattern. Notice how this narrowed the possibilities quickly. Causal hypotheses about digestive disturbances and dental problems were pursued later, one by one. Different hypothesis-testing procedures yield different costs and benefits. For example, one procedure may ensure maximum information but strain memory capabilities. Another procedure may control memory strain but may be too time-consuming.

It may be useful to summarize at this point. When no information is available at the beginning of an assessment, the first thing one's strategy should do is narrow down the possibilities. Having a list of 11 pattern areas to be assessed is one aspect of a diagnostic strategy that does this. If these patterns are the focus of concern in nursing, then they circumscribe the important areas of assessment. Already, the universe is narrowed. Problem spaces are defined for retrieving clinical knowledge from memory.

The pattern areas can be used as broad hypotheses or questions to guide assessment. For example, when a client's role-relationship pattern is assessed, the question is: Does the client have any problems in the area of role-relationships? This question focuses assessment and increases sensitivity to cues.

Data collected before assessment of a pattern may suggest some diagnoses to investigate. Thus the use of preencounter information and a predetermined sequence of assessment can influence sensitivity to cues and suggest hypotheses.

Lastly, as data are collected broad questions and hypotheses give way to more specific diagnostic hypotheses. These are retrieved from memory stores. As the currently identified nursing diagnoses are learned they can be used during assessment as hypotheses about dysfunctional patterns.

The preceding aspects of a strategy are designed to increase sensitivity to cues. The easier the search and retrieval of previously learned possibilities, the less cognitive strain the diagnostician experiences. On the basis of expectations about which problems amenable to nursing intervention are likely to occur, one can make predictions. The next step is to test hypotheses in the "real world" of clinical data.

Perhaps strategies, hypotheses, and decisions about data collection and utilization seem to be foreign concepts. They are important to learn. Diagnosis is something used continuously in a nursing practice career. The introduction to the next section on hypothesis testing, or hypothesis investigation, should dispel any ideas that hypothesis generation and testing is an unfamiliar process.

Retrieval of Diagnostic Hypotheses When immediate identification of some phenomenon is not possible, people construct hypotheses about what the phenomenon could be. These hypotheses direct a search for cues to identification. As previously stated, research has demonstrated that hypothesis generation and testing is a good model for explaining even children's behavior in concept attainment or identification tasks (Levine, 1975).

Consider an example. It will demonstrate hypothesis retrieval and prediction on the basis of past knowledge. The child in play shouts: "It's a bird; it's a plane; it's Superman!" This provides a commonplace example of hypothesis retrieval. Interesting to note, this children's expression is consistent with *likelihood estimates*. In real-life experience a bird is the most frequently seen thing in the sky. Thus *bird* is a good tentative hypothesis to raise first. Planes are the second most frequent possibility to explain the distant speck in the sky. Estimates of the likelihood of events suggest that the least likely hypothesis (outside the world of fantasy) is Superman.

Predictive Hypothesis Testing Questions can be asked to elicit information that can be used to narrow the possibilities. When combined with clinical knowledge, the information elicited permits prediction. For example, what hypotheses should be investigated when an elderly client says her appetite is poor (disease has been ruled out)? These cues, *elderly* and *poor appetite*, suggest hypotheses related to role-relationships, self-perception, nutrition, elimination, and other patterns. Cues that generate multiple hypotheses are predictive cues. Other cues may be so specific, that is, so diagnostic, that they suggest only one possible diagnosis.

When starting assessment of a pattern area, the nurse should collect predictive cues first. They indicate what hypotheses should be investigated. Collecting predictive cues to test several diagnostic hypotheses at once is called *predictive hypothesis testing* (Gordon, 1980).

This procedure utilizes clinical knowledge of the *incidence* of dysfunctional patterns, or nursing diagnoses. It has the tremendous advantage of conserving time. Yet as we shall see this advantage is countered by a higher cognitive strain and risk of error.

In predictive hypothesis testing, contextual information is useful. Recall that this information describes situational characteristics. The *historical context* of a hospitalized client's situation would include such things as diagnosis at admission, type of surgery performed, or medication history. *Current contextual* information includes age, sex, and the presence of therapeutic procedures such as intravenous infusion or oxygen administration.

Contextual information is particularly useful in predicting possible diagnoses. Expectancies about the probability, or likelihood, of events can be retrieved and utilized. All that is needed is a few contextual cues.

Although *not* involving nursing diagnoses directly, an example drawn from research findings should further clarify predictive hypothesis testing (Gordon, 1980). Nurses were given a task of determining whether or not a client was developing any post operative complications (assessment task). All they were told was (1) that they could have any information they wanted and (2) that the patient had had general surgery. The list of things to be assessed (hypotheses) included: thrombophlebitis, wound infection, atelectasis, urinary retention, and hemorrhagic shock. They were also told that it is possible that the client does not have any complication. Obviously, if one knows only that the client has had general surgery, one hypothesis is as likely as the other, and it is equally likely that the patient has no complications. This is an anticipatory assessment task with a pool of pregenerated hypotheses in its pure form.

The nurses had to ask for each piece of information about the patient. Before getting any information, they had to state how it would help them identify the presence or absence of the complications. This requirement permitted the researcher to observe how information was used to test hypotheses about surgical complications. In two simulated cases their strategies were essentially the same. What they did first is of interest in this discussion.

The information they collected in their first two questions was either *time lapse since surgery, type of surgery performed*, or both of these cues. These are situational cues about the *historical context*. They have nothing to do with the current state of the patient, such as blood pressure or urine output. Even when limited to only 12 pieces of information in one task, they asked these same two questions first.

To know whether any surgical complication is present *now*, shouldn't one collect information on the *current* state of the client? Maybe so, but other information may be important first.

How shall we understand the efficiency of these nurses' approach?[4] In their first two questions they found that the patient had had gallbladder surgery and that it was done at "12 noon today" (in the second task, "11 a.m. yesterday").[5] For the experienced clinician this is meaningful information. Using a network of interrelationships stored in memory permits various problem-identification activities. One can restructure past events or predict future events. For example, *if* the cues *short time lapse since surgery* and *gallbladder surgery* are present, *then* hemorrhagic shock is probable. Or, in the second case, *if* the cues are *15 to 18 hours postsurgery* and *gallbladder surgery*, *then* atelectasis is highly probable.

---

[4] Accuracy was very high when the information was limited and the correct judgment was hemorrhagic shock. When information was unlimited and the correct judgment was atelectasis, 52 percent were inaccurate; errors were attributed to information overload and other aspects of their strategy (Gordon, 1980).

[5] The current time when they "did the assessment" was known to be between 2 and 5 p.m. Subtraction could be done to find how many hours had elapsed since surgery.

The nurses' behavior indicated that they used contextual information to test several hypotheses simultaneously. That is, they used a predictive hypothesis-testing procedure. Contextual information about the client's situation made it possible to set the probabilities of the surgical complications. By inferring the probability of each complication from the cues, the nurses were able to focus on the most likely ones and still have sufficient questions left to assess the *actual* presence of the complications.

Predictive hypothesis testing may also increase confidence in the final diagnostic judgment. It is important to remember that clinical information usually has an element of uncertainty. In this type of situation confidence in reliability of data and validity of reasoning and judgment may be increased if things "fit the picture." That is, if things turn out as experience or knowledge indicates they should, confidence increases.

Is this procedure useful only in the area of inferring surgical complications? Probably not. Logically it seems useful in all anticipatory diagnostic situations. The universe of possibilities cannot be tested, so events have to be forecast on the basis of likelihood estimates. Elstein and his colleagues (1978) have found that physicians dealing with uncertainty-based medical diagnoses also begin their task with predictive hypothesis testing.

Let us consider how information, cognitive strain, and risk of error are influenced by this procedure. Predictive hypothesis testing is used to zero in quickly on the most likely hypotheses among those generated. Using contextual cues to investigate several hypotheses at once permits a large amount of information to be extracted from the assessment of one client characteristic. For example, in the surgical complications study, five bits of information could be derived from assessment of one characteristic. That is, the cues *time lapse since surgery* or *type of surgery performed* provided information about the likelihood of the five possible complications. A current state cue, such as blood pressure, provides only one bit of information on a single hypothesis, hemorrhagic shock. Obviously, the benefit of predictive hypothesis testing is that maximum information is derived from each piece of data collected.

One drawback is the high inferential and memory strain. Consider the inferential requirements in the previous example. Information was obtained that surgery occurred at 12 noon today; it is now 3 in the afternoon. Through subtraction it is learned that the client had surgery 3 hours ago. By inductive inference, this is the early postoperative period.

Knowledge from memory suggests that thrombophlebitis, urinary retention, and wound infection are unlikely; they would not be clinically manifested at three hours. Atelectasis also is relatively unlikely. Hemorrhage (or, alternatively, no complications) is the most likely hypothesis during the early postoperative period. In the *second* task the time lapse was 30 hours after surgery; more of the hypotheses were probable.

When nurses learned what type of surgery the client in the research study had had, the same inferential processes were required to relate the cue to each hypothesis. Certainly the inferential strain far exceeds that of testing each possibility one by one. Memory strain is also high. The hypotheses that have been tested and retained or discarded, and the probabilities of each, have to be remembered. The payoff is that the universe of possibilities is narrowed quickly. *Type of surgery* and *hours postoperative* reduced the set from four possibilities to one for some of the nurses. It is often possible to eliminate several hypotheses at once with a few pertinent questions or observations. Then only a few likely hypotheses remain, so that memory strain is reduced.

If hypotheses are eliminated on the basis of a few historical cues that do not represent the critical, defining characteristics of the condition, what risk of error is present? Clearly there is some, unless likelihood estimates perfectly match the real incidence of occurrences. This kind of predictive knowledge is not available in the uncertainty-based world of health care. Thus, predicting that a diagnosis has *no* probability of being present (and hence doing no tests for its actual presence) involves a risk. Alternatively, if the risk is not taken, the universe of problems and all defining characteristics have to be assessed. The risk in this alternative is that time will run out before the diagnosis is made. How often do nurses predict the absence of a nursing diagnosis with only contextual information? This question would make an interesting study that would provide an indication of the extent of risk taking in clinical judgments.

To summarize, the data indicated that the assessment of surgical complications was approached in this way:

1 The client has had general surgery. This information was used to infer that the client was subject to postoperative complications. Five complications were used as the first universe of physiological hypotheses (atelectasis, thrombophlebitis, wound infection, urinary retention, and hemorrhagic shock).

2 What information would narrow the universe? The *type of surgery* and the *time lapse since surgery was performed* were useful in determining probable complications. This information was collected.

3 Data and inferences were combined. What complications are most likely at this point? (Inferential reasoning and holding five hypotheses simultaneously increase cognitive strain, but it is transitory. The number of possibilities will be decreased quickly.)

4 Data were collected about each of the possible complications likely to occur in the designated postoperative period after gallbladder surgery.

This study was done in a structured situation in which hypotheses were given to the nurses. In the next section a more realistic example will demonstrate that if contextual, or predictive, cues are used early, the universe can be narrowed and the probabilities of various diagnoses can be set.

Predicting Probabilities The previous section introduced the idea of generating multiple hypotheses early in assessment of each pattern area. Background data can be used to do this. Hypotheses can be investigated simultaneously by obtaining a cue or cues that contain information relevant to each hypothesis in the set. Contextual information is usually useful.

The procedure was called *predictive hypothesis testing*, that is, multiple hypothesis testing using contextual cues. Information obtained is used to set probabilities of the possible diagnoses (which in the previous example were far fewer than in an admission assessment). The objective of predictive hypothesis testing is to obtain a lot of information quickly to reduce the number of hypotheses; this objective can usually be accomplished with one or two questions. The inferential and memory strain will be transitory.

The name of each pattern area can define the "problem space" and possible diagnoses. Let us consider an example of setting probabilities early in the assessment of a pattern area. The client is a 40-year-old, single, female executive who is being admitted with a medical diagnosis of gastric ulcer.

Assessment can begin with the health-perception–health-management pattern. The first question posed could be "How has your *general* health been in the last few years?" Or the nurse might say, "I noticed from the doctor's note that you've been having problems with . . . " (insert client's report); "How has your *general* health been in the last few years?" This is a lead-in to discussion of health perception by posing a broad question. What has been communicated is (1) the nurse knew something about the problem that initiated the client's contact with health services, and (2) the focus of discussion at the moment was general health in the last few years. The purpose was to communicate interest in *more than* current symptoms.

The client's current pattern of health perception evolved from a previous pattern in which she perceived herself as "healthy." For the last 5 months she has gained weight and says she looks "terrible." Severe abdominal pain unrelieved by milk, cream, or antacids caused her to visit a physician on the same day she was admitted. She delayed seeking treatment because of her busy work schedule. "I guess women have to work twice as hard to succeed," she added.

The tentative hypotheses that could be generated from the one question are many. There are indications of a *health management deficit* and some probable causes. Delay in seeking health consultation and self-medication for 5 months are supporting cues. Furthermore the client's beliefs about "work" and "schedule" may predispose to *noncompliance* if a therapeutic regimen for the ulcer is indicated. Cues to *altered body image* and perhaps to some conflict regarding work were present. Further data are needed.

The previous example illustrates a decision that often must be made. Should the client's verbal reports or the nurse control the sequence of history taking? Some conflict can be generated by this situation. Does the client desire to talk about looking "terrible" or about women in executive positions, or were these just explanations that can be pursued in the relevant pattern area later? What happens if the nurse refocuses on health managment in the example above?

One reason for refocusing on health management, or the area under discussion, is to keep the cognitive strain of information processing under control. Jumping back and forth among pattern areas produces strain, especially for the novice. It also can produce cognitive disorganization leading to diagnostic errors. When information relevant to other pattern areas is mentioned "in passing," the nurse may acknowledge the communication but not shift focus from the area. This decision is made by evaluating whether or not the client has a strong desire to relate further information immediately. The emotional tone of the communication should be considered. A client's repeated refocusing on a subject is a cue to a problematic area.

In the example above the following could have been said: "It's difficult to have these symptoms when your work keeps you so busy. Have you been able to have time for regular checkups?" This acknowledges the point the client has communicated but immediately refocuses specifically on the hypotheses related to delay in seeking care. It is, in a sense, not really a direct question, because the purpose is to return smoothly to discussion of health management. Note the nurse's *recognition* of the client's work situation and the *transition* back to health management.

The cues and hypotheses that arise from these peripheral comments should be followed up later. They provide initial, introductory questions for discussion in other areas. When the role-relationship pattern is discussed, the nurse might say in an inquiring way: "Earlier you mentioned that women have to work twice as hard to succeed. What is it like to work in your company—the people and . . . " (pause).

While proceeding through the health pattern areas, make sure "abnormal" or "unexpected" findings are explained. It may be necessary to retrieve low-probability hypotheses that were initially discarded. If a cluster of cues signifying a problem is not explained by any diagnostic hypothesis, ask for consultation. Consultation sets up a reciprocal relationship. When a colleague (nurse, physician, or other) has difficulty, she or he may consult with you.

To summarize, early cues may suggest a possible dysfunctional pattern and, thus, diagnostic hypotheses. Several hypotheses can be tested simultaneously by collecting contextual cues. Contextual information is the background in which functional health patterns exist. Like *time lapse since surgery*, contextual information is applicable to a large number of hypotheses. This procedure of testing more than one hypothesis at a time, predictive hypothesis testing, involves predicting the probabilities of each hypothesis in order to narrow down the pool. The specific diagnostic hypotheses that are highly probable for the particular client and situation then become the focus for cue search.

The specific steps of predictive hypothesis testing are: (1) begin assessment of a pattern area with a broad hypothesis such as, Does this client have a health-perception-health-management problem? and any background data that are available to direct the initial cue search; (2) ask a question that will elicit cues that permit focusing on a set of hypotheses; (3) use the data to generate specific diagnostic hypotheses if initial cues seem to indicate dysfunction; (4) use predictive, multiple-hypothesis–testing procedure and contextual cues to obtain information about the set of diagnostic hypotheses; and (5) use the information obtained to estimate probabilities of each of the hypotheses, thus (6) eliminating highly unlikely diagnoses early in the process. With one or two diagnostic hypotheses remaining, the cue search can be focused. The few high probability diagnostic hypotheses are then tested and information integrated. Generating and testing hypotheses and integrating the information collected continues throughout assessment of the pattern areas.

Let us explore a more basic level of information processing that seems to explain what is occurring during the diagnostic process. This basic level is clinical reasoning.

CLINICAL REASONING

Underlying diagnostic strategies, hypotheses, and actions made during assessment is clinical reasoning. "Good" clinical reasoning is critical thinking, as described in Chapter 1. In this section the discussion will focus on how clinical, or inferential, reasoning is done and how it is used in hypothesis generation, hypothesis testing, and (subsequently) nursing diagnosis.

Clinical reasoning results in an inference about an identity (inference as category) or a relationship (inference as proposition, or proposed relationship). These are important cognitive processes used in practice. They can be a source of truth or a source of error.

Inferential error may enter any phase of the diagnostic process and influence all further reasoning, including the eventual diagnoses. Two inferential errors rather commonly occur: (1) errors in cue recognition (perceptual categorization), and (2) errors in reasoning from cues to inferences about the meaning and the clustering of cues.

Accuracy is jeopardized when inferences are substituted for data collection, when they outweigh observations, and when they are not validated or examined for logical error. On the other hand, it is virtually impossible to refrain from using inferences when information is incomplete, unavailable, unreliable, and less than totally valid. The situation is quite familiar in everyday life. Is that person friendly? Is it a bird, a plane, or Superman (differential categorization)? Is it going to snow (prediction)?

Inferential reasoning is the process by which the unknown is tentatively inferred or predicted from the known. Where perception is involved the inference is usually immediate. For example, having seen many syringes, the nurse can glance at another one and immediately infer that it is a syringe. (When the same nurse was a freshman nursing student the inference might not have been so immediate and a "long, close look" might have been required.) More complex inferences involved in diagnosis require chains of reasoning. They are usually deliberate, that is, within awareness.

Bruner et al. (1956) suggest a useful way to grasp the meaning of inference: Inference is going beyond the information given, that is, information given in a sensory stimulus. How far beyond the information given should a diagnostician go? Essentially, the question is: To what degree should a nursing diagnosis represent perceived facts about reality as opposed to the nurse's own interpretation and "creation of reality" through inference?

During the diagnostic process the nurse goes beyond the given information in: (1) cue recognition; (2) interpretation of the meaning òf cues; (3) prediction, or hypothesis generation; (4) evaluation of cues as supporting or rejecting a hypothesis; and (5) making diagnostic judgments. It is important to appreciate that inference is involved in each of these five cognitive activities. Even a decision to undertake a nursing intervention or to project an outcome is based on an inference about the effect of nursing action.

The simplest inference used in the diagnostic process is *perceptual* inference, or immediate cue recognition and naming. This type will be discussed first. Then the more complex inferences, which are built on perceptual inference and require reasoning, will be considered.

Perceptual Inference

As discussed in Chapter 4, cue recognition involves coding a sensory stimulus into an appropriate category. One makes the inference that (1) the features of the stimulus and (2) the defining features of a category are sufficiently similar. As an example, look at the visual stimulus in Figure 5-1 and name it (identify it).

You have just made a perceptual inference. The visual stimulus was probably inferred to be equivalent to a certain memory image, and so you applied your category name for that image. Did you call it (1) lines on a graph; (2) a rhythm strip; (3) a heart beat tracing; (4) atrial fibrillation; or (5) an irregular ventricular rhythm strip with absent P waves, small and irregular fibrillation waves, and an irregular QRS complex? Only number 1 is actually correct. All the other responses require the addition of information, not just identification and naming. Figure 5-1 is a line graph. It could represent many things, such as consumer buying trends with peaks at holidays each year. There were no cues to indicate specifically what the graph represented; or were there?

The example, if you were led astray, demonstrates two things. One, you added information on the likelihood of occurrence of a cardiac rhythm strip in a nursing book. Similarly, you inferred identity from your own perspective. Consider these two explanations and see whether you agree.

Likelihood Estimates The context in which a stimulus occurs can have a pronounced effect on categorization. Having learned that certain things are likely to occur at certain times and in particular places, people use this knowledge to anticipate.

Anticipation, or expectancy, activates a set of appropriate categories so that sensory stimuli can be quickly identified. Estimates about the likelihood, or probability, of events have to approximate the actual occurrence of events in the world. Otherwise, perceptual inferences can be inaccurate. With the line graph in Figure 5-1, using expectations paid off. Your estimate that what you saw was most likely an electrocardiogram was correct. It was more likely than not that this kind of graph would appear in a nursing book.

Learning when certain cues are to be expected is important in diagnosis. Yet one must realize that expectations are estimates. Pay attention to the situational context that permits anticipation, but also pay attention to the cues.

Redundant Properties Once categorization has occurred, further inferences can be made about unobserved properties of the stimulus. With a correct categorization it may be inferred that the phenomenon observed shares all, or most, of the properties of the category into which it has been placed. This includes the word-label, or name. For example, it is common to infer that *if* this object is an orange *then* it will, by definition, have juice. The psychological expectation is evident in a surprised reaction if the so-called orange is juiceless when cut. Similar inferences are used clinically. Inferring unobserved properties can be risky, for example, inferring that the quiet, cooperative client is also calm and coping effectively.

On the other hand, many properties are *redundant*. This means that there is a very high possibility that if one or two features are present the others will also be present. As Bruner and his colleagues remark, if a thing has feathers and wings you can *infer* that it also has a beak and legs (1956, p. 47). In other words, one goes beyond the information given when it is safe to do so—when features are *known* to be redundant.

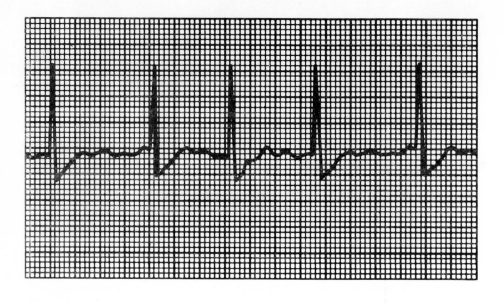

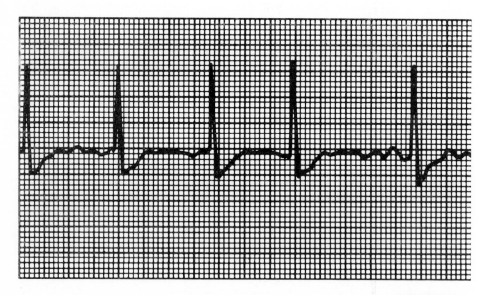

FIGURE 5-1
Visual stimulus.

Fine Discrimination The reader whose identification of Figure 5-1 resembled options 4 and 5 is capable of fine discriminations. No doubt this reader has multiple memory categories for arrhythmias. This accumulation of memory categories is what occurs in specialized learning. The world is coded very specifically. A nurse experienced in the care of acutely ill clients subject to arrhythmias would recognize many stimulus features in the tracing. Others may not pay attention to these features because they do not have categories for coding them. Additionally, they may not have learned the different nursing responses to each arrhythmia category. Their category systems are less complex and their recognition less accurate.

Fine discriminations are learned when they are important for actions. The Eskimo have many words for snow; we have one. Arabic has more names for camels than English, and the Hanunoo people of the Philippines have 92 descriptions for rice but only 1 for automobiles (Bourne et al., 1979, p. 125). Similarly, the cardiac nursing specialist uses more terms to describe arrhythmias than the specialist who does not need to discriminate among heart rhythms.

Categorizing may lead immediately to an interpretation of the stimulus. Interpretation is the activation, in some way, of a category network that produces meaning. For example, from a nursing perspective what does it mean for a client to have atrial fibrillation? How meaning is derived and how it is used in prediction is the subject of the next section.

Humans are amazingly accurate in perception, provided that their system of expectations is congruent with the actual probability of events. In perception the use of clinical inference may be summarized as (1) sensing stimulus features, (2) making an inference regarding identity, and (3) making an inference about properties not observed which, if it is congruent with reality, involves low risk of perceptual error. In regard to risk, the *consequences* of error in perceptual inference enter into the decision between taking a "glance" and a "long, close look."

Propositional Inference

A more complex form of inference than observation and perceptual categorization is demonstrated in the human capacity to derive meaning from cues. The derivation of meaning employs a network of categories and propositions as a basis for inference.

Interpreting the meaning of cues is a critical part of nursing practice. It involves linking one idea to another by a propositional inference. The ideas related can be abstract, such as a proposition about values, or concrete, such as the link between skin color and oxygen levels.

Propositions are learned or personally constructed relationships that join one concept to another. They usually take the form of statements or conclusions. Propositions are constructed from personal experience, research findings, or reasoning.

Propositional knowledge is a network of relationships joining what is isolated by perception and is categorized. It is the basis from which meaning of cues is derived and, in turn, from which expectations and predictions are formed.

Consider as an example a proposition that is used in practice: *Psychological disturbance in one family member will disturb the psychological equilibrium of other members.* Two broad concepts are being related, psychological disturbance and psychological equilibrium; the context is the family. Suppose cues to psychological disturbance were noted in a child admitted for surgery. What diagnostic hypothesis would be generated about the parents? When talking with the parents it would be important to assess for the presence of anticipatory anxiety or a more general ineffective coping pattern. The structure of the reasoning that led to this decision about assessment will take the entire next section to discuss, although the mind performs the reasoning process in less than a second.

Inductive and Deductive Inference   Going beyond identification to derive meaning or to predict events requires inferential reasoning. A person is usually conscious of reasoning processes in a situation that is either new, ambiguous, or complex. In such a situation it takes time to reason, and thought processes are deliberate.

In contrast, when a situation is familiar, inferences or conclusions are drawn quickly and "automatically." The "thinking through" was done at a previous time and conclusions stored in memory. In a situation judged to be equivalent, all that is required is retrieving from memory the meaning of the present cues. Previously learned meanings are then used in interpretation and prediction.

The problem that can arise with "jumping to conclusions" or the "inferential leap" is that (1) previous reasoning was not accurate, (2) the client and situation are not equivalent, or (3) repeated use of routine responses to situations negates new learning, stifles creativity, and is basically boring. For these reasons it is valuable to learn how logical conclusions about the meaning of cues are made. Take a "long, close look" at the familiar and examine those inferential leaps that tend to become so automatic in practice. Going beyond the information in cues is necessary, but it is also necessary to ascertain that the pathway is fairly logical.

The previous example of the child and parents will illustrate how cues and propositional knowledge stored in memory are combined. To analyze the thought process that would cause the nurse to infer that anticipatory anxiety and ineffective family coping are possible, it is necessary to discuss inductive and deductive reasoning.

Inductive reasoning results in categorization or classification of cues. Past learning says that if it has a beak, body, feathers, and wings, it is a bird. This categorization is concept attainment. Reasoning is from the particular case to the general class, bird. Nursing diagnosis, or problem identification, requires an inductive inference but is more complex; cues are ambiguous and contain an element of uncertainty. Multiple inductions and deductions are usually required before a diagnosis can be stated.

Deductive reasoning proceeds from propositional knowledge to an inference about a particular circumstance. Deduction creates information by reasoning from the known to the unknown. If it has a beak, small body, feathers, and wings (known), then it's probably soft to touch (unknown). Predictions about behavior, future events, and things not yet observed are based on deductive inferences.

With this overview let us return to the example about the effects of psychological disturbance on a family. If the situation was unfamiliar, here is the structure of reasoning:

1   This child belongs to the class *family member* (inductive inference)

2 This child belongs to the class *psychological disturbance* (inductive inference)

3 If the child has a family (assume parents or siblings), then (maybe) their psychological equilibrium is disturbed

4 *Anticipatory anxiety* and *ineffective coping* are two categories within the general class *disturbed psychological equilibrium*

The first two operations above are necessary. If the child does not have the characteristics of family member and psychological disturbance, the wrong proposition has been retrieved from memory. The general proposition from which a deductive inference is made has to be applicable to the situation.

Note that in number 3 the word *maybe* is inserted. Inferences are constructed to go beyond the information given in cues. They lead to predictions or hypotheses, *not facts*. Predictions and hypotheses that are derived from them must be tested. This testing is how fact is separated from fantasy about a client.

Inductive inference, or identification, is commonly used in combination with deductive inferences that generate predictions. Consider an example. A nurse, having experienced *multiple* instances, drew this general conclusion by inductive inference: Elderly clients in the hospital get confused at night. Generalizations are useful, as long as the sample of patients is sufficiently representative and negative instances are considered. Sometimes conclusions are drawn on the basis of too small a sample; or elderly patients who are *not confused* at night are ignored. People tend to pay more attention to confirming evidence than to evidence that challenges their beliefs. Can you predict what this nurse did the next time an elderly client was admitted?

First, if observations of a new client were similar to the defining characteristics of "elderly client," he or she would be placed in this category. This is classification, or inductive inference, and generates meaning from cues. It can be useful if good, sound clinical knowledge (not negative stereotypes) is retrieved by using the memory probe, elderly clients. Deductive reasoning proceeds from this categorization if the nurse thinks about what can be predicted about elderly clients. If the previous proposition is employed, then:

Elderly clients in the hospital become confused at night (previous generalization from experience);

This client is elderly;

Therefore, this client will (may) become confused at night (deductive inference).

Obviously, this deduction *cannot* be treated as truth because being elderly is by no means always accompanied by being confused. If the deduction is acted upon as a "fairly good" assumption, all clients categorized as elderly will probably have side rails on their beds at night because:

Nocturnal confusion increases the potential for injury;

This client has (may have) nocturnal confusion;

Therefore, this client has a potential for injury.

Decision: Put on side rails.

On the other hand, if a deductive inference is treated as a hypothesis, *as it should be*, (1) elderly clients will be assessed for nocturnal confusion and (2) the question of why confusion occurs will be raised. Age is insufficient information for diagnosing a potential for injury and putting on side rails. Further cues are needed to determine whether a potential problem exists. More important, not all elderly clients will have to be enclosed by side rails on their beds if care is based on well-formulated nursing diagnoses.

Clinical inferences are so common in the diagnostic process that it is important to grasp differences between inductive and deductive inference. Consider another example. Does this approximate deductive or inductive inference, or both?

1 Early mother-infant separation may predispose to decreased bonding
2 Ms. A's new baby has had to remain in the hospital after her discharge
3 Therefore, Ms. A and her baby are (may be) predisposed to decreased bonding

Statement number 2 is considered equivalent to the category *early mother-infant separation*. This presumed equivalence represents a classification of cues, therefore an inductive inference. The general proposition in number one applies to this clinical situation, and it may be inferred that Ms. A and her baby are possibly predisposed. This possibility is a deductive inference. It sensitizes the nurse to raise a hypothesis or question, "Are Ms. A and her baby showing bonding?"

Another example will demonstrate the uncertain nature of predictions based on inference. It will illustrate also that judgments have to be made under probabilistic conditions. A client was observed to have a bluish cast to his skin, and this sign was categorized as cyanosis.[6] This cue may indicate an emergency or it may not. Cells cannot tolerate acute oxygen deprivation for very long. What inference would you make if you knew nothing else about the client? Is the blood oxygen low? Should oxygen be given?

Other information is being withheld to demonstrate a point: Cyanosis and low blood oxygen saturation are related in a probabilistic manner. Thus you are being asked to make a judgment with no contextual cues to why the client is cyanotic. You should feel uncertain about administering oxygen—at least a little uncertain.

Cyanosis can occur with (1) actual low blood oxygen saturation, (2) certain drugs, or (3) an abnormally high hemoglobin level (false cyanosis). Let us say that the respective probabilities of these occurrences in a population of cyanotic clients are (1) 88 percent, (2) 5 percent, and (3) 7 percent. With these probabilities an inferential error would result in 12 (5 plus 7) of 100 cases if the proposition and reasoning were: Cyanosis is a sign of low blood oxygen saturation; this patient is cyanotic; therefore, this patient has low blood oxygen saturation.

This example demonstrates the risk entailed in inferring unobserved properties. If oxygen therapy was started every time cyanosis was observed, 12 percent of the recipients would not need it. One group within the remaining 88 percent, who had *chronic* low oxygen saturation, might be harmed by the usual dose. The remaining clients might develop brain damage without it. The example illustrates a situation

---

[6]Cyanosis is defined as slightly bluish, grayish, slate-like, or dark-purple discoloration of the skin (Taber, 1980).

where the *risk of inferential error* has to be *weighed*. The consequences of not acting until a blood test is done are weighed against the consequences of administering oxygen.

In the above example *if* the bluish cast to the skin is correctly categorized as cyanosis, *then* blood oxygen saturation should be low most of the time and most clients with cyanosis would get oxygen. This example was chosen to demonstrate the uncertainty that underlies many clinical judgments. Nurses compensate for uncertain data by knowing their clients, learning the probabilities of events, and using this knowledge to interpret the meaning of cues.

The context in which an observation or verbal report occurs influences its interpretation. Attention to the situational context increases the probability that appropriate meaning will be derived from cues and appropriate hypotheses generated. These can then be tested by collecting information.

At this point in the discussion the reader will be sensitive to inductive and deductive reasoning and to prediction on the basis of likelihood estimates, or probability. Now consider an example of information interpretation and hypothesis generation:

A home visit was made to a family in which the 11-year-old child and mother are being seen regarding (1) the child's diagnosis of nutritional deficit related to family meal planning and (2) the mother's dysfunctional dependence related to perceived lack of competency. On return to the community agency office, the visiting nurse charted, among other things, that the mother is going for gallbladder surgery. It was noted that the mother "exercised responsibility for getting a reliable person (her own mother) to provide child care." One of the care objectives had been to increase the mother's independence and sense of responsibility.

In conversation with the clinical specialist, the nurse mentioned that the mother said, "You know it's been hard for me since my husband died. You know he died having surgery, an appendectomy; well, at least he wasn't sick long. I've got my mother to take care of Annie; she's so good with her."

The clinical specialist asked the nurse whether she had any further thoughts (inferences) about the meaning of the communication. The nurse replied that she already knew the client's husband was dead. She also knew assuming responsibilities was hard for the client, but she "was coming along" and demonstrated responsibility lately.

The nurse had a set of observations, derived from the client's verbalizations, which are summarized in Table 5-1. These were shared with the clinical specialist. Each sought to derive meaning as a basis for interpreting the cues. As may be seen in Table 5-2, their inferences differed. Why did one use an explanation involving the client's personal sense of responsibility and the other an explanation that was based on the client's identification with significant others? While examining the contrasts in Table 5-2, try to identify what specific data carried most weight and what data seemed to "slide into oblivion" while being processed. Note also the differences in the two ways the information was put together in cue clusters. Discrepancies between the specialist's and nurse's clustering of cues, reasoning, inferences, and cue search depicted in Table 5-2 can be explained by using the notion of sensitivity to cues and readiness to infer.

Categories and propositions (category relationships) become accessible in a situation because of an expectancy (anticipation, or disposition). Was the nurse "set" to

TABLE 5-1

CUES THE NURSE SHARED WITH THE CLINICAL SPECIALIST

Mother of 11-year-old is going for gallbladder surgery

States husband died having surgery

States husband wasn't sick long

States mother (client's) is to take care of the child

TABLE 5-2

INFERENCES MADE BY THE NURSE AND THE CLINICAL SPECIALIST
ON THE BASIS OF THE CUES THEY SHARED

Visiting nurse's reasoning		

Cue cluster 1
    States husband died having
        surgery
    States husband wasn't
        sick long
	Reasoning
	    None
		Inference
		    None (client is telling me
		        something I already
		        know)

Cue cluster 2
    Mother of 11-year-old is
        going for gallbladder
        surgery
    Client's mother to take
        care of 11-year-old child
	Reasoning
	    Responsible people take
	        action to solve problems
		Inference
		    Client has exercised responsi-
		        bility: reliable person to
		        care for child (my inter-
		        ventions are working)

Clinical specialist's reasoning		

Cue cluster 1
    Mother of 11-year-old is
        going for gallbladder
        surgery
    States husband died having
        surgery
    States husband wasn't
        sick long
    Client's mother to take care
        of 11-year-old-child
	Reasoning
	    Lacking personal experi-
	        ences, people may iden-
	        tify vicariously with the
	        experiences of others
	    Things mentioned together
	        may be related in the
	        speaker's mind
	    Impending surgery can be per-
	        ceived as a threat to the
	        self
		Inference
		    Client thinks she could die
		        during surgery as hus-
		        band did
		    Client has mother to take
		        care of child (1) during
		        her surgery and (2) if she
		        should die

		Hypothesis
		    Fear of dying—impending
		        surgery

		Cue search
		    Ask client how she thinks
		        "the surgery will go"

interpret cues as *responsibility/irresponsibility* only? Had the nurse previously inferred that the nutritional deficit of the child was due to an irresponsibility of the mother in child care? If so, this could explain a sensitivity to this type of cue interpretation. Suppose that she had been working long and hard to help the mother deal with problems, and here was a cue that pointed to increased sense of responsibility and self-confidence, therefore, nursing care success!

It may have been noted that the cues *died having surgery* and *care of 11-year-old child* seem to be clustered and weighted differently by the nurse and the clinical specialist. *Cue-weighting*, as will be seen in subsequent discussion, refers to the emphasis the diagnostician places on any particular cue, or the power of a cue to influence the observer. The differential weighting in the example was probably related to the nurse's psychological set to reason in a particular way.

It may also be possible that the nurse had not learned the propositions the specialist used in reasoning. If they were not stored in memory, then these propositions would not be available for data interpretation. Or both may have had the propositions available for inferring meaning, but differences existed in the accessibility of propositions in memory. The nurse had one explanation "come to mind" and the specialist another.

When the attempt was made to explain the data using the *personal responsibility* idea, the cue *died having surgery* could not be encompassed. It was irrelevant. The nurse's attention was on child care responsibility. The specialist's reasoning accommodated the cue about child care but offered a different explanation because this cue was combined with *husband died during surgery*. Note that the specialist inferred on the basis of a cue cluster; the information was put together. The nurse isolated and then interpreted the child care cue out of the context of the possible meaning of the whole.

Who was right? That is not the most important question; insufficient information is given to make a judgment about accuracy. The question is Which person took account of all the possibilities? Neither did. If the nurse's inferences and the specialist's were combined, the two hypotheses could be tested. We shall give the specialist a plus; she was going to collect more data.

When information is ambiguous and not clear-cut, hypotheses are generated that provide alternative possible interpretations of the data. These alternatives direct the search for further cues to support or negate the several diagnoses being considered. One key to effective clinical reasoning is the generation of alternative explanations. A second is clinical knowledge, a prerequisite for generating explanations.

In analyzing cues, one must learn to guard against permitting highly accessible "sets" of inferences to take over. Although not evident in the above example, it is also essential to avoid making illogical conclusions. Last—and more will be said about errors of this type—the diagnostician must avoid bias and personal prejudices; they lead to the acceptance of invalid conclusions.

Considering Alternatives Explanations that immediately come to mind are useful. Yet it is wise always to search memory stores for alternative explanations, even when everything appears "obvious." One way to get into this habit is to take a behavioral or environmental cue or set of cues and explain their meaning in three totally different ways, that is, from three different frameworks or perspectives. Try a physiological explanation of a cluster of cues, a psychological explanation, and then a sociological explanation. This exercise should provide alternatives, especially for those who have classified their knowledge in memory along these three lines.

Consider an example of using multiple frameworks for interpreting cues that were observed following visiting hours: A cardiac patient had an increase in heart rate of 20 beats per minute, moved about frequently in bed, and had a furrowed brow. How shall the cues be interpreted? What line of questions or further observations should be pursued, and on what hypotheses (inferences) should they be based?

A physiological framework would generate hypotheses regarding cardiovascular function, such as chest pain. A psychological framework might take into account the possibility of a subjective feeling regarding self-perception related to emotional discomfort. A sociological framework might suggest that something could have occurred during interactions with a visitor. Within each area of propositional knowledge stored in memory, deduction using available cues can lead to an inference; this is converted to a hypothesis to guide the search for further cues.

These three areas—physiology, psychology, and sociology—are familiar. Many nurses' memory stores of basic knowledge are organized around the three. Thus the three frameworks make a usable approach to analysis of information. The names of the 11 pattern areas could also be used as a source for generating alternative hypotheses. The cardiac patient's cues may signify a problem in the area of self-perception or role-relationships. The pattern areas provide another type of framework, one that integrates biopsychosocial knowledge.

Applying different explanatory frameworks to clinical data overcomes a psychological set to categorize the data prematurely. Taking alternative viewpoints prevents distortion of data by highly accessible ideas. Readiness to interpret information in habitual ways may yield (1) very accurate predictions and interpretations because one has learned the *real* probability of events in practice, or (2) errors because one has forgotten that wherever people are involved cues are ambiguous and there is always an exception to the general rule. To reduce risk of error, one should always consider alternative explanations and search for a few cues. These cues will indicate which diagnostic hypotheses are worthy of attention.

Now that examples of different frameworks for interpreting data have been considered, a descriptive, easily remembered term can now be introduced. The term makes the processes just learned more concrete.

Branching Discussion of things that cannot be seen, heard, or touched is sometimes hard to understand. This is the case with the processes involved in human thought. Branching is a concept that may help the reader to *imagine* the processes of inductive and deductive reasoning, hypothesis generation, and even strategies. Aspinall's (1979) study suggested that performance in the diagnostic process may improve with consciousness of the idea of branching. Little and Carnevali (1976) have also discussed the concept in regard to cue interpretation.

Branching means the generation of multiple hypotheses that direct the search for cues. It involves use of propositional knowledge, deductive inference, and hypothesis generation. The hypothesis is turned into a question to direct the cue search. When multiple, alternative hypotheses arise, the process can be visualized as branches of a tree—in fact, branches of a decision tree. Consider the following data:

> Ms. J is a 45-year-old, white, married woman with cancer of the liver and jaundice.[7] She is going home in 2 days and is physically able to resume all activities. She states she doesn't know how friends will react to her color.

[7] *Jaundice* is a yellow coloring of the skin and whites of the eyes associated with a high level of bile pigment in the blood, in this case due to changes in liver cells or obstruction.

Figure 5–2 depicts three hypotheses, or branches, generated from considering the cues and pattern areas (role-relationships, self-perception–self-concept, and health-perception–health-management). All three branches represent viable hypotheses, given the clinical data available. Underlying the branching are propositions, deductions, and inferences, all of which are probabilistic statements. The reasoning in two of the areas of branching is as follows:

If jaundice, then abnormality in skin color;

If abnormality in skin color, then change in outward appearance;

If change in outward appearance, then feelings of being different;

If feelings of being different, then negative perception of body or self, and

If feelings of being different, then decreased family and social contacts.

Check client's perception of self.

Check for social isolation.

The experienced clinician rarely needs to go through this reasoning process. Having cared for many patients with jaundice, he or she probably thinks:

Jaundice → altered body image perception

Jaundice → social isolation

Information is then collected to support or reject the hypotheses. If one were pressed to explain the above reasoning, Goffman's (1965) conceptual model of stigma and social identity could be cited.

Consider another example of branching. In an emergency room a nurse has done a screening for problems in the 11 pattern areas of human function. When the role-relationship pattern (work role and relationships) was being assessed, the client said he

FIGURE 5–2
Branching hypotheses that guide cue search.

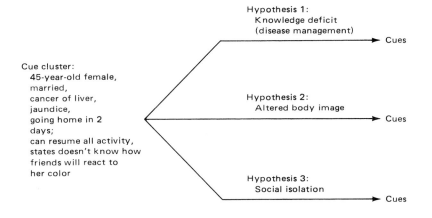

was a plumber. While dressing the severe laceration of his right hand, the nurse asked him how he will manage at work. This branching question was based on a reasonable inference that the laceration would interfere with use of the right hand. The inference was being checked in a nondirective manner to elicit the client's ideas or plans. The basis for the question was the proposition that plumbers work with their hands, lifting and twisting things. The nurse could also question whether or not this man lives alone. How is he going to manage self-care, such as dressing, bathing, and cooking? These questions represent branching from a set of cues, background knowledge, and a sensitivity to human needs for self-care.

Imagine the branching that would direct the search for cues if a plumber's work activities became impossible or contraindicated because of neuromuscular, cardiac, respiratory, or psychiatric problems. To anticipate or predict functional problems from a set of situational or contextual cues is an ability that in many instances makes care effective or ineffective. The ability to branch from a set of cues requires cognitive sensitivity to the likelihood of events. Clinical knowledge and logical deduction are employed in branching. Conclusions are inferences, or hypotheses; when turned into questions, they direct further cue search.

Words sometimes unify several ideas into one neat conceptual package. This is the case with the word *branching*. Learning the term as it has been used here is worthwhile; the process should be used with every cluster of cues. The words *branching from cues to hypotheses* are similar to the previously described "chunk." The idea can be stored and used to retrieve what has been learned about generating hypotheses during data interpretation, prediction, and estimating the likelihood of possible diagnosis.

Points of Reference

The interpretation (analysis) of information has been described as a fairly logical process of reasoning from knowledge (references) stored in memory. Branching from cues using deductive reasoning was compared to the branches of a tree. At times the roots of propositional knowledge are underground.

The preceding analogy is partly correct; propositions used in clinical inference may be silent assumptions as well as fully conscious ideas (Sarbin, Taft, and Bailey, 1960, pp. 48–49). Needless to say, with silent, unconscious propositions or inferences, reasoning cannot be examined for sources of logical error. Although inferences should be validated, at times they slip into data or are used because data cannot be obtained. For these reasons a close look at *points of reference* used for cue interpretation is in order. There are four basic sources for generating inferences: experience, construction, authority, and initial impressions (Sarbin et al., 1960).

Generalizing from Experience Propositions derived from experience are based on the *recognition of similarities* in repeated events. When considered to be similar, repeated events are combined by induction to yield a generalization. Various characteristics of clients and situational events are used as a basis for induction. For example, a nurse makes an observation: When one client in a unit gets very ill or dies (manifested to other clients as a lot of doctors and nurses around the bed), other clients are anxious and upset. Repeated observations of this phenomenon are generalized to the proposition: Critical illness or death on a unit produces anxiety in other clients on the unit. Having created this knowledge from practice, the nurse uses it in the next similar situation encountered. (Notice that no data are used to indicate whether the clients are anxious when the situation is absent!).

When the preceding generalization is used in deduction to explain behavior of the next client encountered, the conclusion is: Mr. J is anxious because of Mr. B's cardiac arrest. If this deduction is treated as a hypothesis to direct cue search instead of an assumption about the *cause* of anxiety, the questions will be: Is Mr. J anxious? If so, is this because of Mr. B's arrest? What did that mean to him? Mr. J is viewed as an example of "other clients"; placing him in this category makes applicable the general proposition about anxiety in the unit following critical illness or death. The proposition then can be used in deduction and hypothesis generation.

The key to accuracy when generalizing from experience is not to rush into action before testing the hypothesis. Collecting information will determine the "truth" of the deduction. Unvalidated assumptions are risky; in this example, anxiety regarding Mr. B's arrest may not be the correct, nor the only, hypothesis to explain Mr. J's behavior. What explanations would have been proposed if Mr. J was anxious and no cardiac arrest had occurred? Other hypotheses would have to be generated.

One can generalize not only from repeated experiences with a particular *situational context*, such as the cardiac arrest situation just discussed, but also from repeated similar experiences with the *same person or persons*. For example, the people in a community may be repeatedly resistant or hostile to developing needed health care services. The nurse *infers* that today the same reaction will occur (and perhaps responds to them as if it is occurring). Generalizations from past behavior to expectations of present or future behavior can be risky. When used as rigid assumptions, inferences may close out cues signalling change. Yet generalizations about a person's behavior can sensitize the nurse to important changes from base line. The key is to be open to cues and remember that most cues have an element of uncertainty.

Consider another example. A clinician, having cared for a number of families in a particular community health nursing district, noticed similarities in their knowledge of preventive health measures. He generalized about the neighborhood: Families in neighborhood A know of the need for immunizations for children. A young family that has lived in this small neighborhood for 10 years encounters some very complex health problems and is added to this nurse's caseload. He is very busy; what is his risk in inferring, versus assessing, their knowledge and practices regarding their small children's immunizations?

Generalizing from experience is useful if the relevant factors producing the similar events are identified. A risk is taken if (1) the new family does not have the same characteristics as the families on which the general proposition was built, (2) important factors producing the relationship are not identified, or (3) overgeneralization occurred initially. Living in the same neighborhood may be totally irrelevant to preventive health measures. On the other hand, it may be relevant because social interactions permit sharing of information about immunizations.

The use of induction from experience, as described above, requires that one have a grasp of the likelihood of events. Repeated experiences can suggest to the person making the inference (1) that things are about to change (the gambler's fallacy) or (2) that a "run" is occurring, that is, when a relationship between certain events has been observed 10 times it is safe to infer that the same relationship will exist the eleventh time. Both rules can lead to error unless one is sensitive to the risks they entail.

People tend to *overestimate* the probability of *impressive events*, thinking more have occurred than was actually the case. For example, cardiac arrests produce an impression emotionally and cognitively. As a second example, when students begin the study of pathology they become impressed by the seriousness of some illnesses and begin to think they and their classmates have the symptoms. These examples describe *salient* (highly striking) experiences. The nurse in the first example may be more sensitive to cues because of the cardiac arrest experience. The students are sensitive to interpret symptoms using the new, impressive, readily accessible categories. In both cases there is increased readiness to infer because of experience.

Recall that anticipation facilitated sensitivity to cues and inferences. It can also lead to "systematic and predictable errors" (Tversky and Kahneman, 1974, p. 1131). Past impressive, salient events may be highly accessible in memory and because of this may appear to be more likely to recur than they actually are.

Generalizing from experience (inductive reasoning) is one reference point for deriving inferences. Sweeping generalities from one emotionally charged situation may be made, or sensitive reflections on multiple experiences and many years of practice may be the source of propositional knowledge. Generalizations may represent great clinical wisdom or totally fallacious statements.

Generalizing from Personal Theories In addition to single propositions, complex systems of propositions are sometimes constructed to interpret cues. Health care providers may have their own personal theories of health and disease and even an implicit theory of personality. This is particularly true in areas where science is "fuzzy." These personal theories can reflect reality or contain many illusions. Most have at least a portion of truth (Jones, 1977).

These so-called theories are constructed during social learning. They are based on experiences in living with other people. Generalizations can be made about human traits, dispositions, and actions. Jones states:

> One way to sensitize people to the existence of such beliefs is to pose a question such as "What do you think of a wise, cruel man?"—a jarring inconsistency for most people. For most people, wise men are generally kind, old, and perhaps jaded, but never cruel. (Jones, 1977, p. 3)

Implicit theories about what people are like, what personality characteristics go together, and what causes behavior can be firmly entrenched. In a study of nurses' inferences of suffering, Davitz and Davitz (1980) found differences between the inferences of Puerto Rican and American (white or black) nurses. The Americans inferred less suffering. In general the disease, age, and socioeconomic class of the portrayed patients influenced inferences of all the groups of nurses studied. Sociocultural learning was probably influential.

In brief encounters, a person's physical characteristics, a situation, or a patient's disease may be sufficient basis upon which to infer traits, dispositions, or secondary health problems. For example, "a high forehead goes with intelligence," "self-confidence predicts a successful and happy person," or "psychiatric patients will be violent" (Dion, Berscheid, and Walster, 1972). These stored "theories" and related propositional "knowledge" are implicit assumptions whose construction has been worked on since childhood.

It is easy to see how these systems of perceiving or classifying used in everyday interaction could create a readiness or disposition to interpret clients' behavior independently of actual cues. In fact, if one already "knows" self-confident people are happy, why collect cues to a self-confident client's emotional state? This tendency to make inferences without factual data is referred to as *bias* (Kaplan, 1973). It can influence interpretation of cues and even perception.

Beliefs about *groups of people* can also be incorporated into implicit theories (Jones, 1977, p. 52). The term *stereotype* describes an inference that all group members are alike. On the basis of one or two cues, a client is classified as a group member and then assumed to have all other attributes of the group stereotype. Stereotypic categorization ignores individual differences, as is evident in the group stereotypes about nurses, physicians, various cultures, races, and people of particular religions or nationalities.

Stereotypes are essentially expectations. They are constructed with minimal actual knowledge of the group and sometimes no experience with group members. Stereotypes generally are based on hearsay evidence that is culturally transmitted. Presumably they are not *directly* related to prejudice (negative attitudes toward a group of persons) (Jones, 1977, p. 61).

A lack of information, a low degree of interest, and limited contact combine to increase anonymity and subsequent sterotypic classification (Berger and Luckmann, 1966, p. 33). Overemployment of stereotypes on the basis of insufficient information "appears to be a sign of rigidity, occasioned partly by lack of intelligence and insufficient familiarity" with persons (Sarbin et al., 1960, p. 196). (Nursing diagnoses meet the definition of stereotypic classification but are not used without valid, reliable, and sufficient data.)

Biases, errors, and misperceptions result if inferences derived from stereotypes are not subjected to validation. Stated differently, the use of sterotypes or attributions *as if they were observed data* ignores the uniqueness of the individual. A designation such as "the gallbladder in 321" encourages anonymity and extremely broad classification of the client.

When *negative* stereotypes are used without knowledge or rational thought, they can have unfortunate consequences. Merton defined these consequences as "self-fulfilling prophecy" (1957, p. 423). False definition of the situation can evoke new client behavior that makes the originally false conception come true. Simply, "if men define situations as real, they are real in their consequences" (Thomas and Thomas, 1928, p. 1104). Extreme caution has to be exercised not to draw negative inferences about clients and their behavior from propositions that have no basis in reality.

Consider an example of negative stereotyping (at least negative in terms of its social value): the *cancer-patient-as-terminal prophecy*. Sometimes implicit "rules" exist in the hospital regarding how terminal patients should behave. One such rule is that they certainly should not be doing future-oriented planning or asking for a podiatrist to treat a bunion or corn! (This kind of behavior on the part of a "terminal" patient is sometimes labeled denial of terminal illness.) With the great uncertainty in prognosis, many times there is no valid reason for the patient not to expect to survive for months or years. Hypotheses derived from pessimistic propositions or beliefs about death, coping, personal worth, and general ability to control events can be communicated unintentionally to clients during assessment. The potential then exists for the self-fulfilling prophecy to occur.

Patterson and Zderad recognize the dilemma of having developed presuppositions, interpretations, labels, categories, and judgments in the everyday world and having to put these aside in the world of practice:

> Man is an individual; he is a unique here and now person. So naturally, *necessarily*, he has his own particular "here" and his own particular "now" . . . each man must have *some* perspective of the phenomenon being experienced. However, by recognizing and considering the particular perspective from which he is experiencing it, a person may become more open to the thing itself. (Patterson and Zderad, 1976, p. 86)

This quotation suggests that rather than trying to ignore personal stereotypes, preconceptions, and biases, one should put them "out on the table" and ask What am I taking for granted? Rather than imposing definitions of the situation, the nurse should observe client and the situation as they are. Reflection and analysis follow observation. The nurse then "mulls over, sorts out, compares, contrasts, relates, interprets, gives name to and categorizes" (Patterson and Zderad, 1976, p. 76).

Sterotyping is actually based on analogy. "*Known*" characteristics and behavior of a reference group (for example, a cultural, national, racial, or religious group) are used as a model to infer or predict *unknown* characteristics or behavior of a person, family, or community. Stereotyping is a risky way of generating information about a client if the stereotype is used as data in diagnosis. Asking questions, observing, and validating the meaning of observations provide far more reliable data. This preferred precedure requires testing preconceptions and biases as if they were hypotheses.

Another form of analogy, and by far the most commonly used, is *empathy*. One's own feelings and intentions are used to infer the feelings and intentions of a client. In using the self as a theoretical reference point, the nurse assumes that all (or many) people share *human* characteristics and behavior. Therefore the nurse's expectation is that he or she and the client will experience things similarly. The client's behavior is thought to be understood or predicted because it is the way the nurse would feel, behave, or act. Inner experiences of the self plus assumed similarity are the bases for empathy (Sarbin et al., 1960, p. 15). In contrast to stereotyping without adequate information, empathy is a form of analogy that is highly valued.

In everyday conversation, people can understand each other because they share the meaning of the symbols (words) they use to communicate. Empathy, in contrast, depends on the shared meaning of reactions to human experiences. Empathy is a nonintellectual, nonlogical understanding of unspoken feelings resulting from active concern and involvement with another person. Empathy cannot be attained without personal concern and involvement.

Empathic understanding appears to be an ability closely related to imagination. It requires attention to situational cues and the *temporary* projection of oneself into the situation the client is experiencing. Resulting perceptions are used as hypotheses to direct cue search. Inferences generated by empathic understanding increase sensitivity to cues, particularly cues about feelings and intentions.

Bieri and his colleagues suggest that the use of the self as an analogy is more likely when one or more of the following are present: (1) similar beliefs, attitudes, and personality, (2) acceptance and liking of the person, and (3) similar social status (Bieri, Atkins, Briar, Leaman, Miller, and Tripoldi, 1966, p. 228). Considering these, it is understandable that one cannot use empathy to generate hypotheses about feelings when knowledge of the client and situation is scanty.

Sensitivity to the feelings of a person in distress depends heavily on the capacity to imagine how the person feels. Understanding is communicated when a clinician begins to inquire (test hypotheses) about feeling and intentions. It may sound too "cold and calculating" to combine the concept of empathy and hypothesis testing. Without the combination, there is a tendency to act without validating empathic inferences.

Personal theories develop as a result of experience in living. They can influence a data base by two routes: information collection and information interpretation. It is essential to be aware that this influence can occur. Although personal theories can lead to sensitivity to cues and the ability to generate hypotheses, a high risk is taken if hypotheses that are based on implicit theories, stereotypes, and empathic reference to the self are not tested and validated by data.

Generalizing from Authority   Teachers, textbooks, research journals, and experienced colleagues are frequently used as reference points for inference. The propositions gleaned from these sources may be research conclusions, clinical lore, and experiential wisdom.

Inferences drawn from research conclusions are highly valid and useful if situations and clients are similar to the research subjects and setting. One has to be aware that conclusions are probabilistic, that is, they may be predicted to apply in 95 out of 100 cases. The risk is that a particular client may have a critically dissimilar characteristic or may be within the other 5 percent rather than the 95 percent to whom the research findings apply. Again it should be noted that information deduced from any propositions should be treated as constructions of the mind of the observer, not as clinical data. Validation in the real world is required if at all possible.

Other nurses also may provide a source of general propositions. Through a process of socialization and instruction, nurses share pooled experiences and probability estimates for certain signs and symptoms.

The orientation period for a new clinician provides opportunities for staff to communicate the nature of the client population in both formal and informal ways. New personnel are told—explicitly and implicitly—what cues are important; they are given feedback about their perceptions and socialized into the norms for assessment and diagnosis.

Socialization into a new role influences expectations. In turn, expectations activate categories and systems of propositions for identifying cues and interpreting data. By activating categories in memory and making them more accessible, socialization increases sensitivity to particular cues.

Bieri and colleagues suggest that the type of setting and type of clients influence perceptual sensitivity and cue search (Bieri et al., 1966, pp. 211–212). For example, if an increased heart rate and restlessness were encountered in a psychiatric nursing setting there might be a tendency to search for cues to self-concept or role-relationship problems. In contrast, the same signs in a surgical setting might influence the nurse to check the client's temperature, the dressing, and the perception of pain or discomfort. Would there not be greater sensitivity to parenting cues in pediatric and obstetrical settings than in medical-surgical nursing settings? Are not intensive care nurses highly sensitive to physiological cues? Indeed they should be, when physiological instability is the major factor requiring admission to this type of unit.

Soares has described an aspect of knowledge that is taken for granted in an intensive care unit; this research illustrates that certain norms exist among "inside nurses" (regular staff) and other norms among "outside nurses" (float staff):

> Inside staff nurses have been exposed to the informal rules of interaction within the particular unit, and they have learned the taken-for-granted meanings that are known to the members of the inside group. Since outside nurses do not appear to understand the meanings conveyed in the unit, as seen by the lack of response to action messages, it seems feasible that these messages and meanings are peculiar to this particular unit. (Soares, 1978, p. 203)

The degree to which the lore transmitted by nursing and medical colleagues influences an individual's thinking depends in part on that individual's professional confidence and experience. A high level of personal need to become part of the belief and value system of the group may be expected to facilitate acquisition of group norms. Studies of Tajfel (1969) and Schutz (1966) suggest that a person who is uncertain how to behave in a situation (possibly a new staff member or a new graduate) seeks information that can be used to respond in a "professionally appropriate" manner.

Caution must be exercised in accepting statements such as "Oh, yes, all the old people in this community act like that"; "We don't bother with that here; they're only in this unit for 3 days"; or "Just do a quickie assessment; the clients here are pretty healthy and don't have any problems." The key is to reflect on the expectancies and probabilities of events communicated by colleagues. Treat the information obtained as hypotheses, not facts. The information may contain gems of wisdom or may lead to perpetuation of errors. An "anchoring point" in theory, research, and one's own values is the best protection against unwisely adopting others' points of view.

Textbooks and teachers provide the most common anchoring point for propositions and likelihood estimates about what occurs when and with what. Yet critical, logical examination of any reference point, including self-constructed propositions and ready-made inferences, is always in order.

Authoritativeness is a characteristic conferred by the receiver of a message. In this section we have considered research, colleagues, teachers, and books that may be perceived as authoritative. They can be, and generally should be, a source of propositional knowledge to use in deducing the possible meaning of cues. As with all other reference points, caution needs to be exercised. Hypotheses generated should be tested by collecting further information.

Generalizing from Initial Impressions People, including clinicians, seem to need some overall reference point from which to begin to assess what a particular person or group is like. Why do they want to know? There are two reasons. The idealistic one is that in order to be very helpful one has to know the client as a person (or group) rather than as an object. One observes objects, but one interacts (or transacts) with people. The interpersonal relationship through which diagnostic information is obtained requires understanding of people as people, not assessment of functional patterns in isolation. The second reason is merely the other side of the coin. Realistically, to perform the clinician role one must have some understanding of the feelings and intentions of the other.

An *initial impression* of a client and his or her general health and situation is formed early in an interaction.[8] It can influence assessment and diagnosis whether or not the nurse is aware of the influence. Therefore it is important to understand how people form initial impressions of others, what peculiarities of practice influence impressions, and what suggestions can help one get around biased impressions. It should be noted that the following ideas apply particularly to cues about *personal attributes* and the *social inferences* that result from their interpretation. These are a "backdrop" which can color further assessments, diagnosis, and even intervention.

People learn through experience to make quick inferences about others' abilities, attitudes, interests, physical features, traits, and behavior. Category labels such as wholesome, friendly, cold, or hard-working are used to describe global impressions of people. Value-belief systems "explain" how these personal attributes are related and whether they are to be positively or negatively valued. (What is being described here is a form of implicit theory about personality and social interaction.)

An initial impression is formed when one meets a person or family or enters a community. In fact, it can be formed even before any words are spoken. The reader who wishes to test the truth of this statement can try sitting on a bus or train, observing others, and as diversional activity imagining what the others are like. Functionally, the initial impression or quick social evaluation permits one to choose one's words and behavior in an initial interaction. Forming impressions quickly is part of the social skill everyone develops.

In addition, but related to the preceding discussion, people may have *general* tendencies to infer social characteristics of others. The extremes are the "Pollyanna syndrome" of extreme optimism and the negative disposition that "people are no darn good." In general, reports of impressions contain more positive than negative descriptors (Jones, 1977). Extreme dispositions to infer are usually modified, at least to some extent, by professional education. They do not disappear entirely, as is evident in studies of clinicians' dispositions toward judgments of maladjustment (Weiss, 1963) and judg-

---

[8]The client is probably also picking up an initial impression of the nurse. Frequently this impression is generalized to all staff and the agency. Clients, like nurses, go beyond the information given to reach inferential conclusions: "She's nice"; "He's a considerate nurse"; "She'll know what to do if something happens."

ments made in clinical assessments (Schmidt and Fonda, 1956). These global tendencies probably color initial impressions.

Theories of impression formation (Anderson, 1968; Asch, 1946) suggest that personal attraction and a conglomerate of evaluative judgments are integrated into an impression. The early impression seems to be a holistic grasp of a *cluster* of cues about the person. Personality (e.g., assertiveness and nonassertiveness); physiognomic (body and facial) features; level of education or intelligence (indicated, for example, by speech patterns); and activity level (e.g., activity and passivity) are personal attributes that can make up the cluster (Hamilton and Huffman, 1971).

Nurses' initial impressions most likely are influenced also by the client's health state. If a health problem exists, the medical diagnosis may produce some social judgments as well as other impressions. For example, some conditions may be viewed as simply happening to a person (cancer) and other conditions may be thought of as the person's or family's fault (obesity or a child's growth delay).

Like other points of reference for interpreting cues, initial impressions can act as a framework, or reference point. Impressions can be useful or can lead to erroneous conclusions. If they slip into the data base without validation, diagnositc errors can occur.

To summarize this section on reference points for inference, it may be said that people, diagnosticians included, interpret ambiguous, uncertainty-based information by using both explicit and implicit propositions. Their interpretations are sometimes colored by what they "know" is true or at least usually true.

Ordinarily people survive quite well on the basis of unexamined and, sometimes, untested inferences. Perception, as Neisser (1978) has said, is self-correcting in the long run. The difficulty in clinical nursing practice is that the "long run" may be too late. Harm or discomfort can occur from interventions that are based on unexamined and untested assumptions. Professionals need to set up a system of checks and balances.

Because at times information is insufficient, imagination fills in. The picture is clarified and gaps are filled. Inferences based on some data and some imagination are usually the fillers. Checks and balances have to be built in to avoid the risk of error; they can be summarized as follows:

1 If at all possible, inferences should be treated as hypotheses to be tested. Validate inferences with the client and recheck inferences about the environment.

2 The roots of inferences (expectations, assumptions, propositions, dispositions, and impressions) should reflect the likelihood of events in the world so that hypotheses are reasonable. Beware of overgeneralizing from experiences that are not representative. Ask for explanations and be curious so that a self-correcting process is established.

3 The process of inferring from incomplete data and previous knowledge should be checked for logical consistency. Avoid inferential leaps.

4 When inference and imagination are used in diagnosis, get feedback. Obtain this by further observation, follow-up, or colleague review. Always keep in mind the risk of acting with incomplete data. Build in safeguards.

5 Inferences tend to enter the data base used in diagnosis when the data base is incomplete. The more data, the less need for creating information by inference.

SUMMARY

When a new client is admitted, a nursing care plan has to be developed. This requires an assessment. The purpose of the admission assessment is to identify nursing diagnoses; if present, these provide a way to organize the care plan. This chapter began a discussion of strategies used in identifying nursing diagnoses.

A strategy is an approach to assessment. It describes the set of decisions a nurse makes about what information to collect and how to use the information. Although an assessment tool, or guideline, determines what clinical data *must* be collected, nurses have to go beyond that minimum. Information obtained from the client usually needs to be clarified or the meaning has to be verified. Also, if cues signify that the client does have problems, decisions have to be made about what information is needed for diagnosis.

Decisions are guided by diagnostic hypotheses. These are ideas about what nursing diagnoses might be present when one or more cues are present. Hypotheses determine the questions to be asked and the observations to be made during the nursing assessment.

In the first section of this chapter, discussion focused on what a hypothesis-testing strategy should accomplish: accuracy, efficiency, and control of cognitive strain. The first objective early in assessment is to narrow the possibilities. Prior to the admission of a client, no information exists; any nursing diagnosis may be a possibility.

As information is collected, diagnostic hypotheses are generated. Hypotheses may arise from preencounter information and from data about functional pattern areas. These hypotheses then define the problem space to be used in formulating questions to be asked or observations to be made. Generating hypotheses involves predicting what problems the client may have and using these predictions as hypotheses to guide the search for cues. The cues enable the diagnostician to zero in on likely possibilities in each pattern area.

The second section of this chapter probed more deeply into the process of hypothesis generation. This exploration revealed that clincial reasoning was the process underlying strategies, hypotheses, and decisions about the collection and use of information. Clinical reasoning is based on inferences from cues and from knowledge stored in memory.

Perceptual and propositional inferences were explored. It was seen that these reasoning processes led to inferences, or hypotheses, about the possible meaning of cues. Hypotheses about possible diagnoses direct the search for further information. In turn, the information obtained is used to clarify and verify the client's responses or the nurse's observations. As this occurs hypotheses are supported, changed, or discarded.

Ways of reasoning have been learned since childhood. Clinical reasoning requires that these skills be sharpened. It also requires that knowledge from experience, personal theories stored in memory, authorities, or initial impressions be examined carefully. Knowledge from all these sources is used in reasoning and can lead to brilliant clinical insights or diagnostic errors.

The discussion of diagnostic strategies will continue in Chapter 6. It will be seen that diagnostic hypotheses generated through prediction have to be tested. Having narrowed the possibilities, the diagnostician has already begun problem identification.

Taking problem identification to completion will result in problem formulation, or nursing diagnosis. The diagnoses formulated can then be used to direct nursing care activities.

BIBLIOGRAPHY

Anderson, N. H. A simple model for information integration. In R. P. Abelson, *Theories of cognitive consistency: A sourcebook*. Chicago: Rand McNally, 1968.

Asch, A. E. Forming impressions of personality. *Journal of Abnormal and Social Psychology*, 1946, *41*, 258–290.

Aspinall, M. J. Use of a decision tree to improve accuracy of diagnosis. *Nursing Research*, May-June, 1979, **28**:182–185.

Berger, P. L., & Luckmann, T. *The social construction of reality*. Garden City, N.Y.: Anchor Books, 1966.

Bieri, J., Atkins, A., Briar, S., Leaman, R., Miller, H., & Tripoldi, T. *Clinical and social judgment*. New York: Wiley, 1966.

Bourne, L. E., Jr., Dominowski, R. L., & Loftus, E. F. *Cognitive processes.* Englewood Cliffs, N.J.: Prentice-Hall, 1979.

Bruner, J. S., Goodnow, J. J., & Austin, G. A. *A study of thinking*. New York: Wiley, 1956.

Davitz, L., & Davitz, J. *Inference of patients' pain and psychological distress.* New York: Springer, 1980.

Dion, K., Berscheid, E., & Walster, E. What is beautiful is good. *Journal of Personality and Social Psychology*, 1972, *24*, 285–290.

Elstein, A. S., Schulman, L. S., & Sprafka, S. A. *Medical problem solving: An analysis of clinical reasoning.* Cambridge, Mass.: Harvard University Press, 1978.

Goffman, E. *Stigma: Notes on the management of spoiled identity*. Englewood Cliffs, N.J.: Prentice-Hall, 1965.

Gordon, M. Manual of nursing diagnoses. New York: McGraw-Hill, 1982.

Gordon, M. Predictive strategies in diagnostic tasks. *Nursing Research*, January-February 1980, *29*, 39–46.

Hamilton, D. L., & Huffman, L. J. Generality of impression-formation process for evaluative and non-evaluative judgments. *Journal of Personality and Social Psychology*, 1971, *20*(2), 200–207.

Jones, R. A. *Self-fulfilling prophecies: Social, psychological and physiological effects of expectancies.* Hillsdale, N.J.: Lawrence Erlbaum Associates, 1977.

Kaplan, M. F. Stimulus inconsistency and response dispositions in forming judgments of other persons. *Journal of Personality and Social Psychology*, 1973, *25*, 58–64.

Kim, M. J., & Moritz, D. A. *Classification of nursing diagnoses: Proceedings of the third and fourth national conferences.* New York: McGraw-Hill, 1981.

Levine, M. *A cognitive theory of learning*. Hillsdale, N.J.: Lawrence Erlbaum Associates, 1975.

Little, D., & Carnevali, D. The diagnostic statement: The problem defined. In J. Walter, G. Pardee, & M. Molbo (Eds.), *Dynamics of problem-oriented approaches: Patient care and documentation.* New York: Lippincott, 1976.

Merton, R. K. *Social theory and social structure* (rev. ed.). New York: Free Press, 1957.

Neisser, U. Perceiving, anticipating, imagining. In C. W. Savage (Ed.), *Perception and cognition: Issues in the foundations of psychology, Minnesota studies in the philosophy of science* (Vol. 9). Minneapolis: University of Minnesota Press, 1978.

Newell, A., & Simon, H. *Human problem solving.* Englewood Cliffs, N.J.: Prentice-Hall, 1972.

Patterson, J. G., & Zderad, L. T. *Humanistic nursing.* New York: Wiley, 1976.

Restle, F. Selection of strategies in cue learning. *Psychological Review,* 1962, *69*, 329–343.

Sarbin, T. R., Taft, R., & Bailey, D. E. *Clinical inference and cognitive theory.* New York: Holt, Rinehart & Winston, 1960.

Schmidt, H. O., & Fonda, C. P. Reliability of psychiatric diagnosis: A new look. *Journal of Abnormal and Social Psychology,* 1956, *52*, 262–268.

Schutz, W. C. Interpersonal underworld. In W. G. Bennis, K. D. Benne, and R. Chin (Eds.), *The planning of change.* New York: Holt, Rinehart & Winston, 1966.

Soares, C. Low verbal usage and status maintenance among intensive care nurses. In N. L. Chaska (Ed.), *The nursing profession: Views through the mist.* New York: McGraw-Hill, 1978.

Tajfel, H. Social and cultural factors in perception. In G. Lindzey and E. Aronson (Eds.), *Handbook of social psychology.* Reading, Mass.: Addison-Wesley, 1969.

Thomas, Clayton, L. (Ed.). *Taber's Cyclopedic Medical Dictionary.* Philadelphia: Davis, 1981.

Thomas, W. O., & Thomas, D. S. *The child in America.* New York: Knopf, 1928.

Tversky, A. & Kahneman, D. Judgment under uncertainty: Heuristics and biases. *Science,* September 1974, *185*, 1124–1131.

Weiss, J. H. Effect of professional training and amount of accuracy of information on behavioral prediction. *Journal of Consulting Psychology,* 1963, *27*, 257–262.

CHAPTER 6

DIAGNOSTIC STRATEGIES: TESTING POSSIBILITIES AND STATING DIAGNOSES

Human beings have the marvelous ability to think about things they cannot observe. They construct by inference what has been, what may be, and what could be. This cognitive capacity has led to great contributions to humanity. Having this ability, people also use it to construct "what is." Constructing diagnostic hypotheses is useful. Yet untested hypotheses, used as a basis for care planning, can lead to errors. The best way to avoid errors is to test ideas in the real world. This chapter deals with how hypotheses are tested and how those supported by data are stated as nursing diagnoses.

The first section will continue the discussion of diagnostic strategies. We are at the point in the diagnostic process by which the most likely hypotheses for describing and explaining a dysfunctional pattern have been identified. Now the question is, Which possibility is correct? The answer is determined by collecting more information through questions and observations. Information is collected to test each diagnostic hypothesis. As we shall see, hypothesis testing requires a focused search for critical defining signs and symptoms. Few in number, these signs and symptoms are the cues that distinguish one diagnosis from another. If these cues are present, they are the basis for the clinical judgment that a problem or etiological factor is present.

During hypothesis testing, cues are clustered. To do this, one must make decisions about how information is to be combined. Does *this* cue support a possible diagnosis? Does *that* cue suggest the problem is not present? Frequently these are not simple judgments to make. Inconsistencies among cues have to be resolved. In discussion of information clustering it will be seen that one cue can influence the interpretation of other cues in the cluster and that some cues influence judgment more than others.

When sufficient supporting information exists, the problems formulated are stated as nursing diagnoses. A section will be devoted to how diagnoses are stated after assessment findings are reviewed. The important understanding in this section is that problems formulated during assessment have to be reviewed in the context of the whole.

Human beings are not perfect information processors. Diagnostic errors can occur during data collection, during interpretation, or in clustering. In the final section sources of error will be considered. Awareness of potential errors will clarify why double checking has been emphasized in discussion of the diagnostic process.

FOCUSED CUE SEARCH

Chapter 5 showed how to process early data until a few highly probable diagnostic hypotheses are identified. These hypotheses then provide a focus for further cue search. Now, the presence or absence of diagnostic cues has to be determined. *Diagnostic cues* are the critical defining signs and symptoms of a nursing diagnosis that *will* be present *if* the problem is present.

A focused cue search requires a different hypothesis-testing procedure than prediction of possibilities. The focus has to be on assessing what is, now that prediction has narrowed the universe of what could be. If predictions were correct, one of the current diagnostic hypotheses being considered should describe and explain the cues. Let us briefly reconsider what has already occurred in early hypothesis testing in order to note how and when change in hypothesis testing occurs.

Hypothesis-Testing Procedures

When assessing the client and situation, a cue to a dysfunctional pattern may be obtained. This requires a diagnostic strategy for identifying the problem. A diagnostic strategy describes the sequence of decisions that are made about how information is to be collected, interpreted, and utilized. Decisions about information collection and processing are reflected in the hypothesis-testing procedures a nurse employs.

Two major hypotheses-testing procedures, identified by Bruner and his colleagues (1956) are *multiple* and *single hypothesis testing*. These terms mean that either a *single* diagnostic hypothesis such as sleep-onset disturbance is tested, or *multiple* hypotheses are tested simultaneously, such as sleep onset, early awakening, sleep pattern reversal, and other sleep pattern disturbances. Each procedure influences information intake, cognitive strain, and risk regulation in different ways.

Multiple-Hypothesis Testing In Chapter 5 it was seen that when a pattern area is assessed, background information and early cues are used to *predict* likely possibilities. Although every known diagnosis in a pattern area could be tested one by one, a more reasonable decision is to obtain predictive or contextual cues and test multiple hypotheses simultaneously. This hypothesis-testing procedure was called predictive testing. It is a form of multiple-hypothesis testing that employs contextual or predictive cues. As discussed, predictive testing of several hypotheses simultaneously ensures that maximum information is obtained at a point in assessment of a pattern area when information is needed to narrow the possibilities.

Obtaining information to test several diagnostic possibilities at once may still be appropriate after the most likely diagnoses have been identified. This is because some diagnoses share the same defining characteristics. Discrimination among the diagnoses is possible because the value of the shared characteristic differs in quantity or quality. The multiple-hypothesis–testing procedure is useful (1) if a number of possibilities exist, such as occurs early in assessment of a pattern area and (2) if diagnoses in the set share the same defining characteristics but the characteristic has different values when different diagnoses are present.

Cognitive requirements are high when multiple hypotheses are tested simultaneously. This is because the number of hypotheses to which information has to be related increases. Inductive and deductive inferences are required to relate the cues obtained to each hypothesis being tested and to increase or decrease hypothesis probabilities as a result of the information obtained. As experience increases these reasoning processes usually happen in less than a second; unlikely diagnoses are eliminated and the memory and inferential strain is reduced quickly.

Cognitive strain can occur if memory and inferential requirements exceed the diagnostician's capacity. Strain on cognitive capacities is manifested by forgetting information and by inferential errors. One reason for cognitive strain is prolonged holding of a large initial pool of hypotheses because of poor selection of predictive cues. Unlikely diagnostic hypotheses cannot be eliminated when good predictive information is lacking.

Examples of poor selection of predictive cues occurred in the research study involving surgical complications previously discussed (Gordon, 1980). A few nurses sought cues that did not provide maximum information; their strategy did not meet the objective of narrowing possibilities early in the task and thereby reducing memory and inferential strain. They sought cues such as amount of time spent in the recovery room or the units of blood administered. These cues contain much less information about surgical complications than time-lapse since surgery and the type of surgery performed. To identify highly probable diagnostic hypotheses quickly requires clinical knowledge of predictors and optimal decisions about the sequence of information collection.

A second, but related, reason for cognitive strain is prolonged multiple testing of hypotheses. This is manifested as continued collection of information that predicts the likelihood of a set of diagnostic hypotheses. Highly valid predictors may have been collected but the diagnostician attempts to further reduce uncertainty. Usually the continued search for predictive cues is due to a lack of understanding of the probabilistic nature of clinical information. Recognize that uncertainty in prediction cannot be totally eliminated. Rely on good predictive cues and begin to test likely diagnostic hypotheses; one can always return to the unlikely possibilities if necessary.

Multiple-hypothesis testing can be expected to decrease or be absent after (1) the most probable diagnoses to explain a dysfunctional pattern have been identified and (2) values of defining characteristics shared by two or more diagnoses have been obtained. After possibilities are generated and an estimate of the probability of each hypothesis is made, a decided shift in procedure is required (Gordon, 1972, 1980). Thereafter, the data sought are specific to the remaining hypotheses and each is tested, one by one.

Collecting information that differentiates among the remaining hypotheses requires a search for diagnostic cues. These are the critical cues that define and differentiate among diagnoses. Single hypothesis testing is appropriate at this point.

Single Hypothesis Testing   Assume that a judgment has been made that the client's description of a pattern area indicated some type of dysfunction or potential dysfunction. Second, assume that early data provided a base for generating possible diagnostic hypotheses to explain the data. Assume also that further data permitted probabilities to be set and unlikely possibilities discarded. Now a few highly probable hypotheses remain and provide a focus for cue search. A focused search requires a switch in hypothesis-testing procedures.

Each diagnostic hypothesis has to be investigated, one by one (if cues do not overlap), using the single-hypothesis–testing procedure. *If* the problem is present, signs and symptoms that define the diagnosis will be present.

A *single-hypothesis–testing procedure* involves assessing a client or situation to test one hypothesis at a time. This is a reasonable approach when critical, differentiating cues apply to only one diagnosis. Moreover, if only one or two hypotheses remain, they can be tested one by one.

The main advantage of testing hypotheses one by one is that *memory strain and inferential strain* are not increased over the basal level. This ease is welcomed if the generation of hypotheses, predictive testing, and testing of overlapping cues were prolonged early in the assessment of the pattern area. Another advantage is that the potential for forgetting or inferential errors is low when only a few hypotheses exist.

As long as one obtains valid, relevant information, the use of cues to test single hypotheses one by one ensures accuracy. No risk is taken, because *all* hypotheses in the set are tested. For this reason, confidence in the results of assessment should be high.

To use single hypothesis testing exclusively throughout the entire admission assessment would be an inefficient diagnostic strategy. Maximum information is not obtained from each question with this procedure. If only one hypothesis is generated and tested at a time, and if cues are shared, information relevant to other possibilities is lost. On the other hand, the information could be held in memory; but this approach removes one of the major advantages of this procedure, which is low memory strain.

Single testing is a costly procedure if used exclusively. It increases total time for assessment. In addition it would require repetitious questioning and observation, which would create the impression of disorganization. Yet when memory and inferential strain are high and when time and resources for testing are unlimited, this procedure is useful. If the assessment situation is problem-focused, as occurs after diagnoses are established, the procedure is certainly ideal. In emergency situations single hypothesis testing is not applicable. The successive investigation of single hypotheses is a "safe but slow" way of proceeding (Bruner et al., 1956).

The major shift to a single-hypothesis–testing procedure within a strategy appears to occur when the diagnostician is confident (for the moment) that the most probable tentative diagnoses have been identified. Consider an example. The sleep-rest pattern of a 40-year-old client is being assessed. A question has been posed and the client has responded that she has not been sleeping too well. This cue indicates a sleep pattern disturbance; a diagnostic strategy for investigating the cue is needed. The change to a dysfunctional pattern occurred about 2 weeks before hospital admission. Background information and the pattern areas already assessed suggest one etiological cue: This client has realistic health concerns; about 2 weeks ago she was told she may have cancer.

The diagnostic hypotheses generated were (1) sleep onset disturbance, (2) sleep pattern disturbance—early awakening, (3) sleep pattern interruption, and (4) sleep pattern reversal. Interventions for these four are different; thus it is important to identify which is the problem. The only causal hypothesis at the moment is broad and vague: health concerns—cancer.

A cue to predict the probabilities of the multiple hypotheses generated was sought. The client was asked for a specific description of her sleep pattern. Simultaneous predictive hypothesis testing of the four diagnostic hypotheses revealed that sleep onset disturbance and early awakening disturbance were most likely. Data about the hours she was sleeping did not support either hypothesis 3 or 4. The client sleeps 3–4 hours per night. The etiological hypothesis (concern about having cancer) and two of the four hypotheses about the problem remain at this point. A focused single hypothesis-testing procedure is appropriate. Sleep onset disturbance and early awakening disturbance are the diagnoses still under consideration. Now the critical differentiating cues must be obtained. Early awakening decreases in probability when the nurse asks a clarifying question: The client says the reason she awakens early is that the whole household always retires at 10 p.m. and arises at 5 a.m. The next question asked is designed to elicit data to support or reject the remaining diagnostic possibility, sleep onset disturbance.

What type of data should be collected to test this single hypothesis? The focus is on the here and now. Critical cues are found *within* the components of the pattern area. (Etiological factors are not, necessarily, as will be discussed later.) Current state characteristics and current contextual (situational) characteristics are the types of data that indicate the actual presence or absence of a problem.

It is important to remember that most clinical judgments require historical base-line data. Obtain historical state or contextual cues if they have not already been collected. Compare these to the current findings to judge whether or not *change* has occurred in the pattern or aspect of the pattern. Also compare the current data to the range of normal values for the client's age, sex, culture, and so forth in order to guard against the risk of overlooking a *stable* but *dysfunctional* pattern.

The cues diagnostic of a sleep onset disturbance are: (1) perception of difficulty falling asleep, (2) a 15-minute or longer sleep delay after attempt to go to sleep, and (3) consecutive episodes of delayed sleep onset (Schwartz and Aaron, 1979, p. 27). Knowing this, the nurse can formulate questions to elicit the pertinent data. As previously discussed, measures of client characteristics must be reliable and valid. Which of the following would elicit the most reliable and valid data:

1 When you have difficulty getting to sleep, how many minutes would you estimate it takes to fall asleep? Does this occur frequently?

2 When you have difficulty getting to sleep, how long do you lie awake? Is this every night?

The first option focuses in on the data needed, whereas the second is less specific— the client could respond, "A long time." A time-consuming second question would then have to be asked. Moreover, the question about consecutive episodes is leading the client to a particular response in the second option. As experience is gained in formulating good questions, the time required for assessment decreases. In this case, the client responded that most nights it takes 3 or 4 hours to fall deeply asleep. The diagnostic hypothesis of sleep onset disturbance is supported. Now the probable cause of this sleep problem has to be determined.

Etiological Hypotheses   A clear grasp of the problem has to be obtained before the reasons for its existence are purposefully explored. During exploration of the problem, cues to etiological factors may have been communicated. The client with the sleep pattern disturbance had already mentioned learning of her medical diagnosis 2 weeks before admission. Recalling this cue from a previous pattern area suggests one etiological hypothesis. The client's problems in sleeping also began "about 2 weeks ago." The two cues were combined under the hypothesis, health concerns—cancer.

Alternative causal hypotheses need to be generated as they were during exploration of the problem. Asking the client *her* explanation of the sleep disturbance may be useful. Sleep onset disturbances can be related to presleep routine, noise, anxiety, decreased activity, indigestion, hunger, problem-solving activities (working out plans), fear of death (primitive fear that sleeping is like dying), and other factors. Given the information available regarding this woman, what are the probabilities of each of these hypotheses? Pay attention to the inductive and deductive reasoning used and to the applicability of propositional knowledge retrieved from your long-term memory. What procedure would you use for testing these hypotheses?

The data available are: pattern change 2 weeks ago; knows possible diagnosis of cancer. This is certainly not much to go on. Most of the hypotheses above are at a 50:50 probability. Perhaps deductive reasoning from the proposition that laypersons view cancer as fatal might increase the probability of anxiety and fear of death. How shall etiological hypothesis testing be pursued?

The client was asked why, in her opinion, the change in sleep pattern had come about. She considers her sleep disturbance to be caused by "thinking through problems," bedtime being a quiet time to do this. The nurse must make a decision at this point. Eight etiological hypotheses previously have been identified (indigestion, noise, presleep routine, and so forth). Should the nurse (1) pursue this branch (the client's statement aabout thinking through problems) by inquiring about the problems, (2) branch to other hypotheses, or (3) consider *thinking through problems* the etiology because it is consistent with previous data on health concerns?

A decision to seek more cues about *thinking through problems* may be wise. A sensitivity to the trust and rapport established at this point in the interaction influences the decision. The decision may be influenced also by the nurse's inference about what "problems" may exist. Is it the possibility of having cancer that is being "thought through?" Silence for a moment may elicit more cues.

If the client is not open to sharing information, the nurse should hold the cue. As patterns such as self-perception and role-relationships are assessed, more cues probably will be elicited. In its present form the etiology is still too vague and suggests that other diagnoses may be present. Thus the third option the nurse might have chosen—to accept *thinking through problems* as the etiology—is not advisable.

An alternative decision is to find out whether presleep routine, noise, daytime activity, late or heavy meals (indigestion), hunger, or any symptoms related to her disease are contributing factors. If not, a comment that her idea must be right may lead to further elaboration of the problems she is thinking through.

Note that soliciting the client's perception of the cause employs a multiple-hypothesis-testing procedure. When information was obtained it supported one hypothesis, presleep problem-solving activities, but did not directly contribute to resetting the probabilities of the other hypotheses (unless the "problems" the client mentioned are related to fear; this is not known).

Very commonly the etiology of a problem in one pattern area lies in another pattern area or in environmental factors influencing patterns. The hypotheses above were in the nutritional (indigestion, hunger), self-perception-self-concept (fear, anxiety), activity-exercise (decreased daily activity or the by-product of activity—noise), and cognitive-perceptual (problem solving and plans) patterns. One would expect problems in one pattern to have causes in others when a group of functional patterns are interdependent and interactive. A problem in one area frequently results from other dysfunctional patterns.

Predisposing Etiological Factors   Etiological factors may be present in the absence of any actual health problem. In this case they are referred to as *risk factors*. These are factors in the client or situation that predispose to a dysfunctional pattern. The potentially dysfunctional pattern or pattern component is labeled. Diagnostic terms indicating potential problems are used (Appendix A). For example, disturbance in the thirst stimulus mechanism predisposes to potential fluid volume deficit. Similarly, impaired physical capacities such as inability to obtain fluids without assistance increases the risk for this problem. Identifying potential problems involves predicting what could occur in the future. On the basis of that prediction, preventive nursing action is taken.

Predicting susceptibility, or risk, employs predictive hypothesis testing, described in Chapter 5. Information is obtained and inductive inferences are made from cues. Deductive conclusions are drawn and formulated as diagnostic hypotheses about a possible problem. What would be the next step?

The next step is to test the hypotheses generated. Cues to the state of the client which have to be present if an actual problem existed are *absent*. Thus, a current problem is ruled out, but risk factors (cues predicting a problem) are still present. A diagnosis of a potential problem is made based on the judgment that risk factors are present. A flow chart depicting the process of diagnosing potential and actual health problems is shown in Figure 6-1. If diagnostic cues to a problem are absent, either there is no problem or a potential problem exists. Risk factors in the client's present situation, predictive cues in the history, and future projections are three types of information that support the diagnosis of risk (also called susceptibility, or potential for a dysfunctional health pattern).

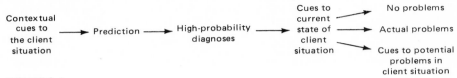

FIGURE 6-1
Actual and potential problem identification.

How does one "look into the crystal ball" and say at some level of probability that *this* client will develop *this* problem if the course of events is not altered? One proceeds by combining and weighting three kinds of data in clinical judgment.

First consider the client's current functional patterns and their stability. A current pattern may be optimal because of the situation. For example, severely disabled people can function optimally in a supportive and compensatory environment. Are there any historical data that would predict instability of this environment? If not, the prediction can be made that optimal function will continue. No risk is present and no potential problems. Notice that historical and current data were used to evaluate stability in the client's situation.

Now, let us tip the balance. A disabled client is going home from the hospital and lives alone in a rural community with automobile-based transportation, and two-story houses. The potential problems due to environmental change are probably obvious; if not, scan the nursing diagnoses in the 11 pattern areas of Appendix B. For example, without good nursing discharge planning the client is at risk for problems such as social isolation, impaired home management, and perhaps total self-care deficit. Notice that the future (going home) had to be projected before a set of possible problems was anticipated.

A story may illustrate good and not so good "crystal ball gazing." Once there was a nurse whose vision was fair. She noticed that the respiratory tract secretions of an alert 10-year-old client were increasing in amount and thickness. The child had a tumor on the right side of his neck that caused irritation of the trachea and generalized weakness. It was known that the child had had one episode during which his lips and nail beds had become bluish (cyanotic). She inferred, correctly so, that thick secretions had partially blocked his respiratory passages. In anticipation that the boy was at risk for another such episode, the nurse immediately wrote a nursing order for frequent suctioning! Not liking the term *nursing diagnosis*, she ignored that whole idea and did not really formulate the potential problem.

This same client had another nurse who had studied nursing diagnosis and was becoming adept at the diagnostic process. This nurse observed the same cues but went a step farther. As seen in Figure 6-2, cues were clustered under a tentative diagnostic hypothesis: potential ineffective airway clearance. Logical deductive reasoning about (1) the relationship between fluid intake and viscosity (thickness) of secretions and (2) generalized weakness and ineffective coughing suggested a search for risk factors (low fluid intake and ineffective strength of cough). The second nurse proceeded like a detective. After cues were collected, the nursing diagnosis of potential ineffective airway clearance was made and risk factors were stated.

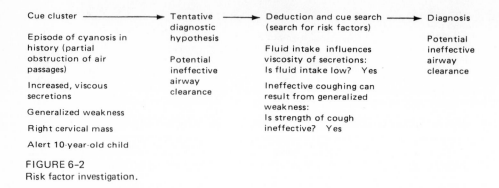

FIGURE 6-2
Risk factor investigation.

This nurse immediately wrote orders: (1) for frequent suctioning with periodic reevaluation of need; (2) to encourage fluids and determine the child's favorite drinks (low fluid intake noted and high viscosity of secretions); (3) to increase coughing effectiveness by abdominal support (child was taught the game "press stomach in and out with hands" and then "press stomach, cough, and feel what happens"); and (4) to monitor for signs of respiratory distress. The orders were *diagnosis-specific*; the first nurse's orders were *symptom-specific*. To every fable there is a moral: Nursing care is more effective when one knows what one is treating.

In the first case there was action, correct but insufficient; in the second case, the diagnosis suggested a creative design for care. Nursing diagnoses provide a cognitive resting point. Stop, think, and plan how to reduce the risk of ineffective airway clearance. In the first case the cyanotic episode plus increased viscous secretions suggested *one* intervention. When, in the second case the question was raised, What can be done for potential ineffective airway clearance, the nurse's thinking was broad, open, and creative.

It is important to note that the data and predictions contain some uncertainty. A potential problem diagnosed by a nurse in a hospital may be viewed as an error in diagnosis by a visiting nurse. For example, age, marital status, parity (number of live births), and mother-baby interaction are four assessment parameters that appear to influence hospital nurses' judgments regarding postpartum clients' susceptibility to parenting problems (Nicoletti, Reitz, and Gordon, 1981).

A combination of cues such as 35 years old, married, first baby, anxiety in baby care, and impending discharge can suggest a potential for parenting problems. When living arrangements and support systems are unclear, a decision to refer the client to a visiting nurse may be made. A home visit may reveal a totally different mother-baby interaction from those observed in the hospital. The visiting nurse may not agree with the diagnosis.

Short hospitalizations may not permit sufficient data collection and verification about some clients and their situation. Equally true, the setting may influence behavior. Judgments have to take into account the risk of error in underestimating or overestimating risk factors and the costs incurred in referrals. Most importantly, *early* collection of highly predictive cues places the hospital nurse in a position to anticipate postdischarge problems that may occur. Of course, if referrals flowed from prenatal to postpartum to postdischarge care providers, the data needed for identification of babies and families at risk might be more readily available.

Some guidelines may be helpful in formulating potential problems:

1 Generate possible problems from probability estimates and cues.

2 Assess and combine predictive cues.

3 Determine (1) whether overall risk can be reduced by *nursing* intervention and (2) which risk factors will lower risk, or lower risk most quickly, in a particular situation.

4 Consider timing. Risk factors may signify an immediate problem because of the client's situation (e.g., disease, scheduled surgery, or life situation). Risk factors may also indicate that there is a potential problem but the decision is made to postpone treatment until situational factors change (such as postoperative recovery).

In summary, hypothesis testing procedures differ from hypothesis generation procedures. This appears to be the case in both actual and potential problem identification as well as in identification of etiological factors. After likely diagnoses have been identified, procedures within a strategy shift. The most probable diagnostic hypotheses become the bases for a focused cue search. Unless diagnostic cues overlap (have differing values that distinguish one diagnosis from another), the procedure of choice is to investigate the remaining hypotheses one by one.

A single-hypothesis–testing procedure is useful when only a few hypotheses are being considered or when there are no overlapping cues. The type of data sought is specific to each diagnostic hypothesis. These data are the diagnostic cues that constitute the critical defining signs and symptoms of each nursing diagnosis. Without the presence of these specific cues, the diagnostic category name should not be used. (As previously stated work is in progress to identify critical signs and symptoms. The current status of signs and symptoms for each category can be seen in Kim and Moritz (1981), or in the manual that accompanies this book (Gordon, 1982).

Critical diagnostic cues are usually few in number and differentiate one diagnosis from another. Supporting data may also be sought. Supporting data influence confidence in a diagnosis when cues are uncertainty-based or available measures are only partially reliable.

Hypotheses permit cues to be related and clustered as they are collected. This clustering process goes on in short term, or working, memory. Simultaneously, data under each pattern area are recorded on paper. Going from no information to a well-supported diagnosis is not always a smooth process. Inconsistencies and conflicts in the data are sometimes observed. How to resolve these, and the process of weighting information to make judgments, will be topics considered in the next section.

INFORMATION CLUSTERING

Putting together the information obtained from assessment is a critical activity in the diagnostic process. It is referred to as *clustering of cues*. Clustering of information appears to occur as soon as the information is perceived, meaning assigned, and hypotheses generated. Thus it is artificial to call clustering a step in the diagnostic process.

Like collecting and interpreting information and naming, information clustering is continuous throughout the process of nursing diagnosis.

This section will discuss how to resolve inconsistencies and conflicts in data as the data accumulate. Weighting of clinical cues in making diagnostic judgments will also be discussed. *Weighting* refers to the power of a cue to influence judgment. The respective weight given a cue by a diagnostician influences which information gets clustered under a diagnostic hypothesis and which information is discounted as not useful.

Resolving Inconsistencies

Previous information, irrespective of its source, sets up expectations for new information. Expectations are based on the nurse's past knowledge and experience or previous data from the client. When new information conflicts with expectations, one becomes aware of inconsistency. To inquisitive clinicians, such inconsistency creates a dilemma. They know that ignoring inconsistencies increases the risk of diagnostic error and can also result in harm to the client. Attention has to be paid to resolving the dilemma.

Through expectations we "know" how things *should* appear, come about, or be related. Inconsistencies represent an inability to fit data together. To recognize inconsistencies, first a comparison is made between what was expected and what has been observed. Then the nurse reasons deductively using "If . . . then . . ." statements. For example, *if* a client reports not eating much, *then* obesity should not be present. When "things don't turn out as they should" the question of why arises. Resolution of inconsistencies must take into account possible sources for the apparent conflict: measurement error, expectations, and conflicting or unreliable reports.

Inconsistencies Caused by Measurement Error When inconsistencies arise, a measurement error should be considered. During a nursing history, verbal reports of the client can be misunderstood. At times this occurs because of inattentive listening. Misunderstanding can also result from lack of clarity in a client's communication. If there is any doubt as to whether a client's statement was heard correctly, the client should be asked to validate or repeat the information. Care must be exercised to explain the reason for the repetition, because rephrasing or requesting repetition is also a technique for confronting a person or focusing attention on statements.

During examination of a client, measurement errors can produce apparent inconsistencies. Observations should be repeated if doubt exists. Instruments, for example, blood pressure machines, should be checked, as well as the technique used to obtain the measurement.

Inconsistencies Caused by Expectations What appear to be inconsistencies in data may be merely a nurse's incorrect expectations. Inadequate knowledge or inexperience can produce faulty expectations. In addition, expectations are based on interpretations; thus errors in previous or current reasoning may be the basis for apparent inconsistencies. Sometimes an understanding of the client's personal intentions, values, or beliefs provides a logical interpretation of the client's behavior and resolves what had seemed to be inconsistencies in the data. This is in contrast to viewing behavioral data from one's own inferences and perspective.

Inconsistencies Caused by Conflicting Reports Clients' and families' verbal reports may conflict. This produces apparent inconsistencies among various people's reports. Or the same person may give inconsistent reports at different times.

It is not uncommon for conflicting or contradictory reports to be given by a client and family member, by different members of a family, or by different groups within a community. The question arises, Whose information is to be taken into account and whose discounted? A number of hypotheses can be raised. Do biases or cognitive deficits explain the conflicting reports? Is it a matter of different perspectives, such as objective (others') versus subjective (client's) points of view?

Resolving conflicting reports requires caution and tact. The strategy has to be well thought through. Direct confrontation may serve only to induce guilt or defensiveness. If conflicting reports are discussed only with one party, interpersonal conflict between the two parties could arise later when they become aware of differing reports. In some instances it may be wise to discuss the differences in perceptions with both parties together. A major factor in the decision is the current mental or physical health of the people involved.

Conflicts may also be apparent when a client's previous and current verbal reports differ. For example, a client may report an event or set of symptoms that is not consistent with the report the client gave to another health care provider or at another time. Temporary memory lapse, the interpersonal milieu in which the client felt the need to report things differently, or the way questions were formulated may explain the conflict in data. The client can be asked in a gentle manner about the apparent inconsistency.

Inconsistencies Caused by Unreliable Reports A client's verbal reports during a nursing history may be judged unreliable. Extreme caution must be exercised in making this judgment if errors are to be avoided, because information considered to be unreliable will be discounted and therefore given minimal weight in diagnostic judgments. Assumed incompetency is one reason verbal reports are judged unreliable. The presence of cognitive or sensory deficits can suggest to the care provider that verbal reports should be used cautiously. Yet errors can result if a client's reliability has been incorrectly assessed. For example, many times elderly clients are stereotyped as incompetent or cognitively deficient because they look old, whereas in fact no deficit may exist.

A well-publicized case of psychiatric stereotyping was reported by Rosenhan (1973); it dealt with "being sane in insane places." Behavior of a group of persons was interpreted as manifesting psychosis because psychotic behavior was what was expected in the setting, a psychiatric hospital.

Concluding that information is biased is a second reason for discounting it as unreliable. Situations can occur wherein clients or family members consciously or unconsciously provide biased reports. For example, a strong motivation, and perhaps a realistic need, to leave the hospital may influence a client to bias reports of his or her health state. Moreover, family members may overemphasize or underemphasize certain symptoms because of basic anxieties or needs. These situations are usually easily recognized because the reported information is inconsistent with other observations. The nurse needs to focus on discovering the underlying problem.

A third reason that some observers discount information as unreliable is their prior classification of the character, or personality type, of a client or relative. Consider the following client classifications: drug addict, alcoholic, hospitalized prisoner, hypochondriac, malingerer, sociopath. These negatively valued client classifications may predispose health care providers to question clients' verbal reports and can lead to very serious error.

Reasonable and respectful consideration should be given to any client report without discrimination on the basis of character stereotypes. Health care providers may infer that five instances of complaint without a basis predict that the sixth complaint is of the same type. Sometimes this is the instance when the appendix ruptures or the client acts in desperation.

Resolving, as opposed to ignoring, inconsistencies decreases the risk of error. Awareness of inconsistencies prevents fitting the data to hypotheses. Rather, hypotheses should be generated to fit the data actually present.

Weighting Cues in Judgment

Much research and rhetoric has occurred in order to explain how clinicians put information together. Do they add one cue to another, or are cues weighted? Some resolve this controversy by demonstrating that clinicians can do either (Anderson, 1972; Elstein, 1976).

When cues are added together to make a diagnostic judgment (Dx) the procedure is merely $a + b + c + d = Dx$. The whole (Dx) is merely a sum. For example, the following cues could be added together:

1 Two-centimeter-wide break in skin over coccyx
2 Demarcated border
3 White and glossy lesion
4 Minimal depth
5 Redness at borders and in adjacent skin
6 History of long periods of lying on back
7 Verbalized pain and discomfort
8 Left-sided paralysis

The problem would be decubitus ulcer. (Etiological factors will be ignored for the moment.) Do you think all pieces of information should be weighted exactly the same? In the above list, are some cues not as important *for diagnosis* as others?

The highest weighting would be given to *two-centimeter-wide break in skin over coccyx*. This is an ulcer. The term *decubitus* refers to lying down; the cue *history of long periods of lying on back* should be given weight equal to the skin break in diagnosis of a decubitus ulcer. *White and glossy lesion, minimal depth,* and *red at borders and in adjacent skin* are cues to severity (grading) of the lesion. They permit a finer discrimination and would be of equal value in judging severity. The cue, *demarcated border* would be weighted and valued lower; it is not as influential in judgment. *Verbalized pain and discomfort* is of low diagnostic value; it supports the observation, but the diagnostic judgment could be made without it. The verbal cue would not be available if the patient was comatose. (Actually, this cue points to another problem, that of pain management.)

Consider another example in which the judgment is not as clear. The setting is a community clinic. The client is being treated for hypertension. These cues are present:

1 Tense posture
2 Flat, low tone; slowed speech; dull, depressed facial expression
3 Lost job (company closed plant)
4 Depressed thoughts but no thought of suicide
5 Perceived himself as self-made success in past
6 Perceives self as self-made failure now
7 Wife is poorly controlled diabetic
8 Cannot discuss problems with friends: "They would think I was a failure."
9 Does not know what to do: "The job market is so bad"; "I just sit all day"; "This never happened to me before."

Consider the above cues and the following diagnoses; which is the best diagnostic judgment of the four?

- Self-concept disturbance/role change
- Ineffective coping/role change
- Potential for suicide
- Situational depression/role change

The selection of self-concept disturbance/role change suggests that cues 5 and 6 were weighted most heavily in judgment. Cues 8 and 9 may have been most impressive to some readers, who would then have chosen ineffective coping/role change. Cues 2, 4, 7, and 9 may have been most influential, thus leading to the conclusion that situational depression/role change was present. Selecting potential for suicide suggests that the reader discounted the cue *but no thought of suicide*; this verbal report must have been weighted very low or considered unreliable as a predictor.

Now let us see whether adding two other cues can influence judgment. One is a situational cue and the other is historical information. The clinic is a community mental health clinic and the client has a history of suicide attempts. Did these additional cues influence your weighting of previous cues?

The example demonstrates that different people can be influenced differently by information. This is especially true when data are uncertain, as clinical data are. Second, the example suggests that pieces of information are not always judged independently of one another. One cue can influence the weighting of another. Weighting and clustering information differently is probably the reason experts may differ in their diagnoses.

The third point demonstrated was that information can be discounted in making a diagnostic judgment. Care providers make an estimate of the quality of information. Their estimates can be affected by other information or inferences about the client and situation.

PROBLEM FORMULATION

In this and the previous chapter we have considered a strategy for going from no information to a diagnosis. The purpose of this section is to summarize the process. The summarization will trace the process of problem formulation, *which begins with the first cue to a dysfunctional pattern*. Consideration will be given to how problems formulated during the diagnostic process are stated as nursing diagnoses.

Irrespective of a nurse's conceptual framework for practice, certain cues are important. These are cues to the client's functional health patterns. When signs of a dysfunctional pattern appear, the need arises to describe and explain them. This need motivates the nurse to collect information beyond that which is elicited by a standardized assessment tool. To go beyond the predetermined format for assessment, a strategy is needed. First the universe of possibilities has to be narrowed. Second, after likely diagnoses are identified, a strategy is necessary to determine which diagnosis best describes the dysfunctional pattern.

A strategy describes a sequence of decisions about (1) what information to collect, (2) the sequence of collection, and (3) how to use the information. As we have seen, these decisions are guided by hypotheses about what the client's problem might be.

A diagnostic hypothesis is a tentative formulation of a health problem. It answers the question What could these cues mean? Early hypotheses may be as general as *nutritional problem* or as specific as *protein deficit*, depending on the background information available and the early cues elicited from the client.

Early information, such as medical disease, age, or initial impressions, usually includes cues to the client and situation. Although not specific to a particular nursing diagnosis, these cues can be used to predict a set of diagnostic hypotheses. For example, initial information and observations may reveal a thin, tense, elderly client admitted to a nursing home for long-term care. Cues like these can generate a number of tentative hypotheses early in the assessment of patterns.

The key to success in diagnosis is to generate alternative possibilities. This prevents settling too early on a favorite hypothesis. As discussed in Chapter 5, the nurse creates hypotheses by interpreting the possible meaning of a cue or cue cluster.

Meaning is derived from cues by clinical reasoning, both inductive and deductive. The particular meaning a nurse derives depends on the network of categories and propositions stored in that nurse's long-term memory. This network of propositions and categories includes clinical knowledge about how one cue relates to another, how cues relate to diagnoses, and the relationships among diagnoses. An example is knowledge about the relationship between cues to tension and the inference that the client is frightened. By deduction, the nurse may apply this knowledge to the tense, elderly client described previously. The broad hypothesis *fear* could then be generated.

Also stored in memory are estimates of the likelihood that particular cues are related to certain diagnoses under certain conditions. For example, the nurse has to calculate (1) the probability that the observed posture and muscle tone mean the client is tense, (2) the probability that being tense means the person is frightened, and (3) the likelihood that fear would occur in the context of a nursing home admission.

The reasoning involved in generating alternative hypotheses about the meaning of cues is called *branching*. Inferring that there could be four or five sources of fear would be an example of branching in the nursing home admission situation. The multiple hypotheses generated are then tested by obtaining data that predict which are most likely. This procedure permits narrowing the possibilities.

A strategy should permit the diagnostician (1) to narrow the universe of possibilities quickly and (2) to determine which hypotheses are most likely. Likelihood can be tested by obtaining contextual cues that are predictive. Using predictive cues to test multiple hypotheses *simultaneously* was referred to as *predictive hypothesis testing*. Inferential and memory requirements are high when this procedure is used, but maximum information is obtained from each question or observation. The other approach to hypothesis testing is *successive* testing of each hypothesis. Inferential and memory requirements are not as high, but neither is maximum information obtained from each cue with single-hypothesis testing.

Predictive hypothesis testing is a "risky but fast" strategy. Hypotheses judged to be extremely unlikely are eliminated. This reduces the number quickly, but risk is involved. The decision to eliminate hypotheses has to be based on reliable knowledge of the likelihood of a diagnosis in situations similar to the client's. Also, reliable predictive cues have to be used. On the other hand, not every nursing diagnosis (currently 44 have been identified) can be fully investigated.

When a few diagnostic hypotheses remain, a shift in hypothesis-testing procedure occurs. Now the objective is a focused search for specific cues. The most probable diagnoses are tested first. They serve to direct decisions about what information to collect and how it is to be used. Data are collected to determine whether the critical signs or symptoms that define each diagnosis are present.

When critical defining signs and symptoms of each tentative diagnosis are the focus of information collection, a single-hypothesis–testing procedure is appropriate. Obtaining data to test each hypothesis one by one should reveal which hypotheses are supported and which are not. As information is obtained it is clustered under the remaining hypotheses. The hypothesis which is supported is judged to be the diagnosis.

Studies suggest that human beings, having generated hypotheses, *seek* confirming evidence of their hypotheses. Could this mean that they discount diagnostic cues that do *not* support their hypotheses? Overdiagnosing could be the result, especially when dealing with ambiguous, uncertainty-based information.

Bourne and his colleagues argue that seeking confirming cues is an *appropriate and useful strategy* (1979, p. 289). Assessing signs and symptoms that should be present if the diagnosis is present will determine immediately whether the hypothesis is correct or not. The alternative, collecting data that would *disprove* a diagnostic hypothesis, requires too much cognitive work (Wason and Johnson-Laird, 1972). The end result would be that one would know which diagnoses are not supported but not which ones are (Bourne, Dominowski, and Loftus, 1979, pp. 289–290). This is a poor position to be in when having to plan care. Thus the best procedure is to test hypotheses by looking for signs and symptoms that would be present if the diagnosis was present. At the same time one must be alert to the possible tendency to seek support for favored hypotheses.

When signs and symptoms of a problem are not present but contextual cues and commonly associated etiological factors exist, the diagnosis of a potential problem should be considered. Etiological factors in this case are considered risk factors. The diagnosis of a potential problem is based on prediction and on a cluster of cues signifying susceptibility, risk, or potential for a dysfunctional pattern.

In summary, problem formulation begins with the first hypotheses generated to explain cues that are indicative of a dysfunctional pattern. The diagnostic strategy employed in admission assessment should:

1 Narrow the possibilities by identifying a problem space
2 Determine likely diagnostic hypotheses
3 Allow investigation of the most likely hypotheses first
4 Permit a focused cue search to test, modify, or discard hypotheses
5 Ensure confidence and accuracy in judging which diagnostic hypothesis is sufficiently supported

Discussion has focused on how to begin assessment and how to formulate a diagnosis when a dysfunctional pattern exists. The strategy is the same for *each* pattern area. As information accumulates, generating hypotheses becomes easier. Similarly, the focused cue search is more efficient as familiarity and trust begin to develop between the client and nurse.

With experience, tentative diagnostic hypotheses can be constructed during assessment. Rather than a review of 11 pattern areas, assessment becomes a flow across topics. Information is combined as the nurse proceeds. Possible problems are viewed in the context of previously accumulated data.

Because of a basic interest in people, most nurses derive satisfaction from getting to know their clients. Perhaps this is why assessment is one of the most interesting aspects of practice. Even more satisfaction is derived from being able to help. In the next section we will consider how the results of assessment are stated so that diagnoses can be the focus for the helping relationship nurses establish with clients.

Statement of Diagnoses

Following assessment of the 11 pattern areas, the nurse concisely records the data from the nursing history and examination and also the nursing diagnoses. A concise way of expressing a diagnosis on a record is to use a slash. Examples are lowered self-esteem/incomplete integration of body image change, and noncompliance (activity prescription)/knowledge deficit. (The format is problem/etiology.)

There has been discussion in the literature about how etiology should be expressed. Mundinger and Jauron (1975) suggest this format: lowered self-esteem *related to* incomplete integration of body image change. This approach is consistent with Henderson's idea of a relational concept (1978, p. 81); the concept of etiology, or cause, is related to the nurse's concept of the problem.

At the present time we do not have research to support the hypothesis that A, a set of interacting factors, *causes* B, a problem. Etiological factors are *probable causes*. They are arrived at by the best means and judgment at the time. Dictionary definitions of the terms *due to, related to,* or *associated with* do not provide clear guidelines for choosing one term over another; they are similar, although *due to* does appear more "certain" than the others.

Currently, not all diagnostic categories accepted for clinical testing (Appendix A) have etiological factors listed. Furthermore, the listed etiologies may not fit data you have collected. In these instances, formulate an etiological statement that best describes your data. Keep it clear, concise, and descriptive.

Accepted diagnostic categories can be used as labels for both problems and etiological factors. For example, one category name may describe signs and symptoms of a problem. Another category on the list may include the signs and symptoms of a probable cause of that problem (etiological factor). A client may have low self-esteem and the predominant cause may be altered body image. Or impaired home maintenance management may exist because of a mobility deficit. The listed diagnostic categories are combined as problem/etiology in the way (1) that best describes the clinical data one has and (2) that is most useful for planning intervention.

Depending on the supporting data available at the end of assessment, problems and etiological factors may be recorded as (1) a cluster of signs and symptoms, (2) tentative diagnostic or etiological hypotheses, or (3) nursing diagnoses. Let us consider first the two options that are available if the data available are insufficient for diagnosis.

A *cluster of signs and symptoms* can be recorded if insufficient data are available. A good rule is never to state a diagnosis unless critical defining characteristics are present. This rule prevents diagnoses based on inference rather than supporting data. On the other hand, remember that diagnoses are not statements of logical certainty; certainty may be impossible to attain even with additional data.

The admission assessment may support only *tentative hypotheses* about the client's problem or etiological factors. Record these as possibilities and continue assessment later.

The goal of assessment is to state *nursing diagnoses* that provide a clear basis for planning nursing care. As experience accumulates, the nurse will usually be able to state well-formulated diagnoses by the end of admission assessment; when that is possible, plans for dealing with problems can be discussed with the client. When the interaction among diagnoses in various pattern areas is not immediately clear, a review of findings is necessary.

Review of Findings The client's situation as a whole is the basis for all behavior observed during history and examination. Pattern areas are only a way of organizing data and coping with the complexity of the human situation. Therefore a review of findings is necessary to ensure that diagnostic judgments are not made in isolation. Interaction and interdependence of pattern areas have to be considered.

Each problem identified is reviewed in the context of the whole client-situation (environment). Is a problem really an etiological factor? Also consider the opposite—is an etiological factor really the basic problem? For example, is self-care deficit probably a result of the client's decreased activity tolerance? Suppose *sleep onset disturbance* is used to describe a dysfunctional sleep-rest pattern: Is this problem maintained by the ineffective coping pattern that also exists? A client can have current signs and symptoms that are not conclusive enough to support a diagnostic hypothesis.

Could they be predictive cues that signify a risk state? If so, does a potential problem exist?

A second consideration also requires a holistic view of the client-environment situation. Could the "problems" identified be optimal for the client and situation as a whole? For example, data may indicate noncompliance (dietary regimen) related to denial of illness or denial of prognosis of a disease. When all health-related data are considered, denial may be an optimal health perception pattern. No treatment may be indicated if the denial represents an effective coping pattern at the time. In other situations, the client may need help integrating new information. The problem may be formulated as delayed readiness to accept information/denial of illness. Situations such as these require thought. Discussion with colleagues is also useful when one is learning to state diagnoses.

Other Findings Few specific comments have been made about using the client's total data base, that is, data from physicians, nurses, and others (consultants). The writer has purposefully avoided including these other data sources in order to convey the idea that a nursing assessment is appropriate whether or not the client has a disease. Nursing diagnoses are identified by assessing *the client*, not just the client's *response to a disease.*

Considering the client-situation (environment) as we have done, prevents omission of factors such as disease, age, health history, or environment. All of these factors influence functional patterns. It is unlikely that shortness of breath, leg cramps, intolerance of foods, or sexual difficulties after neurological trauma could be missed in a functional pattern assessment. In a well-done nursing history and examination, dysfunctional patterns associated with disease will be apparent. What should be just as apparent are other contextual factors in the life of the client. These include developmental changes and environmental factors.

The client's disease, treatment, and prognosis are predictive cues. When combined with other contextual cues, they suggest possible dysfunctional patterns. For example, consider acute loss of hearing caused by an infectious disease. Uncompensated hearing loss can produce many functional problems. Predictions have to take into account the client's developmental level. The child who has not learned speech will have different problems from those of the 50-year-old, who has. Disease states can be used to predict dysfunctional patterns, but the predictions cannot be made in isolation from the client-situation as a whole.

Treatment of disease is a second factor that can be used to predict changes in functional patterns. Complete bed rest is a medical treatment that imposes almost total activity restriction. Obviously, this situation suggests potential problems requiring preventive nursing care; two examples are potential skin breakdown and potential joint contractures.

Imagine what it would be like to find out you have a chronic disease and that treatment will require changes in nutritional pattern, activity-exercise pattern, and others. Initially there may be a coping pattern disturbance. A knowledge deficit may produce noncompliance in disease management. These few examples emphasize the need to consider medical treatment as a situational factor influencing patterns.

The third factor used in prediction of dysfunctional patterns is the client's *prognosis.* A medical prognosis is a prediction about the course and outcome of a disease, including a prediction of the likelihood of recovery. All aspects of a prognosis can influence functional patterns. Particular effects on patterns depend on the organ or system involved. Prognosis for a stormy course, poor outcome, and poor likelihood of recovery has a generalized effect on the client-situation as a whole.

Is Disease an Etiological Factor? Theoretically, a disease, its treatment, and its prognosis can produce dysfunctional patterns. Observations of clients, at least in the acute care setting, appear to substantiate this theoretical possibility. Actually, there is no research either to support or to challenge these observations. Could the observations be slanted (biased) toward a conspicuous subgroup rather than representative of all people who have the disease? Are there people who have diseases but maintain optimal function for their situation? If so, then the generalization that a disease is the probable cause of a dysfunctional pattern will lead to error in some situations.

This issue of disease as the cause of a dysfunctional pattern is important. If a disease is specified as the etiology in a nursing diagnosis and if intervention is directed at etiological factors, do nurses treat diseases? Treatment of the disease would be necessary to remove the cause named in the nursing diagnosis. The question can also be raised: If a client's disease is cured, does the cure always produce optimal functioning within the patterns? It does not. Accordingly, one must consider whether dysfunctional patterns in people with disease may have multiple causes. Could it be that etiological factors other than disease are the focus of diagnosis and treatment by nurses?

Let us consider an example. The client has a fractured hip and is permitted no weight bearing. One nurse diagnosed impaired mobility due to fractured left hip. Designing a care plan *specific* to this diagnosis was difficult. A second nurse viewed the "real problem" as a self-care deficit (bathing-feeding-toileting) related to an uncompensated mobility impairment. (The latter problem formulation combines two accepted diagnostic categories.) The intervention then can be logically derived: Help the client to compensate for the mobility deficit.

Rewording Medical Problems Nursing diagnoses do not describe the total focus of nursing practice. Nurses carry out medical treatments and evaluate clients' responses to those treatments. They treat physiological problems (such as arrhythmias) and diseases under protocols. They also provide 24-hour observation of a client's responses to therapy. These types of treatments and observations are directed toward the disease process. Accepted terms are available for describing diseases; these can be used *after* the medical diagnosis is made. There is no need to relabel diseases.

Consider the following signs and symptoms: (1) confusion, (2) somnolence, (3) restlessness, (4) inability to move respiratory secretions, (5) decreased blood oxygen, and (6) increased blood carbon dioxide. This cluster of cues is labeled *impaired gas exchange* and is accepted for clinical testing as a nursing diagnosis (Kim and Moritz, 1981). Other nursing diagnoses of this type are *fluid volume deficit, alterations in cardiac output, ineffective breathing patterns,* and *chronic abnormal tissue perfusion.* These are pathophysiological conditions to be referred to a physician, not true nursing diagnoses, as *currently defined*. Actually, these descriptions are substitutions of patho-physiological terms for disease labels. Interestingly, each of these suggests the possibility that nursing diagnoses may be present that *are* amenable to nursing care.

Consistency among Care Providers' Diagnoses Some would argue that nursing diagnoses should be consistent with medical diagnoses or those of other care providers (American Nurses' Association, 1973). *Consistency* by definition means compatible, noncontradictory, or conforming to some principle or course of action.

The first point to be made is that there may be no medical diagnoses. Thus consistency is unattainable. The second point presents more difficulty. Problems diagnosed by physicians, nurses, or social workers are in three different domains: disease, functional patterns, and personal-social matters. Clients can have various problems in each area and in many combinations. Is a nursing diagnosis of unresolved grieving/loss of wife consistent with a medical diagnosis of appendicitis? A client could have both of these diagnoses, yet neither consistently predicts the other.

Apparent inconsistencies may arise in regard to assessment data collected by different professionals. Although used in different ways, many of the same data are gathered by the various health care providers. If the data are inconsistent, discussion among the professionals and reassessment can usually resolve any contradictions. If apparent inconsistency occurs at the level of diagnosis, disagreement on a diagnosis that is *well supported by data* is also resolved by discussion. The opinion of that care provider who is expert in the problem area and most knowledgeable about the client should be weighted most heavily.

Statement Modifiers In some cases modifying terms may be used in stating diagnoses. This is done to facilitate care planning. For example, a level of acuity may be specified. Terms such as acute, chronic, mild, moderate, and severe are useful.

With diagnoses such as impaired mobility or self-care deficit it is necessary to describe the client's position on a continuum. These problems range from level 1 (the client requires the use of equipment or a device) to level 4 (the client is totally dependent and does not participate in self-care). Level 4 is most often applicable to a client with extensive paralysis or one who is unconscious.

In this section a diagnostic (problem-formulation) strategy was summarized and factors to be considered in stating diagnoses were reviewed. Problem formulation begins early in the admission assessment. Gradually, as data accumulate, the "picture" of the client's functional health patterns emerges. As this occurs diagnoses are used to describe (by naming the problem) and explain (by identifying etiological factors) any dysfunctional patterns that are present.

After the assessment is completed, the findings are reviewed in the context of the picture that has emerged. This review requires taking a second look at all problems and etiological factors in the context of the client-situation as a whole.

Physicians' or consultants' findings, if available, are integrated as predictors during assessment. A client's disease is a superficial etiological factor; usually it is not used in stating a diagnosis for directing nursing care. It was recommended that diseases not be relabeled as nursing diagnoses. The section concluded with a discussion about difficulties in determining whether medical, nursing, and social casework diagnoses are consistent. Consistency across disciplines is complicated by the fact that the problems of interest to nurses, physicians, and social workers are in different domains.

When stating nursing diagnoses one must remember that the currently accepted list includes diagnoses at various levels of description and precision. New diagnostic categories may have to be created. Ten years hence diagnostic terms will be better defined; in the meantime the following guidelines may be useful for formulating a client's nursing diagnosis:

1 Ask yourself, Is *this* really the problem? Show other nurses the data base and see whether their diagnostic judgment is the same.

2 Are the problem and etiology identified in the diagnostic statement likely to be resolved with nursing care? (Using nonnursing consultation does not mean the problem is not a nursing diagnosis.)

3 Are the problem and etiological factors stated so that they can be used as a focus for planning nursing care? Currently identified nursing diagnoses need to be tried in practice. If they are not found to be useful in a particular instance, the nurse can and should come up with another concise descriptive term. Remember that the client's problem is not to be fitted to the diagnosis: The diagnosis is to be fitted to the client's problem.

With increasing experience in stating nursing diagnoses, the nurse may notice that certain clients' *problems* seem to cluster. In the next section some speculations will be offered about the idea of problem clusters.

Problem Clusters Currently the identified nursing diagnoses describe clusters of related *signs* and *symptoms*. A cluster of related diagnoses would be a *problem cluster*. Very little work has been done on problem clusters; in fact, there has been only speculation.

Some clients' diagnoses seem to be related by one broad etiological factor that could be the basis for all the specific problems. This common etiology is an overriding dysfunctional pattern similar to what is called a life pattern. In Roy's (1980) conceptual framework it would be a *general* pattern of maladaptation. Orem (1980) might call this a *general* pattern of impaired self-care agency. Rogers (1970) presumably would view it as a pattern and organization of the life process. What relevance does clustering specific diagnoses under one broad diagnosis have for nursing care?

If a composite pattern is identified as the *basis* for specific problems (including diseases), intervention may be needed at two levels. If a client has a nutritional problem, specific intervention is needed for that problem. Yet the nutritional problem and a coexisting cardiac disease may be just one part of a general life pattern. If a broad pattern is judged to be unhealthy, intervention is needed also at that broad, general level. In fact, perhaps all the specific problems could be resolved if the general life pattern changed.

Interventions at the level of broad life patterns may require more nursing skill than some beginning practitioners have acquired. First there is a need to validate with the client the general pattern the nurse has constructed from assessment data and diagnoses. This validation has to be undertaken with awareness that value-laden areas are going to arise. Human beings have freedom of choice about the way they live their lives, at least to a large extent. They may or may not wish to discuss the bases for their choices. Even when provided with health-related information, they may not wish to change. These wishes have to be respected.

Will diagnoses at the level of general patterns be identified? If identified will they be a useful focus for planning nursing care? Answers are not yet available. At present, intervention is at the problem level in most cases; perhaps this is the level that nurses believe is most useful. In a later chapter we will consider some work that relates to the general pattern level.

RETROSPECTIVE EVALUATION OF DIAGNOSES

When uncertainty in diagnosis can be reduced but not eliminated it is helpful to have ways of checking judgments. Checking that critical defining cues are present is one way of validating a diagnosis before intervention begins. A second way is to evaluate change in signs and symptoms of the problem after problem-specific intervention has been initiated. This second check involves retrospective evaluation of a diagnostic judgment.

Nursing care is directed at the probable cause, or etiology, of a problem and effectiveness of care is measured by client outcomes. If the outcome of nursing care is a positive change in the status of the problem, then the nurse may assume that the previously identified etiology was at least one probable cause. This procedure of evaluating the correctness of the etiology by observing the effectiveness of the intervention is a *retrospective test* of the cause of a problem.

Consider an example. If (1) knowledge deficit is *correctly* viewed as the predominant factor causing noncompliance and (2) the intervention is designed to increase the client's knowledge, then (3) the outcome assessment should indicate a change from noncompliance to compliance. What if this expected outcome does not occur, as shown in Table 6-1?

As may be seen in Table 6-1, one cannot make clear-cut assumptions about etiology from outcome data. If there is no change in signs and symptoms, several possible reasons have to be considered. Returning to the example about knowledge deficit, let us assume the intervention was the best possible for the diagnosis. Four questions can then be raised. Was knowledge deficit the correct etiology? Could there have been other, unidentified etiological factors? Were some events or situational factors overlooked? Was noncompliance just a sign of another problem? These are possible reasons why nursing care did not produce a change.

Now let us assume that the etiology is correct but the intervention was ineffective. As can be seen in Table 6-1, either the choice of intervention or its implementation (or both) may not have been correct. Knowledge deficit may indeed have been the predominant etiological factor, but teaching methods may have been ineffective—maybe the client's readiness for learning new information was not considered. It is useful to think about intervention as a test of the accuracy of nursing diagnosis.

The questions for consideration when the expected outcomes *are* attained (again see Table 6-1) will benefit future clients. Asking these questions enables the nurse to

TABLE 6-1
OUTCOME EVALUATION OF THE PROBLEM–ETIOLOGY
IDENTIFIED

Outcome evaluation	Considerations
I Change in problem status not as predicted (e.g., signs and symptoms of problem still present)	1 Were the assumed etiological factors (cause) not correct? 2 Were other unidentified factors, etiological or otherwise, operating? 3 Was the intervention inadequate to produce change in the problem? 4 Were the intervention methods applied correctly?
II Change in problem state as predicted (e.g., signs and symptoms of problem not present)	1 Are there any other explanations for the change in the problem? 2 Was the intervention influencing only the assumed etiological factors or others also?

learn from practice experiences. For example, was knowledge deficit the predominate cause of the client's noncompliance? Could it be that the human concern and rapport established during teaching influenced the client's *motivation*, and that that, rather than learning, produced change? Perhaps the intervention influenced other unspecified factors as well and the combined effect produced the result.

Unless these questions are considered, the previously effective combination of problem, etiology, and intervention, when applied in a future situation, may not produce the outcome. Why? Mainly because a *group* of etiological factors may be operating, not just the one or more that have been identified (in the present example, knowledge deficit). By chance, the intervention dealt with these unrecognized etiologies and hence produced the desired outcome.

Conclusions from unexamined judgments cannot be applied to future clients' problems. The kind of reflection just discussed is necessary. Essentially, this is called "learning from practice." Future clients benefit from the nurse's past experience. (This is probably why employment advertisements specify "experience required"; the implicit assumption is that past experience has been used to increase clinical judgment and skill.)

As one's diagnostic skills and clinical knowledge base increase, inferences or hypotheses will come quickly to mind and will guide data collection. Both diagnostic ability and clinical knowledge take time to acquire. The beginner should not be discouraged about failing to consider some factors the clinical specialist identifies but should instead use the specialist to increase his or her own clinical knowledge.

Reflection on the accuracy of diagnoses is an important part of learning. In addition it is always useful to know in advance the errors that can occur. This section dealt with hindsight; the discussion of sources of potential error in the next section deals with foresight.

SOURCES OF DIAGNOSTIC ERROR

Diagnostic errors lead to undertreatment or overtreatment of clients. If a problem is not diagnosed, harm may result or quality of life may be impaired. This failure to diagnose an existing problem is an error of *omission*. Harm and impairment of the quality of a client's life can also result from overdiagnosing, or diagnosing nonexistent problems. These diagnoses would be errors of *commission*. Both errors can occur during data collection, data interpretation, and data clustering. Discussion in this section will focus on potential errors in these areas and how to prevent them. It will be seen that clinical knowledge, inferential reasoning, and the ability to put information together are major influences on diagnostic accuracy.

Is it more serious to diagnose a problem when no problem exists or to judge the client "healthy" when a problem is present? In nursing diagnosis uncertainty and doubt will arise. It is usually said that clinicians must avoid errors. Because of the probabilistic nature of the information upon which diagnoses are made, it is more realistic to say that the error rate in diagnosis should be kept very low. To return to the question, Are certain errors more tolerable than others in doubtful situations?

Perhaps errors of omission and commission are not equally tolerated by clients, colleagues, and society. To determine which error is more serious, we need to look at the values practitioners hold and the social factors that influence values. On the basis of certain values, professions develop implicit but persuasive ways of dealing with uncertainty in judgments. Let us first discuss sources of error in nursing diagnosis and then consider how to prevent them.

Errors in Data Collection

The information collected during assessment influences the *entire* diagnostic process. If data are omitted, diagnoses can be missed. If large amounts of data are collected in an unorganized manner, cognitive processes can be overwhelmed. Irrelevant data can produce the same effect. Thoroughness is important. Yet data must be relevant to areas of nursing concern if the purpose of data collection is nursing diagnosis.

Inconsistencies and errors can enter into the history and examination. The particular data that are sought and the way the data are collected both influence accuracy. Methodological errors can be caused by inaccuracies in measurement of a client characteristic. Questions asked during history taking may lead the client to say what seems to be expected. Or the nurse may not listen attentively. Perceptual errors, such as underestimating the depth of respirations, or faulty equipment can also be a source of measurement error.

Neglecting to collect critical data is another source of potential error. The nurse may overlook critical cues because of distraction, lack of organization, or inadequate clinical knowledge. For example, lack of knowledge about coping deficits or about risk factors in potential skin breakdown can lead one to miss cues. Too narrow a concept of nursing may cause one to exclude some material from assessment (for example, coping patterns). Data collection errors result.

Failure to obtain client reports in areas about which the client's subjective information is critical is another source of inaccuracies. Similarly, relying on only predictive (contextual) data and inferences increases the rate of error; current data about the state of the client are also needed. Sometimes data are collected but not considered in analysis. Ignoring a critical cue that should have been pursued leads to errors of omission.

Overload of data can also lead the diagnostician astray. When large quantities of irrelevant data are collected, cognitive capacities for processing information can be overloaded. For example, questions may be irrelevant or clients may ramble.

To maintain a low rate of error in data collection, think of what the data collection process involves: (1) perceptual accuracy, (2) organization, and (3) interviewing and examination skills. First, consider *perceptual accuracy*. What may influence this? Clinical knowledge is one factor. People may at times observe without perceiving. Many errors in perception result from not having available categories for classifying sensory information. These categories are based on clinical knowledge. The nurse must be curious and question what is observed; this is how knowledge develops and errors are avoided for both the novice and expert diagnostician.

Perception is a neuropsychological phenomenon. Thus it is influenced by health states, fatigue, and boredom or routine. It is particularly important for perceptual alertness that nurses maintain their own functional health patterns, particularly sleep and rest. One could surmise that extended work shifts may tax perceptual-cognitive processes, perhaps especially in settings where continuous alertness is critical.

A second factor related to data collection errors is *organization*. There are two aspects: (1) preorganization and (2) organization during assessment. *Preassessment organization* has been emphasized in previous discussions. Briefly, one must know one's conceptual focus and the pattern areas. The critical areas for data collection within patterns should be listed. In addition, one must decide how to begin and select a possible sequence.

As data collection begins, *concurrent organization* is needed: that is, as the assessment proceeds, the nurse has to organize the data by generating hypotheses that permit clustering of data. (This has to be supplemented by recording the data also under pattern areas.) The human mind cannot handle large amounts of unorganized data. Some method of keeping track of what has gone before is needed because previous data and hypotheses influence what questions are asked in branching. Probably one of the major reasons for missing critical cues is lack of concurrent organization of data during history taking and examination.

Interviewing and examination skills are critical factors in perceptual accuracy. Data are generated by the things the nurse does. These activities include inquiries, supportive replies, silence, touching, and examination. Characteristics such as physical attributes of the head, face, shoulders, arms, and posture of a client in bed are observable. Actions are required to elicit data about less readily apparent characteristics. If these actions are not taken, not chosen wisely, or not performed correctly, perception suffers.

Errors in Data Interpretation

If the meaning of cues is inaccurately interpreted, diagnostic errors result. Cues signifying a dysfunctional pattern may not be interpreted as dysfunctional; an error of omission will result. Overdiagnosing occurs when a functional pattern is interpreted as dysfunctional. Usually the diagnostic errors occur because of inadequate clinical knowledge. Insufficiently taking developmental or individual norms into account also contributes to errors of interpretation.

Another source of error in data interpretation is overgeneralizing from one observation of client behavior. The behavioral sample can be inadequate (too few observations, or atypical ones) or interpreted outside the context of the situation in which the behavior took place. One episode of hostility does not mean the client is a hostile person. Remember that assessment relies on patterns of behavior, not isolated events. Similarly, a history of mental or cognitive disturbance may be purely history. Current data may be totally different.

To maintain a low rate of error the nurse must validate his or her inferences. Errors occur if hypotheses are not treated as tentative and subject to revision. Furthermore, generating hypotheses early does not mean that early ideas are the only ones considered. Additional data may require additional hypotheses.

When judgments have an element of uncertainty, probabilities have to be taken into account. Errors can result from incorrect notions about the likelihood of diagnoses. As described, an element of forecasting or prediction enters into diagnosis. Adequate testing of hypotheses helps to control errors in prediction.

One technique for examining interpretations of data is *reframing* (Clark, 1977). This is a process of shifting perspectives. A familiar example is looking at the sky and deciding the day is partly cloudy; from another perspective the day is partly sunny.

Behavior can have so many meanings that it is well to consider alternative explanations. Reframing can be applied to one or two cues, a tentative hypothesis, or a cluster of cues in a diagnosis. Try to reframe the following cues:

> This behavior is familiar to nurses who work in pediatric, public health, or school settings with "shy" children. A child who clings to his mother, withdraws, and does not play with other children is apt to make a lasting impression on a nurse. There is a tendency to call this "separation anxiety." (Clark, 1977, p. 840)

After attempting to look at these cues in a different way, read the following. Note that Clark reinterprets data from the perspective of the child's thinking:

> Reframing will enable the nurse to pick out the adaptive portions of the child's behavior from his point of view. The child does not know what the new experience holds. He only knows he has been taken to a strange place for some unclear purpose. He is actually to be commended for sticking close to the one familiar object in the environment, his mother, until he can figure out what is happening. In this sense, the child's behavior is quite adaptive, since it allows for some stability through closeness to mother until information can be gathered on what action is appropriate. (Clark, 1977, p. 840)

The earlier interpretation of separation anxiety may be realistic if the behavior continues. If separation anxiety is ultimately diagnosed, having considered adaptation as an alternative should increase the nurse's confidence that error has been avoided.

Try another example adapted from Clark (1977). For medical reasons a client requires complete bed rest. He is not to get out of bed. This activity restriction has been discussed with him and he acknowledges the need for it. Repeatedly the nurse observes the client out of bed. Obviously, the problem is noncompliance with activity prescription! What might be the reasons for this behavior? Is there a deeper problem? Here is how Clark reframed this data:

> To reframe the patient's behavior from his point of view, staying in bed may seem like an attempt to force him into a dependent, helpless position, and getting out of bed may be an adaptive maneuver. A patient who refuses to accept the "sick role" may harm himself physically in the short term, but he may be taking steps to preserve his long-term self-image. In other words, refusing to accept the "sick role" can be adaptive. (Clark, 1977, p. 840)

Reframing is similar to branching. It is an important concept in reducing errors. Try to see the world from the client's eyes when interpreting cues. Also, as previously recommended, obtain the client's perception of the health problem, its probable cause, and any action that has been taken to remedy the problem. A total reformulation or rejection of a hypothesis may result.

Errors in Data Clustering

Clustering, it may be recalled, is the combination of cues. Three kinds of errors can occur in clustering: A nursing diagnosis may be made prematurely, incorrectly, or not at all.

Premature closure is a common error. A diagnostic judgment is reached before all critical information has been considered or even before all information has been collected. The observations that have been made are inadequate supporting data.

One of the reasons a new charting system, the problem-oriented method, was introduced in hospitals around the country was to prevent premature closure. Problem-oriented recording requires the diagnostician to list the subjective and objective data for each problem. Clearly this form of charting forces the clinician to specify the data base for each diagnostic judgment. Having recorded the cues used in making each judgment, the clinician can examine whether or not sufficient supporting evidence is available. More will be said about this charting system in the next chapter.

Incorrect clustering of cues can occur in formulating the problem, in identifying the etiology, or in combining the problem and etiology. The result of incorrect clustering is that data supposedly supporting the diagnosis clearly contradict it (Voytovich, Rippey, and Copertino, 1980). This error is usually related to inadequate knowledge of critical signs and symptoms. It is similar to labeling a chair as a table. The rules for using any language apply also to diagnostic "language."

Lack of standardization of diagnostic categories used in nursing diagnosis contributes to this type of error. If the difference between a chair and table was not specified in dictionaries, errors in use of the terms would occur. The situation is similar in nursing diagnosis. Try to use currently identified signs, symptoms, and category definitions. The potential for errors will be reduced but probably not eliminated until precise definitions are standardized.

Not synthesizing (not combining cues) obviously leads to errors of omission. Whereas some nurses tend to close prematurely, others delay diagnostic judgment. This delay may represent an attempt to reach absolute certainty when in reality the situation is inevitably based on some degree of uncertainty. Think of a nursing diagnosis as the best hypothesis of the moment; be open to new information that can reject or further confirm judgments: These are the keys to working with uncertainty-based data and judgments.

Sometimes the only clinical data available are ambiguous. Doubt exists; yet a judgment has to be made. Although errors in judgment are to be avoided, some are considered more serious than others. Implicitly or explicitly, rules exist for avoiding errors the profession or society views as serious.

Implicit Rules

In an interesting article about unwritten rules for making decisions, Scheff (1963) examined differences in tolerance for certain errors of judgment. The following synopsis of his ideas will serve as a basis for considering what implicit rules might influence nursing diagnosis.

In a court of law, a person is innocent until proven guilty. The rule is "when in doubt, acquit." Underlying this rule are the assumptions that (1) conviction will do irreversible harm to a person's reputation, (2) the person is weak and defenseless relative to society, and (3) society can sustain some errors without serious consequences.

Note the dilemma. A legal judgment of guilty when innocent has serious consequences for the individual. Yet a judgment of innocent when guilty can have serious consequences for society. An acquitted offender may commit further crimes. Western society resolves the dilemma in favor of the individual; in fact the assumption of innocence is stated in legal codes and accepted by jurists.

What is actually occurring? There are two types of errors a jury could make:

Type I error: The accused is *actually guilty*, but the hypothesis of *not guilty* is accepted.

Type II error: The accused is *actually innocent*, but the hypothesis of *guilty* is accepted.

Before receiving data from witnesses and the interpretations of lawyers, juries are instructed to avoid a Type II error. Society does not tolerate convicting the innocent; if doubt exists, acquit.

In the profession of medicine, the same types of errors are possible when clinical data are ambiguous:

Type I error: The client *actually has a disease*, but the hypothesis of *no disease* is accepted.

Type II error: The client is *actually disease-free*, but the hypothesis of *disease* is accepted.

Colleagues, clients, and the general society generally do not tolerate a Type I error. What implicit rule is followed by practitioners of medicine?

According to Scheff (1963), the rule is not always explicitly stated or as rigid in medicine as in law. Yet it does exist: "When in doubt, diagnose disease." This bias can influence medical assessment. It encourages the physician to consider symptoms as possibly signifying illness until disease is ruled out. When in doubt, it is far more important to continue to suspect illness than to suspect health.

The assumptions that underly this implicit rule are: (1) undetected disease will have serious consequences, (2) diagnoses are not considered irreversible, and (3) society expects disease, if present, to be diagnosed. Physicians are aware that a malpractice legal decision can result from a Type I error. That is, a client may sue if dismissed as healthy when in fact disease was present and subsequently produced harm. Furthermore, if a client remains in society with untreated infectious disease or behavior harmful to others, there may be serious consequences.

A dilemma accompanies the rule "When in doubt diagnose or suspect illness." Calling clients' attention to their bodily state can produce physiological and psychological changes. The client may alter many aspects of life and assume the sick role in work, family, and social situations (Haynes, Sackett, Taylor, Gibson, and Johnson, 1978). Furthermore, psychiatric as well as some medical disease labels carry social stigma. Type II errors are costly to individuals or society, and many people question whether unnecessary surgical and psychiatric treatment is occurring. Yet the implicit rule of "Better safe than sorry" prevails (Scheff, 1963, p. 100).

Scheff suggests that personal biases toward Type I or Type II errors are influenced by the disease characteristics, the physician, the client, and the health care setting in which diagnoses are made. He raises a number of possibilities that are relevant to nursing as well as medical diagnosis:

> Physicians who generally *favor active intervention* probably make more Type II errors than physicians who view their treatments only as assistance for natural bodily reactions to disease. The physician's *perception of the personality of the patient* may also be relevant; Type II errors are less likely if the physician defines the patient as a "crock," a person who ignores or denies disease.
>
> The organizational setting is relevant to the extent that it influences the relationship between the doctor and the patient. In some contexts, as in medical practice in organizations such as the military or industrial setting, the physician is not as likely to *feel personal responsibility* for the patient as he would in others, such as private practice. This may be due in part to the conditions of financial remuneration, and perhaps equally important, the sheer volume of patients dependent on the doctor's time. Cultural or class differences may also affect the amount of social distance between doctor and patient, and therefore the amount of responsibility which the doctor feels for the patient. Whatever the sources, the more the physician feels personally responsible for the patient, the more likely he is to make a Type II error. (Scheff, 1963, p. 104)

It is also interesting to think about whether nurses are influenced by their perception of the personality of the client, for example, in the initial impression. Does perception of personal responsibility for a client versus perception of team responsibility influence diagnostic errors? Do nurses who view nursing as assisting the client make fewer Type II errors than nurses who view nursing as doing things for the client? Answers are not available, but the questions provoke thought.

No research has been published about nursing diagnostic errors. One could imagine that there are rules that bias practitioners toward either of the following errors:

Type I error: The client actually *has a functional health problem*, but the hypothesis of *no problem* is accepted.

Type II error: The client is *actually problem-free*, but the hypothesis of *functional health problem* is accepted.

In doubtful situations are the rules in nursing similar to those of the courtroom? When in doubt, assume health. Or are nurses' implicit rules and assumptions similar to those of their colleagues in medicine? When in doubt, diagnose a problem (or continue to suspect a problem).

Many comments are heard admonishing nurses *not* to be problem-focused. It is said that the client's strengths, not problems, should be emphasized. This is quite true in *treatment*. Focusing on strengths—areas of wellness and capabilities—is an approach that mobilizes the client's resources. In *diagnosis*, a bias toward recognition of health rather than of problematic states can result in diagnostic errors of omission, Type I errors. If symptoms signifying diagnostic hypotheses are not investigated, problems can be missed.

With regard to observing signs and symptoms of disease, nurses are told that when in doubt they should assume these signify complications and call a physician. As Hammond (1966, p. 29) has suggested, nurses have to think for themselves as well as think "as" the doctor thinks; when observing disease states and carrying out medical treatment the nurse is under the "cognitive control of the doctor." Within this cognitive set may be the rule "When in doubt, diagnose or suspect disease complications." Is it difficult to shift to an opposite rule in nursing diagnosis? This question would make an interesting clinical study.

Legal as well as moral responsibilities argue for avoiding errors of omission. It is understandable that one may not wish to diagnose potential for injury or trauma when cues are uncertain. This diagnosis, for example, might necessitate cautioning the truck driver with uncontrolled seizures not to drive although his employment would be interrupted by following that recommendation. Values enter into any judgment. The best thing is to be aware of the potential consequences of diagnosis and treatment when symptoms are doubtful.

Also, be aware of the consequences of delay in diagnosis and treatment. If delay is the action of choice, continue to collect data and attempt to resolve ambiguities. Learn the technique of discussing observations with clients in a nonthreatening, nonanxiety-producing manner. They can help, when psychologically and physically able, to identify their actual or potential health problems. It is very important that the nurse not reinforce the sick role but instead help clients to *feel capable* of handling any health problems diagnosed.

In addition to errors of omission (Type I) and errors of commission (Type II) there is an "error of the third kind," solving the *wrong* problem (Mitroff and Featheringham, 1974). Preparing a care plan for the wrong problem wastes nursing time. Most importantly, the real problem can cause client discomfort if allowed to progress.

Diagnosing and treating the wrong problem can usually be avoided if the meaning of client behavior is explored. The only way to understand the behavior of the client is to ask. It is as simple as that. Inferences made without checking the client's viewpoint can lead to completely erroneous problem formulations and ineffective care plans.

Case Example

The following case will illustrate problem formulation. The setting is a hospital. As you read the *nursing* assessment and take notes, attempt to cluster the cues that signify actual or potential health problems.

Before making this assessment the nurse had background information from the physician's history and physical examination. The client, Mr. K, had a 5-year history of "slightly elevated blood pressure." *One year ago* he had experienced an episode of dizziness for 12 hours. *At that time* he started taking medication for his blood pressure. *Six months ago* he had discontinued medication when he felt better. In the *last 6 months* before his admission, two other episodes of dizziness occurred, lasting 1 to 2 hours and being relieved by rest. Frequent headaches were also reported.

Mr. K's father, now deceased, had had diabetes and hypertension. The client's mother, who died one year ago of a stroke, had also had hypertension. His wife and two children (14 and 10 years old) are well.

An episode of dizziness and numbness of his left arm brought Mr. K to the emergency room. The physician described him as a 55-year-old obese Caucasian male who was head of a Spanish center in a large southern city. The medical diagnosis at admission was hypertension and transient ischemic attack. This diagnosis and his family history placed Mr. K at risk for a stroke.

When the nurse began the nursing history and assessment, Mr. K's dizziness and numbness had gone. The background information suggested the possibility of problems in his health-perception–health-management pattern. The following assessment data were collected; the main diagnostic hypotheses the nurse raised while doing the assessment are added in italics.

Nursing History and Examination

First hospital admission of 55-year-old married, obese, white male administrator of a Spanish center. Sitting upright in bed, tense posture and expression (*fear; obesity*).

Health-perception–health-management pattern: Viewed health as good until 1 year ago when diagnosed as "having high blood pressure." States job "stressful" "but the people need me" (*job stress*). Had headaches for last 6 months and two episodes of dizziness (one at work and one at home) lasting about 2 hours. Rested and symptoms went away. Delayed seeking care because was "too busy" (*job stress*). Thought dizziness was caused by "overwork," not blood pressure (*job stress*). Discontinued blood pressure medication and M.D. visits about 6 months ago "when blood pressure came down and I felt better"; states medicine caused impotence (*potential noncompliance/disease management*). To emergency room today because of left arm numbness and fear of stroke. Mother died of "stroke" 15 months ago. Concerned that he hasn't been taking care of himself; states, "I need to learn about what to do." Wants to know "everything" (*fear of stroke or death*). Asked if OK to do some job-related paper work if someone brought it in (*job stress*). Takes no medicines currently except Alka-Seltzer and laxative; doesn't smoke; social drinking.

During introductions and while stating the purpose of the interview, the nurse's first impression was of a person in fear. Mr. K was sitting upright in bed; his posture and facial expression were tense. It was inferred that he had been very frightened by the loss of feeling in his arm. Was he interpreting his symptoms in the context of his past experience (mother's stroke and death)? The hypothesis of fear influenced the conduct of the interview. It was important to establish trust in care providers to provide some reassurance.

The hypothesis of obesity was also generated from the initial impression. The nurse planned to follow up this topic when nutritional and activity patterns were assessed.

Review of the client's health-perception pattern indicated a change. He had thought his health was good until 1 year ago, when high blood pressure was diagnosed. Although blood pressure had been "slightly elevated" for 5 years, the change in health perception had probably occurred with the first episode of dizziness and start of medication. This was also about the time of his mother's death.

Six months after beginning treatment, Mr. K preceived that his "blood pressure came down" and he "felt better." Sexual impotence had occurred (impotence is common with certain blood pressure medications) and he discontinued medication and medical care. Further symptoms occurred and the client's action was to rest. This action was consistent with his previous interpretation of the cause of symptoms, "overwork" and being "too busy." There seems to have been delay in seeking health care, but today the loss of sensation in his arm could not be ignored.

Previously there may have been denial of change in health state or vulnerability. In addition the client may not have had knowledge to interpret the physical signs. What should the present data suggest to a nurse? One, the present symptoms have had an impact. Two, the client wants to "learn what to do." Yet knowledge deficit may not be the only reason for his past behavior.

The tentative diagnostic hypothesis, potential noncompliance, served to cluster early cues and inferences—past history of not attending to symptoms, discontinuation of medication and care, misinterpretation of symptoms, and possible conflict between his health management and work-related activities. Knowledge deficit may be *one* risk factor, but the cue of "too busy" suggests motivational or time-management factors. The need to "learn what to do" is suggestive; yet readiness for learning and actual knowledge deficiencies need further assessment. Moreover, the client does not yet have medical recommendations for future care, so teaching about self-care in compliance with the medical regimen will have to be deferred.

Mr. K's asking whether he may do job-related paper work could have meaning. Does he need to take his mind off his concerns, need diversion, have guilt about being away from his responsibilities, or need to maintain the self-perception of being well enough to do work?

"Wants to know everything" was tentatively interpreted as either fear, need for control, or motivation toward better health management. This and the cues to dysfunctional patterns cited previously were underlined during note taking for follow-up as other patterns were assessed.

The nurse suggested to Mr. K that he seemed to want and need more information to help him plan how he could take care of himself. Then a smooth transition was made to the next area discussed which was his nutritional-metabolic pattern.

Nutritional-metabolic pattern: Mr. K's diet history revealed adequate protein, excess carbohydrate and fat, minimal high-roughage foods (fruits and vegetables), approximately 3 cups of coffee per day, but a fluid intake of 700–800cc/day (*constipation pattern*). No history of lesions in mouth corners or mucous membranes. Has gained weight gradually last 15 years (*exogenous obesity*); dieting unsuccessful; problem is "probably the stress of my job; I get home and eat a big supper and snacks in the evening"; no food dislikes (*caloric excess*). Takes lunch (sandwich and cake) to work and eats at desk. Restaurants in area not good. Some indigestion and heartburn after lunch attributed to days with multiple stressors (*job stress*); takes Alka-Seltzer.

At this point the nurse reevaluated Mr. K's emotional state. He had begun to relax his body and facial muscles.

Unsuccessful dieting, excessive intake of carbohydrate and fat, "big supper and snacks," minimal high-roughage foods, report of gradual weight gain last 15 years, and the absence of an endocrine disease (medical assessment data) suggested the probable cause of obesity was caloric intake. Intake of both fluid and high-roughage food was low. These cues will have to be followed up when Mr. K's elimination pattern is assessed. The cues "days with multiple problems" and "stress of job" supported the previous hypothesis of job stress. This stress will have to be further assessed. It is influencing hypertension management and the client's nutritional pattern. The nurse then assessed the elimination pattern.

Elimination pattern: Daily bowel movement pattern with 2 or 3 episodes per month of constipation (hard stools and straining) lasting 2 days; laxatives used when constipation occurs (*intermittent constipation pattern/dietary habits*). Attributes constipation to his diet; knows he should eat better.

The data about this pattern supported the hypothesis of intermittent constipation pattern. Was the constipation related to dietary habits (low fluid intake, minimal high-roughage foods) previously reported? Job stress may be a contributing factor. In this pattern there is again evidence of health-management deficit. A picture of conflict between health practices and work "responsibilities" seems to be emerging.

Activity-exercise pattern: Spectator sports, uses car, minimal walking due to time schedule, sedentary job, considers self too old for exercise. Increasing fatigue last few weeks, less energy during the 2 months before admission; no self-care deficit (*decreased activity tolerance* and *knowledge deficit: age-exercise*). Recreation consists of reading novels, watching TV, dining with other couples. Lives in first floor apartment in city and drives 3/4 mile to work (*exogenous obesity/caloric intake-energy expenditure imbalance*).

Activities (work and leisure) suggested a sedentary pattern with minimal exercise. The perception of having less energy was not attributable to anemia (laboratory tests) or heart failure (physician's examination). Yet the perceptions of fatigue and less energy were real; the hypothesis was descriptive of the functional problem, decreased activity tolerance. Again, there was further indication that a busy schedule was conflicting with health management. Knowledge deficit existed regarding age and exercise. Also, note the revision of the hypothesis about obesity; information from two pattern areas was clustered and exogenous obesity/caloric intake–energy expenditure imbalance was formulated.

Sleep pattern: Averages 4 to 6 hours of sleep per night, quiet atmosphere, own room with wife, double bed, uses bed board. Presleep activities include watching TV or completing paper work from job; difficulty with sleep onset 1 month; awakens many mornings thinking about job-related problems (*sleep pattern disturbance/ presleep activities; job stress*).

A sleep pattern disturbance existed. This may have been contributing to the increasing fatigue. A probable cause lay in the presleep activity (paper work from job). Comments about awakening with thoughts of job-related problems supported the nurse's supposition that job stress was an influential factor for this client. Cues were clustered under this etiological hypothesis and presleep activities.

Cognitive-perceptual pattern: Sight corrected with glasses, changed 1 year ago; no change in hearing, taste, smell. No perceived change in memory; "I couldn't take it if I started losing my mind, like with a stroke" (*fear of stroke*). Learning ability: sees self as somewhat slower than in college, alert manner, grasps questions easily. Takes no sedatives, tranquilizers, other drugs. No headache at present.

Again during discussion of this pattern there was mention of stroke. Fear (stroke) was further supported.

Self-perception–self-concept pattern: Sees self as needing to do things well (job, father role, husband role); "Sometimes I don't think I'm doing well with my family, having them live in this area, but in my job you have to be near when people need help" (*role conflict*). "It will be just great [sarcasm] if I get sick and they have to take care of me instead of me taking care of them" (*fear of dependency*).

Conflict between sense of responsibility to family and to job seemed to be present. Now he will have three responsibilities to balance: family, job, and responsibility to self (health). Fear (stroke) was changed to fear (dependency). The cue "just great if I get sick and they have to take care of me . . ." influenced this modification.

Role-relationship pattern: Describes family as happy and understanding of his job commitments; wife former social worker; "kids good." "But I know we'll have trouble as Joe [10 years old] gets older"; "Maybe I should move out of [lower socioeconomic neighborhood]"; 10-year-old assaulted 4 months ago; 14-year-old boy interested in sports and "keeps out of trouble, so far" (*family concerns*). Family usually "sits down together" to handle problems. Social relationships confined to "a few other couples"; finds this sufficient. Job demanding 9 to 10 hours per day; "always trying to get money to keep the center solvent" (*job stress*). Assistant taking over while in hospital. Enjoys job and helping people; coworkers are "good to work with." Wife states the two of them are close; worried about husband's health; states he is more concerned with other people than himself; she admires him for this. Wife able to handle home responsibilities during hospitalization. States she and children had physical exam recently; no health problems; no elevation in blood pressure.

The family relationships elicited were positive and supportive. Concern and indecision were voiced regarding the environment (assault, "know we'll have trouble," and "maybe I should move"). The neighborhood environment could be a source of worry and stress in addition to the job problems (center's financial solvency).

A picture of his work was emerging: indigestion and heartburn on "days with multiple problems"; "stress of job"; "job was cause of high blood pressure"; "too busy"; "overwork"; wants to do job-related paper work in hospital; sedentary job; awakens thinking of job-related problems; financial solvency; presleep activities sometimes job-related; and job demands 9 to 10 hours per day. These data were clustered as job stress. Is he saying that although his work is stressful he enjoys it and his coworkers?

Concern expressed by Mr. K's wife was expected under the circumstances. She and the children were managing, so at present there was no evidence of family coping problems. How did her comment about the client's concern for others fit into the picture? Is this a value that the client and his wife hold?

Sexual-reproductive pattern: Two children; states impotent when on BP medication. When BP "went down," stopped meds; potency returned (*potential noncompliance*). No problems perceived in sexual relationship.

These data generated no new hypotheses. The information about impotency related to blood pressure medication would be a useful aid to the physician in his or her choice of medication.

Coping–stress-tolerance pattern: Feels tense at work (*job stress*); has tried relaxation exercises with some alleviation; doesn't always have time. States the best way to deal with problems is to "attack them." Afraid of having a stroke and being dependent: "This thing today has really scared me" (*fear of dependency*). "I have too many things to think about at work and at home, and now this blood pressure thing" (*role conflict*). Life changes: father died 3 years ago; mother died of stroke 15 months ago; took job at Spanish center 2 years ago to be near mother who "was getting old." Pleased he did this and feels good about it.

The previous mention of job and family stressors led naturally to a discussion of the coping–stress-tolerance pattern. "Attacking" problems seemed to be the predominant coping pattern expressed. The continuing theme of job stress was evident. Job stress was now interpreted as the factor receiving the "blame" for his state of affairs.

Further support for the fear (dependency) hypothesis was found in the cue "This thing . . . really scared me." The tentative hypothesis of conflict received support from the cue "Too many things to think about, and now this. . . ." Questions regarding his mother's death elicited no verbal or nonverbal cues to unresolved grieving.

The life changes as well as the assault on his child placed considerable strain on coping patterns. Yet there were indications of support (family relationships) and a disposition toward finding a solution for present problems.

Value-belief pattern: "Life has been good to me"; feels deeply about "injustices in society" and wants to do something about them (*value conflict*). States family is important to him. Religion (Catholic) important to him; would like to be active in church affairs.

In response to a question about things important to him, "injustices" and family were mentioned. These data prompted a change in the earlier hypothesis of role conflict. A value conflict is more likely present. This hypothesis revision was supported by cues about (1) family concerns and perceived responsibilities, (2) the valuing of the needs of others, and (3) time available.

The nurse performed an examination following the history. The above hypotheses were kept in mind. There was also an openness to further cues.

Examination

Vital signs: BP 205/118; T 37.6°C (99.8°F); P 80, regular and strong; R 18
Nutritional-metabolic pattern:
Skin No redness over bony prominences; no lesions. Dryness, calluses on feet with discomfort when touched.
Oral mucous membranes Moist, no lesions.
Height and weight 180 cm (5 ft 11 in); 104 kg (230 lb) actual weight; 99.8 kg (220 lb) reported weight.
Activity-exercise pattern:
Gait Steady.
Posture Well balanced.
Muscle tone, strength, and coordination Hand grip firm left and right; lifts legs; can pick up pencil; tenseness in neck and shoulder muscles.
Range of motion (joints) Within normal limits.
Prosthesis and assistive devices None.
Absence of body part No.
Cognitive-perceptual pattern:
Perception Hears whisper; reads newsprint with glasses.
Cognition Language—English; grasps ideas, both abstract and concrete; speech clear; attention span good.

Self-perception–self-conception pattern:
General appearance   Well groomed, evidences good hygiene.
Nervous or relaxed   Tense; some relaxation during history taking.
Eye contact   Yes.
Attention span   Good.
Role-relationship pattern:
Interactions   Communications with wife supportive, both somewhat tense; children not present.

Obesity was further confirmed by the height and weight measurements. Tenseness of neck muscles was clustered with other cues to Fear (dependency). Numbness of left arm had disappeared.

The nursing history and examination provide a beginning understanding of the client's health patterns. The history and examination also demonstrate the individuality of clients and show how assessment can identify clients' problems. Diagnostic hypotheses in Mr. K's situation were added, deleted and revised as follows:

Fear → fear (stroke; death) → fear (stroke) → fear (dependency)
Obesity → exogenous obesity → exogenous obesity/caloric intake–energy expenditure imbalance
Job stress → (delete; incorporated under value conflict and responsibilities)
Potential noncompliance (health management)
Constipation → intermittent constipation pattern/dietary pattern → intermittent constipation pattern/dietary and exercise pattern
Caloric excess → (delete; incorporated as etiology of obesity)
Decreased activity tolerance (to be evaluated further after medical treatment)
Knowledge deficit (age and exercise; incorporated under health management)
Sleep pattern disturbance/presleep activity, job stress
Family concerns → (delete; incorporated under value conflict and responsibilities)
Role conflict → (delete; incorporated under value conflict and responsibilities)
Value conflict → value conflict/perceived job and family responsibilities

A final review of findings produced further revision. The following nursing diagnoses, supported by data, were recorded (a slash separates the problem and etiology):

Exogenous obesity/caloric intake–energy expenditure imbalance
Intermittent constipation pattern/dietary and exercise pattern
Sleep pattern disturbance/presleep activity, perceived responsibilities
Fear (dependency)/perceived risk of stroke
Potential health managment deficit
Value conflict/perceived job and family responsibilities

The diagnoses related to obesity, sleep, and constipation became more specific as data accumulated. It can be noted that these represent a problem in one pattern area and etiological factors in other pattern areas.

Fear (dependency) was probably related to the perceived risk of a stroke. A care plan that emphasized developing a feeling of personal control through reduction of risk factors might help this client.

Potential health management deficit was used to describe the history of non-compliance with medication and follow-up care and the client's general neglect of health. The diagnosis *potential noncompliance* could have been used. Yet no evidence was present to suggest there was previous intention to comply.[2] In addition, there were data to support an interest in learning "what to do." The care plan would emphasize teaching and counseling for general health promotion. Special emphasis would be given to correcting misinformation about age and exercise. A podiatry referral will be recommended to Mr. K to relieve his calluses, which may cause sufficient discomfort to prevent walking and other forms of exercise. Specific teaching would be provided about hypertension and other areas of risk factor management.

A conflict in values existed. Mr. K's family was important to him. Also important was his contribution to resolving "injustices" through his work. A sense of responsibility "to do things well" in both areas produced conflict. The cues were: "need to be near when people need help," "maybe I should move . . . ," "sometimes I don't think I'm doing well with my family . . . ," more concerned with others than himself, enjoys job and helping people, and multiple references to demanding responsibilities in his job. The cues were clustered and described as value conflict related to perceived job and family responsibilities.

From the nurse's perspective, the problem is more complex. The client's value system (hence his conflict) should also include responsibility to himself, to protect his own health. A serious illness will not permit Mr. K to realize either set of values or carry out the responsibilities he has chosen to assume. Yet at this time there are few cues that his conflict includes health-maintenance responsibilities to self. The nursing diagnosis has to describe the conflict that exists, not the conflict that *should* exist.

Nursing care will focus first on helping the client to examine the possibility of balancing his life. First, things important to him will be discussed, that is, his perceived job and family responsibilities. It is expected that current health concerns will come to be perceived as a third area of conflict. This insight can then lead to an examination of how a balance of responsibilities can be attained. The nurse must exercise caution during these explorations of Mr. K's personal values and lifestyle, since clients have a right to choose how to conduct their lives. The nursing responsibility is to help them look at alternatives that include health promotion. In the end, the client chooses.

The case of Mr. K illustrates the broad life pattern that was previously discussed as an overriding pattern that encompasses all diagnoses. For example, *all* of Mr. K's health problems seem to be related to the choices he has made and the responsibilities he has chosen, and not chosen, to assume. In fact, a nursing diagnosis could be stated as: health management deficit related to value-choice pattern. Currently, some nurses intuitively grasp clients' life pattern problems and intervene at this broad level. But questions remain. Is this level of problem identification useful for planning intervention? Are both broad and specific levels of diagnosis needed?

---

[2]*Noncompliance* is defined as failure to participate in carrying out the plan of care *after indicating initial intention to comply.*

Could this broad pattern be identified without going through the step of identifying specific diagnoses, such as exogenous obesity, sleep pattern disturbance and the other diagnoses in this case?

The first step toward answering these questions is to have nursing diagnosis an integral part of nursing practice. Then it will be possible to see at what level diagnoses should be formulated. Facilitation of care planning will always be an important criterion by which nursing diagnosis is further developed, and decisions about level of diagnosis will be made in accordance with that criterion.

SUMMARY

The first topic in this chapter was concerned with hypothesis-testing procedures within a strategy. Once the likely diagnostic hypotheses have been generated from cues, these procedures are used to test the hypotheses. The focus is on critical diagnostic cues. If present, these are supportive evidence for the presence of a health problem. Single hypothesis testing was recommended; this procedure permits a search for specific cues to test likely hypotheses one by one.

The second topic discussed was information clustering. As are information collection and interpretation, clustering of cues is a continuous activity throughout the diagnostic process. As information is obtained and clustered with previous data, a judgment is made. Is data consistent or inconsistent with previous information and expectations? Before one judges that information is inconsistent, a double check should be made of measurements, expectations, and interpretation of data. This prevents fitting the information to a hypothesis; rather, diagnostic hypotheses should be generated to describe or explain the data actually present.

In addition to being judged as to consistency, information is weighted while it is being clustered. Weighting refers to the power of a cue to influence judgment that a hypothesis is supported or not supported. It was demonstrated in the discussion and by examples that cues are weighted in the context of other cues. In most situations a cue has more influence in diagnostic judgment if it "fits the picture."

Weighting of information is also influenced by judgments about the source of information. If the client or other informant is thought to be unreliable or biased, information that person supplies may be discounted. This may also occur when reports conflict or a client is negatively stereotyped. Caution should be exercised not to discount information without first investigating the accuracy of the nurse's impressions about the informant.

The third topic was problem formulation. This process begins with the first hypotheses generated and ends with a nursing diagnosis. The important point to realize is that tentative diagnoses are formulated when the first cue to a dysfunctional pattern is observed. When assessment of pattern areas has been completed, a review of findings is necessary. Diagnostic hypotheses, supported by data, are examined in the context of the client's total situation. Nursing diagnoses are then stated and used as a basis for planning care.

Retrospective tests of diagnoses were suggested. It was seen that if anticipated outcomes do not occur both diagnoses and interventions should be examined for error.

Another way of preventing errors was to be aware of the sources of diagnostic error. Data collection, interpretation, and clustering were examined as sources of potential error.

A case example of an assessment illustrated how diagnostic hypotheses are generated and investigated during assessment. The example also showed how findings from the admission assessment are reviewed and nursing diagnoses stated. The next chapter will explore the use of nursing diagnoses in planning care and in other nursing activities.

BIBLIOGRAPHY

American Nurses' Association. *Standards for nursing practice.* Kansas City, Mo.: American Nurses' Association, 1973.

Anderson, N. H. Looking for configurality in clinical judgment. *Psychological Bulletin*, August 1972, *78*, 93–102.

Aspinall, M. J. Use of a decision tree to improve accuracy of diagnosis. *Nursing Research*, May-June 1979, *28*, 182–185.

Bourne, L. E., Jr., Dominowski, R. L., & Loftus, E. F. *Cognitive processes.* Englewood Cliffs, N.J.: Prentice-Hall, 1979.

Bruner, J. S., Goodnow, J. J., & Austin, G. A. *A study of thinking.* New York: Wiley, 1956.

Clark, N. Reframing. *American Journal of Nursing*, May 1977, *77*, 840–841.

Elstein, A. S. Clinical judgment: Psychological research and medical practice. *Science*, November 1976, *194*, 696–700.

Gordon, M. *Manual of nursing diagnoses.* New York: McGraw-Hill, 1982.

Gordon, M. Predictive strategies in diagnostic tasks. *Nursing Research*, January-February 1980, *29*, 39–46.

Gordon, M. *Probabilistic concept attainment: A study of nursing diagnosis.* Unpublished doctoral dissertation, Boston College, 1972.

Hammond, K. R. Clinical inference in nursing: A psychologist's viewpoint. *Nursing Research*, 1966, *15*, 27–38.

Haynes, R. B., Sackett, D. L., Taylor, D. W., Gibson, E. S., & Johnson, A. L. Increased absenteeism from work after detection and labeling of hypertensive patients. *New England Journal of Medicine,* October 1978, *299*, 741–744.

Henderson, B. Nursing diagnosis: Theory and practice. *Advances in Nursing Science*, October 1978, *1*, 75–83.

Kim, M. J., & Moritz, D. A. *Classification of nursing diagnoses: Proceedings of the third and fourth national conferences on classification of nursing diagnoses.* New York: McGraw-Hill, 1981.

Mitroff, I. I., & Featheringham, T. R. On systemic problem solving and the error of the third kind. *Behavioral Science*, 1974, *19*, 383–393.

Mundinger, M. O., & Jauron, D. G. Developing a nursing diagnosis. *Nursing Outlook*, 1975, *23*, 94–98.

Nicoletti, A., Reitz, S., & Gordon, M. Descriptive research on parenting. In M. J. Kim & D. A. Moritz (Eds.), *Classification of nursing diagnoses: Proceedings of the third and fourth national conferences on classification of nursing diagnoses.* New York: McGraw-Hill, 1981.

Orem, D. *Nursing: Concepts of practice.* New York: McGraw-Hill, 1980.

Rogers, M. *An introduction to the theoretical basis of nursing.* Philadelphia: Davis, 1970.

Rosenhan, D. L. On being sane in insane places. *Science*, January 19, 1973, *179*, 250–258.

Roy, C. Roy adaptation model. In J. P. Riehl & C. Roy (Eds.), *Conceptual models of nursing practice*. New York: Appleton-Century-Crofts, 1980.

Scheff, T. J. Decision rules, types of error, and their consequences in medical diagnosis. *Behavioral Science*, 1963, *8*, 97–107.

Schwartz, A. K., and Aaron, N. S. *Somniquest*. New York: Berkley Books, 1979.

Voytovich, A. E., Rippey, R. M., & Copertino, L. Scorable problem lists as measures of clinical judgment. *Evaluation and the Health Professions*, June 1980, *3*, 159–170.

Wason, P. C., & Johnson-Laird, P. N. *Psychology of reasoning: Structure and content*. New York: Harvard University Press, 1972.

CHAPTER 7

USE OF NURSING DIAGNOSIS IN DIRECT CARE ACTIVITIES

The previous chapters have defined nursing diagnosis and attempted to lay before the reader the process of diagnostic judgment. This earlier discussion has been to one end: application of diagnosis to client care.

In a profession with a social responsibility, thinking and reasoning skills have to be applied, not just learned for abstract, theoretical purposes. In fact, it is questionable whether true learning about concepts like diagnosis can occur without application in the real world. The test of an idea is its usefulness in practice: Does nursing diagnosis facilitate direct client care activities? If nursing diagnosis is merely an intellectual exercise, a status symbol, or an ivory tower idea, why learn it?

The reader would not have been led through six chapters if nursing diagnosis had no clinical relevance. In this chapter it will become clear that the effort spent in formulating diagnoses greatly facilitates the planning of effective nursing care. First we shall consider the rightful place of diagnosis, that is, within the nursing process. It will be demonstrated that diagnosis is used as a focus for a chain of interrelated decisions. These include decisions about the care that is needed to attain the desired results.

Besides using their heads, hands, and hearts, nurses communicate. Verbal and written communications are an integral part of direct care activities. How nursing diagnoses enhance the transfer of information about a client's condition and nursing care needs will be a second topic. Examples will demonstrate that diagnoses organize thoughts for purposes of communication.

A third topic, discharge planning, builds on the understanding of nursing diagnosis in nursing process and in communication. The process of care planning is taken beyond a daily activity to planning of continuity between settings and care providers. Again, examples will illustrate how nursing diagnoses are the basis for making and communicating discharge plans.

Diagnosis and the nurse's legal responsibilities and risks are interrelated. We shall consider a way in which diagnostic judgments might enter into cases of alleged professional negligence. By a case example it will be made clear that diagnostic judgments are a "duty" in the legal sense; not diagnosing can be as serious as misdiagnosing. This will lead us to the last topic of this chapter, who should diagnose.

NURSING DIAGNOSIS AND NURSING PROCESS

As currently conceived, nursing process is a problem-identification and problem-solving approach to client care. It is the basis for a helping relationship characterized by knowledge, reason, and caring. Structurally, the nursing process is adapted from the scientific approach to solving problems.

Previous chapters have emphasized the problem-identification phase of nursing process. We have seen that the diagnostic process is used in this phase to evaluate a client's health status, identify problems if any are present, and label these problems with nursing diagnoses. When a sufficient understanding of the client's health problems is gained, a nurse shifts from a diagnostic to a problem-solving process.

Within the problem-solving phase of nursing process, outcomes are projected, plans for reaching the outcomes are determined, actions are implemented, and progress is evaluated. The components can be summarized as follows:

Problem identification using diagnostic process
  Data collection
  Diagnostic judgment
  Diagnostic labeling of actual and potential problems
Problem solving using problem-solving process
  Outcome projection
  Care planning
  Intervention
  Outcome evaluation

The elegance of this approach lies in its broad applicability to reasoning in any domain. Yet clearly the skeletal structure needs to be clothed. Nursing process becomes a process of nursing when the above components are attired in *values*, *concepts*, and *standards* of nursing.

Guiding Values

The way problem identification and problem solving are carried out depends on a nurse's values and beliefs about human nature and helping. Some nurses believe that clients should diagnose their own problems. Others advocate having the nurse act as diagnostician and expert decision maker. Neither approach is applicable to *all* nursing situations. This will become evident as we examine two extremes.

At one extreme a nurse may believe that a client comes to a health care provider for help. What is sought is clinical expertise in the identification and solution of health problems or potential problems the client cannot identify and solve. The nurse serves the client as resource and expert. Strategies for implementing nursing process require that the nurse collect data, diagnose, and intervene. The client provides information and then things are done to improve his or her health.

This belief system and strategy for using nursing process are useful if the client is unconscious or feels too weak to participate; but if applied to all clients and situations this becomes an authoritarian approach.

At the opposite extreme is the position that all nurse-client interactions should promote growth toward a realization of human potential. The nursing role is "helper, assistant, and colleague in a cooperative search" for health (Combs, Avila, and Purkey, 1971, p. 214).

The second philosophy leads to a strategy in which a client is considered the expert in assessing situations, diagnosing problems, and arriving at effective solutions. Nurses operating under this philosophy accept responsibility for creating conditions in which the client carries out these activities, not for identifying problems and solutions. This procedure is similar to the problem-solving method of social work practice discussed earlier.

This approach to nursing process requires that the client have both energy and inclination to develop insight into problems and to engage in problem solving. It is applicable in situations in which change in the client's perceptions and behavior has to occur in order to facilitate healthy functional patterns.

The nurse retains responsibility for labeling health problems the client identifies. The strategy associated with this form of helping requires expert diagnostic and problem-solving skills because conditions must be created in which the client develops insight, considers options, and makes choices.

Guiding Concepts

Problem identification and problem solving are guided by a set of concepts. These concepts provide a way of thinking about (1) what health problems are of concern to nurses, (2) what kinds of solutions are sought, and (3) what types of interventions are used in practice. This triad will be recognized, from the discussion in Chapter 3, as a framework for nursing.

Suppose, for instance, that actual and potential self-care deficits were the focus of concern. The diagnosis nutritional deficit/food selection would be thought of as a discrepancy between self-care agency and self-care demand. An educative and supportive system of care would be designed to assist the client in learning about food selection (Orem, 1980).

A conceptual framework is necessary to guide thinking. Within the self-care agency framework a nurse would think of problem identification as identification of self-care deficits. Problem solving would focus on the design of a nursing system of care. Goals, or outcomes, would be expressed in terms of independent self-care management. Other frameworks, such as the adaptation, life process, or behavioral systems previously discussed, provide different concepts to guide nursing process.

Guiding Standards

A profession derives its authority to practice from society. In return it has a responsibility to be mindful of the public trust. Traditionally, the quality of practice has been monitored by colleagues and state licensing boards. In recent years public pressure for assurance that quality care is being delivered has prompted professions to develop standards of practice.

In 1973 the Congress on Practice of the American Nurses' Association published basic standards for professional nursing practice in any setting. These may be seen in Table 7-1. Since that time other divisions and specialty groups have published their specific standards using the original standards as a model. The question may be asked: Why are standards important and what do they have to do with nursing diagnosis?

Standards are valued and achievable criteria for nursing performance, against which actual performance can be judged (Bloch, 1977). For example, suppose a registered nurse wishes to know whether the way he or she practices is at least satisfactory. A comparison between personal practice and the national standards for practice could be made. Or suppose a nursing student wants to evaluate the progress he or she is making toward professionally accepted nursing standards. The student could make the same comparison, knowing that by the time of graduation the standards should be met.

Standard II is of particular interest in this discussion. It states that nursing diagnoses are derived from health status data. The fact that this standard exists means that nurses have stated a criterion for satisfactory professional practice in the area of nursing diagnosis. Thus consumers can expect nursing diagnoses to be made if they are getting

TABLE 7-1
AMERICAN NURSES' ASSOCIATION STANDARDS OF NURSING PRACTICE

Standard I
   The collection of data about the health status of the client/patient is systematic and continuous. The data are accessible, communicated, and recorded.
Standard II
   Nursing diagnoses are derived from health status data.
Standard III
   The plan of nursing care includes goals derived from the nursing diagnoses.
Standard IV
   The plan of nursing care includes priorities and the prescribed nursing approaches or measures to achieve the goals derived from the nursing diagnoses.
Standard V
   Nursing actions provide for client/patient participation in health promotion, maintenance, and restoration.
Standard VI
   Nursing actions assist the client/patient to maximize his health capabilities.
Standard VII
   The client's/patient's progress or lack of progress toward goal achievement is determined by the client/patient and the nurse.
Standard VIII
   The client's/patient's progress or lack of progress toward goal achievement directs reassessment, reordering of priorities, new goal setting, and revision of the plan of nursing care.

Source: American Nurses' Association (1973).

TABLE 7-2
COMPARISON OF NURSING STANDARDS, NURSING PROCESS,
AND THE PROBLEM-SOLVING MODEL

Nursing standards*	Nursing process	Problem-solving model
Collection of health status data (I)	Assessment	Observation, data collection
Nursing diagnosis (II)	Diagnosis	Problem identification
Plan, goals (III)		
Priorities (IV)	Outcome projection	Problem solving
Client/patient participation (V)	Planning	(methods, goals, outcomes)
Actions (VI)	Implementation (intervention)	Problem-solving actions
Progress determination (VII) Reassessment; revision (VIII)	Evaluation	Evaluation

*Roman numerals refer to particular standards listed in full in Table 7-1.

an acceptable quality of care. Professional nurses have a responsibility to ensure that standards of care are met for clients, since many cannot ensure this for themselves.

Problem identification and problem solving, nursing process, and standards of practice have many similarities. The resemblance is evident in the comparisons presented in Table 7-2. The *collection of health status data* (Standard I) is referred to as assessment in the nursing process. In problem solving, it is referred to as observation and data collection. *Nursing diagnosis* is specified in both the standards (Standard II) and nursing process; it is synonymous with problem identification. The *nursing plan* is described more specifically in the standards than in nursing process, but is the same as designing methods and stating goals and outcomes in the problem-solving model.

Clearly, both the standards and nursing process are similar and both are based on problem identification and problem solving. It is well to appreciate these similarities and not to think three different things are being referred to when the different labels are encountered.

Beliefs about helping relationships, concepts used in nursing process, and standards guide the use of nursing process and its component, nursing diagnosis. Previous chapters have demonstrated how diagnostic categories are used in problem identification. In the following sections the relevance of nursing diagnoses to care delivery will become clear. The objective will not be an in-depth discussion of problem-solving activities; rather the emphasis will be on how to use nursing diagnoses in these activities.

Nursing Diagnosis in Care Planning

The nurse's desire to change the course of events gives nursing care planning its momentum. A health problem may have dire consequence if left to run its course. It also may cause great discomfort even if natural resolution occurs. Nurses attempt to alter these possibilities by thinking ahead, making decisions, and formulating nursing care plans.

Once health problems are recognized and labeled as nursing diagnoses, responsibility for treatment arises and decisions are required. The decisions to be made in the treatment of any nursing diagnosis are:

1 What are the desired outcomes?
2 What plan of nursing care is needed to reach the outcomes?
3 After implementation of nursing care, were the desired outcomes actually reached?

Nursing diagnosis is merely an intellectual exercise unless used in making these decisions.

Let us consider the way nursing diagnoses can help in decision making. During the discussion the nurse will be viewed as the decision maker. If the process is understood and practiced, the important ideas can then be modified for application to those situations in which clients are guided in doing their own decision making and planning. The first step is to decide what health outcome is desired.

Projected Outcomes Suppose you wish to be in San Francisco on Tuesday to meet a friend. Deciding this before starting a trip increases the probability that you will get there. Otherwise, on Tuesday you may be in Louisiana. This failure to specify what outcome is desired can produce inconvenience, additional cost, distress, and delay.

The reasoning is similar in nursing. Being in San Francisco on Tuesday would be called the desired outcome. In health care an *outcome* is a valued health state, condition, or behavior exhibited by a client. It may be, for example, a client's verbalized intention to take some particular health-promoting action, or it may be a behavior or condition observed by a nurse.

Other, similar terms are in use, such as *objectives* and *goals*. *Outcome* is synonymous with *behavioral objective*; both specify observable behaviors of the client. Goals are usually broader statements that require further specification. Measurable outcomes that indicate goal attainment have to be identified.

Adding the term *projected*—projected outcome—means that a prediction, or forecast, of a future behavior has been made. Outcomes are projected in order to guide decisions about care; later they are measured to evaluate the effectiveness of the care that has been given. Projecting outcomes permits the nurse to know when the problem is solved.

Outcomes are projected before nursing actions are planned or carried out. There are two reasons for this. One, the health problem describes the *present* health state of the client; the projected outcome describes the *desired* health state. When the discrepancy is consciously examined, the therapeutic task becomes evident and alternative actions can be considered. The actions most likely to lead to outcomes are selected and implemented.

The second reason for deciding on outcomes before planning and acting is equally important. Basically, when outcomes are attained the client is discharged from care. During the delivery of care, projected outcomes are used to evaluate daily progress toward attainment.

Of what relevance to outcome projection is a nursing diagnosis? Without a diagnosis that describes the health problem it would be difficult even to attempt to specify outcomes. Projected outcomes describe the state of a client after, or at some stage of, problem resolution. Thus a diagnosis is the basis for outcome projection.

Consider the example of a hospitalized client. The gentleman was 25 years old. He had paralysis of the lower half of his body as a result of a car accident in which his spinal cord was severely damaged. A number of risk factors predisposed him to a change in circulation to tissues over the bony prominences of his body; the nursing diagnosis was potential skin breakdown.

Given this diagnosis, what desired outcome of nursing care would you wish to observe at the time of the client's discharge from the acute care setting? Obviously the valued outcome is *skin intact at discharge*. Notice what has occurred. The diagnosis of potential skin breakdown was made, and then the reverse of breakdown, intact skin, was stated as the desired outcome of nursing care.

Converting the diagnosis into a desired health state is a quick method for projecting outcomes. The critical signs and symptoms that define a diagnosis are useful in the transformation. Logically, their opposites define the resolution of the problem. Even positive changes in symptoms would indicate progress toward problem resolution.

Consider another problem. A client with heart failure is unable to bathe; whenever she tries, shortness of breath and fatigue occur. The nursing diagnosis is self-bathing deficit, level 2 (requires assistance) and the probable cause is decreased activity tolerance. Mentally transforming the problem into a desired functional state permits outcome projection. In this case the outcome would be self-bathing.[1]

Notice that outcomes in the previous examples are stated concisely and definitely. Specificity is necessary to guide planning; vague words and statements make it difficult to know exactly where one is going. Furthermore, only with specific outcomes does one know when the nursing goal has been reached. For example, "good skin color" or "good knowledge of . . ." are difficult to measure. How is "good" to be recognized?

Consider the following diagnoses and outcomes; which of these are useful for planning care and evaluating progress (diagnoses are written in the problem/etiology format)?

1 Exogenous obesity/caloric intake–energy expenditure imbalance
Outcome: weight loss 10 pounds; 5-week visit
2 Ineffective airway clearance/decreased energy
Outcome: breath (lung) sounds clear; day 2
3 Low mother-infant bonding/separation
Outcome: parental attachment behaviors present; 3-week visit

In the above examples, numbers 1 and 2 are measurable outcomes that can be used in planning care and evaluating the effectiveness of nursing intervention. The third statement is too broad. What attachment behaviors are to be present? What should be expected in 3 weeks?

Value-Laden Decisions Outcomes are value decisions. In the example above it can be inferred that having intact skin and bathing independently are highly valued by most people. The arguments are numerous: (1) bathing removes dirt, dead skin, and secretions; (2) intact skin prevents infection, and (3) independence is "better" than dependence. Most adults probably would agree. Yet in essence writing an outcome is

---

[1] The diagnostic category of self-bathing/hygiene deficit has four levels. These levels (Table 3–7) can be used to state progress toward independence.

stating a personal value—the profession's value or a social value. The desirability of intact skin would raise little if any controversy, but with many other diagnoses the situation is not as clear.

The client has the right to choose outcomes. In their enthusiasm to promote health, nurses can easily unconsciously impose their own personal or social values on others. Outcomes for problems related to cognition, beliefs, self-perception, or relationships require choices that are best made by the client or in collaboration with the client. Philosophically, if the nurse believes clients should participate in actions to solve their problems, it follows that clients must be involved in deciding outcomes. From a practical perspective, participation in setting outcomes increases motivation toward achieving those outcomes.

In many instances the client says what he or she wishes remedied; listening can enable the nurse to know what that is. On the other hand, clients may not know what outcomes are possible. Additionally, they may have difficulty coping with an event or may be in conflict about making a choice. Their ability to use their problem-solving capacities may be lowered. In these situations a nurse may suggest alternatives.

A 65-year-old woman had a nursing diagnosis of social isolation related to altered body image and fear of rejection. After having a leg amputation and being fitted with an artificial limb, she stayed in her apartment. She told most close friends that she was unable to have visitors and avoided other tenants. The desired outcome for the health problem was: resumes previous level of social relationships.

The nurse took an indirect approach because of the high degree of stress the woman was experiencing. Yet the client was given an opportunity to reject the outcome. In essence, here is how the diagnosis and projected outcome were translated to the client: "You mentioned before that you are trying to avoid your friends because you think they would be disgusted by someone with a leg off. Could we think about how they would react and how you could handle this if you did decide to invite them?" The nurse paused for the client's reaction to the subtly introduced outcome of inviting friends to her apartment. The client looked down and said, "I do miss having people in." The nurse interpreted the statement as a wish to resume previous social contacts. At that time the client could not more directly agree to the outcome because of her fear of rejection by friends.

Some have advocated written, signed contracts for outcomes. It has been demonstrated that contracts with clients have some effect on compliance with needed behavior changes, such as dieting. But contracts produce a formalism in the nurse-client relationship that many nurses reject.

In order to introduce the idea of projecting outcomes by using nursing diagnoses, the concept of problem resolution has been somewhat oversimplified. Transforming indicators of a problem (signs and symptoms) to positive health behaviors is easier to do "in the head" than "in the world of reality." The final resolution of a client's health problem may require steps rather than one leap.

If short-term resolution of a diagnosis is not possible, outcomes representing progress toward resolution are stated. For example, outcomes may be projected for accomplishment by the date of hospital discharge *and* for 3 months, 6 months, or longer if the client is under continuing care.

Time, resources, and costs are factors to be considered in projecting outcomes.

Before one can specify individualized outcomes within a realistic time frame for outcome attainment one must know what interventions will be used. What is done (nursing and client actions) influences the client's progress toward resolution of the health problem. Yet what is done is influenced by clients' choices, capabilities, and resources.

Interventions   Thinking of ideal outcomes such as being in San Francisco on Tuesday motivates a person to find a way of getting there. Realistically, the traveler would have to consider wardrobe, packing, transportation schedules, and finances. With these considerations in mind, outcome attainment may be set for Tuesday 3 years hence! Similarly, in care planning the current state of the client and highly valued outcome are considered first, and then the way of getting "from here to there."

Interventions are the actions taken to help the client move from a present state to the state described in the projected outcomes. They may involve doing for, doing with, or enabling a client to do something to influence or resolve the health problem. The type of intervention selected depends on the nursing diagnosis and outcomes. As Figure 7-1 shows, specific interventions for individual clients depend on the choices, capabilities, and resources of the client and the creativity of the nurse.

A Focus for Intervention   A nursing diagnosis provides a focus for thinking about what interventions may resolve a problem. The alternative approach would be to treat isolated or unorganized signs and symptoms such as frequent crying spells, difficulty in breathing, or inability to bathe self. Interventions at the symptom level may help for the moment but rarely resolve the underlying problem. If the truth of this last statement is not apparent, try to identify interventions by using the above signs and symptoms as a focus. Contrast those interventions with the ones you would use for the diagnoses stated in the following paragraph.

Using a diagnosis and projected outcome as a focus increases the probability of selecting effective nursing interventions. For example, each of the previously listed signs (crying spells, difficult breathing, and inability to bathe) was investigated and clustered with other signs and symptoms. The problem and etiology were formulated

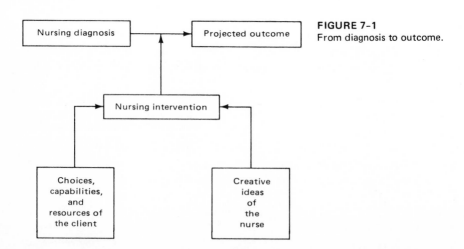

FIGURE 7-1
From diagnosis to outcome.

in each case and labeled as follows: (1) the crying client's diagnosis was ineffective coping/perceived incompetence (parenting); (2) ineffective airway clearance/thick secretions was the statement formulated for the client with dyspnea; and (3) self-bathing deficit (level 3)/decreased activity tolerance suggested many more specific interventions than did the sign inability to bathe self. In the third situation, bathing the client might solve the immediate need, but helping the client to increase activity tolerance gets at the essence of the problem.

Trial and error is a common approach if isolated signs and symptoms are used as a focus for care planning. This method is wasteful of nursing time. It also can prolong the client's discomfort, allow problems to become more severe, and lead to adverse effects. Trial and error is used either because meaning cannot be derived from the un-clustered signs and symptoms or because there are so many possible meanings. Think of the multiple meanings of the sign crying. Each is associated with a different intervention.

Diagnoses are concepts from which a knowledgeable nurse can derive meaning. Consider the diagnosis ineffective airway clearance/thick secretions. Biopsychosocial theories and research about airway obstruction, secretions, and client responses can be used as a framework to determine an approach to care. Specifically, theories provide help in understanding a problem, designing possible interventions, and calculating when intervention may be effective. Thus, conceptualizing and diagnostic labeling of problems facilitates memory or textbook search for theory. This in turn provides meaning and ideas that guide care-planning decisions.

What happens when the nurse focuses on the nursing diagnosis and on the available theoretical knowledge is similar to what occurred in the generation of diagnostic hypotheses during the stage of problem identification. The right problem space opened up multiple possibilities. In problem solving, this occurs when a problem space in memory or a textbook index is searched for alternative interventions.

Although on the surface a routine intervention may appear sufficient, clients deserve thoughtful planning of their care. This requires thinking of alternative methods, their consequences, and the probability that they will be effective for the particular client and situation.

Generating Alternative Interventions   When searching textbooks or memory stores for possible interventions, keep the problem in mind but focus on the etiology. If the probable cause can be influenced, the problematic health pattern should change.

Consider first a basic example: E (etiology) is the probable reason the P (problem) exists. If E is removed, the prediction is that P will be resolved. Intervention is directed primarily at E.

This abstract reasoning is applicable to clinical situations. Recall the 65-year-old woman whose diagnosis was social isolation/altered body image. After leg amputation she learned to use an artificial limb but continued to stay in her apartment and allowed no friends to visit. Before the amputation she went shopping, had friends in for coffee, and was socially active in her church. The outcome desired by the client and nurse was *resumes previous level of social relationships.* What shall be the focus of intervention for the visiting nurse?

Just recommending that the client socialize has a low probability of success. Thus the problem alone does not offer a focus for generating interventions. If body image alteration is the etiology, influencing body image may in turn influence socialization.

Etiological factors identified in the diagnosis are the focus of intervention. If these can be changed, the problem should begin to resolve.

Another example should help clarify the need to focus on etiology in generating alternative interventions. A second client also had alteration in socialization but the etiology was impaired mobility. For this 65-year-old woman who had been, as she described it, "a social butterfly," staying in the house was "confining"; she was becoming despondent. Visiting friends and going to holiday celebrations and the theater were important to her, yet the permanent peripheral vascular changes caused by diabetes impaired her mobility for stair climbing and walking distances.

The intervention for this client was entirely different, although the problem specified in the nursing diagnosis was the same. The focus for thinking about a solution was the etiology, impaired mobility. The nurse generated alternative interventions. Keeping these in the back of her mind, she encouraged the client to think of ways to circumvent the mobility impairment. The choice was to rent a wheelchair for steps (ramps) and distances; friends gladly helped. The visiting nurse arranged for the chair, and the client was delighted that they had found a way for her to resume social activities.

In these examples the alternatives for intervention were rather clear-cut. When more complex situations are encountered, the nurse must stop and think through the situation. The first step in deciding on an intervention is to answer the question, What is the therapeutic problem?

A *therapeutic problem* exists if interventions to attain outcomes either have a low degree of success; are unknown; or, while known, have been unsuccessful in the client's particular kind of situation. Aptly named, this is the *wicked decision problem*.

The nurse must define the therapeutic problem. Is it a behavioral change that is needed? Is it conflict resolution? Are there other ways of looking at the therapeutic problem? Keep the problem/etiology and outcome in mind and then think of offbeat or "far out" ideas; Osbourne (1963) and Gordon (1961) suggest methods such as this to increase creative thinking. Logical analysis is applied only *after* the ideas are generated.

Individualizing Interventions During the process of generating alternative interventions, the nurse thinks about factors related to the problem/etiology and to the particular client and situation. Consideration of these factors enables the nurse to individualize interventions. Individualizing interventions increases treatment success rate.

The areas of information in which data are needed to individualize care are:

1 *Personal client factors* The client, whether an individual, family, or community, has unique characteristics. These influence intervention. If interventions are being considered for an individual, then age, developmental stage, sex, culture, religion, family structure, and other personal characteristics are considered. Some of these are equally applicable in family or community intervention. In some instances further data collection may be necessary.

2 *Client's perception* The client may associate various causal factors with his or her problem even though objectively they are unrelated. Unless correction of misperceptions and faulty associations about the cause of a problem is built into the intervention plan, the intervention may fail because the client considers it unrelated to the etiology and therefore meaningless.

3 *Current level of compensation*   The client may have mobilized some strengths, defenses, or resources to compensate for the problem. Data about compensation help the nurse decide about the degree of nursing assistance required and also allows recognition of the client's strengths. Diagnoses can be classified as compensated (only monitoring is necessary), partially compensated (some nursing assistance is needed), or uncompensated (the client requires full nursing assistance).

4 *Problem magnitude and urgency*   The acuity or severity of a problem influence the type and timing of intervention. Certain conditions are urgent and intervention must be immediate. These are health problems that can result in harm to the client or others.

As an example, a client who is having surgery in 24 hours and who is near panic and not coping effectively requires immediate intervention. Either the surgery has to be cancelled or the anxiety has to be reduced quickly. With diagnoses such as potential for injury or potential for violence, immediate reduction of risk factors is needed.

5 *Extended effects*   Interventions have the potential for extended effects. Indirectly or directly they can influence members of the client's family, work group, or social circle. For example, what effects will a major diet change have on the other household members? Forethought is needed when interventions are planned, so that no additional problems will be created by their extended effects.

Interactions among nursing diagnoses should also be considered in planning intervention. If treatment for one problem is planned in isolation, there can be extended effects on coexisting problems. As an example, the usual treatment for one diagnosis may be contraindicated when another nursing diagnosis is present. Similarly, the treatment for a nursing diagnosis may negatively or positively influence a disease or a medical treatment; the reverse can also occur. Interactions among *all* diagnoses and *all* treatments have to be taken into account in decision making.

6 *Cost-benefit factors*   Consequences of treatments are a consideration in decision making. Each intervention has a "price." The costs can be financial, social, or psychological. *Benefits* are the advantages that accompany (or are expected to result from) the outcomes of treatment in terms of (1) optimum health and well-being or (2) an immediate or long-term life goal of the client. Possible benefits of the results of various interventions being considered are weighed against possible costs.

One dimension of cost-benefit considerations is psychological or social cost related to functional benefit. Before recommending or guiding clients to change their behavior patterns, consider the payoff. Be knowledgeable about the predicted benefits of change so that clients can weigh alternatives and make informed choices. Changing behavioral patterns is one of the most difficult things for people to do, especially during adulthood.

A client may value the expected outcome as a benefit but feel the cost (e.g., stopping smoking or giving up desired foods) is too high. In this situation the nurse and client should try to find a way to reduce the cost of the intervention. Perhaps a less valued outcome (e.g., switching to low tar cigarettes) is all that can be accomplished at present. It may also be possible to increase the client's value-rating of the beneficial outcome enough that the price will be paid.

A second dimension of the cost-benefit factor is financial cost related to the functional benefit of the expected outcome. Given today's soaring health care costs, if two alternative interventions for a diagnosis result in the same beneficial effect, choose the less expensive. Before ordering consultations, equipment, or services for the treatment of the problem consider whether the benefit is worth the cost. Consumers are currently demanding that cost-benefit ratios be considered in treatment planning.

Predicting Effectiveness of Interventions Consideration of the six factors just discussed should narrow down the treatment alternatives for a particular client's nursing diagnosis. The remaining alternatives have to be subjected to final scrutiny. The one that has the greatest probability of being effective is chosen.

The *predicted effectiveness* of an intervention is the probability that it will lead to the projected outcome. For example, suppose the probability that intervention A will lead to outcome C is 60 percent, whereas the probability that intervention B will produce outcome C is 90 percent. If A and B "cost" the same, B will be chosen.

Predicted effectiveness takes into account all of the six previously mentioned factors that are relevant to the diagnosis. Thus the predicted effectiveness is a prediction about individualized interventions for a particular client and situation. Obviously, the intervention with the highest probability of being effective is chosen and implemented.

Priority Setting A client may have multiple diagnoses, not all of which can or should be treated at the time they are identified. Priorities for treatment depend on (1) the urgency of the problem, (2) the nature of the treatment indicated, and (3) the interactions among diagnoses.

Nursing diagnoses that if untreated could result in harm to the client or others have the highest priority for treatment. Examples include potential for violence, potential for trauma, and ineffective airway clearance. In these examples the priority is clear. In many other instances thorough knowledge of the client and situation is necessary before the nurse can be sure what patient conditions *are* urgent.

The type of treatment that is indicated also helps determine priorities in particular cases. If a client is physiologically unstable, as might commonly be the situation in an intensive care unit, treatment of diagnoses requiring learning of behavioral changes would not be given a high priority. Intensive care units are not designed for treating knowledge deficits about postdischarge health management; nor is an emergency room designed for treatment of noncompliance with a weight reduction program. Consideration has to be given to the cost of keeping a client in an expensive nursing care setting for a problem that can be treated in a less expensive setting.

Another factor that influences priority setting is the possibility of interactions among diagnoses. Suppose a 10-year-old client has the following diagnoses: chronic exogenous obesity/caloric intake–activity imbalance; dysfunctional grieving/loss of parent; and compromised family coping. Should priorities be set, and if so, how?

Although the coping and grieving problems are not judged to be probable causes of obesity, they are two problems that potentially can interact. Improved family coping may provide greater support to the child and assist in resolving the grief process. When these problems begin to improve, the child can be helped to lose weight, ideally with family support. Priority setting enhances treatment when the client has multiple problems. Yet priority setting would be impossible without clearly identifying the nursing diagnoses.

Implementation and Evaluation After decisions about interventions and priorities are made, the treatment plan is begun. During implementation of the plan, continued assessment provides feedback that is used to evaluate prior diagnostic judgments and treatment decisions. Assessing the client's progress toward the projected outcomes enables the nurse to evaluate the effectiveness of the interventions. Progress toward outcomes is evaluated during the course of nursing intervention by problem-focused assessment as described in Chapter 4. Data collected about the status of the problem are the basis for evaluative judgments. If the intervention is effective, the signs and symptoms used to diagnose the problem should be changing.

At this point we may summarize the use of diagnoses in problem identification and problem solving. The nurse's first concern is to identify the client's health problems and apply diagnostic labels. Then use of a systematic problem-solving process takes precedence. During this problem-solving phase of the nursing process, diagnoses are the bases for projecting desired outcomes, deciding on interventions by which to attain the outcomes, implementing interventions, and evaluating the attainment of diagnosis-specific outcomes.

After one has completed this process of problem identification and problem solving, it appears in retrospect to have been a *sequence* of steps. In actuality, the entire set of activities is always in mind. Each decision influences other decisions. It is a matter of greatest importance to maintain open-mindedness about observations and new data that are collected during all phases of nursing process. Never be hesitant to consider new data and revise judgments; this open-mindedness is the key to handling probabilistic clinical information.

Nursing Process in Disease-Related Care   Nursing process is a problem-identification-problem-solving process. As such, it is adaptable to domains of problems other than nursing; one domain is that described by medical disease. Although the subject of this book is nursing diagnoses, some consideration should be given to nurses' disease-related care activities and the clinical judgments upon which care is based.

The first judgment when a client is admitted is based on the quick-scan emergency assessment described in Chapter 4. This assessment differentiates between emergency and nonemergency situations. For example, Mr. F. was brought to the emergency room by ambulance after a car accident. Head injury was obvious from his bleeding laceration, minimal spontaneous activity, and sluggish response to verbal communications. The situation was judged to be a medical emergency and a physician was immediately summoned. Judgments about emergencies and the need for a particular health professional are continuously made in nursing. Although the need for medical evaluation was quite obvious in this client's case, judgments are many times uncertainty-based when clinical signs are ambiguous.

Further physical assessment of Mr. F., a 45-year-old man in previous good health, involved the search for cues to his neurological status. The most likely possibility was intercranial bleeding from trauma. The signs observed signified moderate head injury (concussion).

A client from the emergency room with a history such as Mr. F.'s would require immediate assessment upon admission to an acute care unit and continued close observation. Judgments about the level of nursing care required are based on a nurse's medical knowledge. Irrespective of whether or not physician's orders were written, Mr. F. would be observed for increased intracranial pressure, intracranial bleeding, associated spinal cord injury, other undetected injuries, and infection of his head laceration. These hypotheses would be generated from the cues present on admission and the medical diagnosis. Hypothesis testing would involve a search for cues defining these conditions.

Two hours after admission Mr. F. had changes from base-line data collected at admission (decreased level of consciousness, no spontaneous motor activity, reaction only to strong stimuli, increased dilation and fixation of right pupil, and changes in vital signs). The observed physical signs suggested the hypothesis of intracranial bleeding and possibly a subdural hematoma. Having generated this hypothesis the nurse caring for Mr. F. immediately called the physician and anticipated surgical intervention.

Mr. F.'s physiological problems and the nurse's responses demonstrate similarities and differences between nursing diagnoses and disease-related nursing judgments. Assessment, hypothesis generation, and hypothesis testing are similar; only one set of cognitive behaviors need to be learned. Similarly, information used in disease-related clinical judgments has the same characteristics as discussed in Chapter 4; the general principles of assessment also apply. Differences exist in what information is collected and processed; a body of knowledge in medical science is required for assessment and experience must be gained in its application. Differences also exist in the actions taken. When a hypothesis about disease progression or complications is supported, a judgment is made to (1) orally inform the physician, (2) note the information in the client's record, (3) carry out or withhold treatments designated by existing physician's orders or nursing protocols, (4) carry out palliative treatments based on nursing judgment, or (5) execute a combination of these actions. In contrast, the main responsibility after nursing diagnosis is (1) to plan and execute nursing treatment and (2) to facilitate treatment coordination by communication with other health care professionals.

Treatment Coordination　When a client has both nursing and medical diagnoses, treatment has to be coordinated. Otherwise interventions could conflict and outcomes might not be attained. Having regularly scheduled time for mutual sharing of information among the professionals involved in client care is ideal. Regular communication promotes understanding of each care provider's diagnostic judgments and treatment decisions. It increases the probability of integrated care and also promotes working relationships.

It is easy to understand the need for coordination. Yet implementation in certain settings requires ingenuity and initiative. Who shall take the initiative? In acute care settings, such as hospitals, nurses have 24-hour responsibility for implementing client's medical and nursing treatments and for seeing their families. Accordingly, nurses need to be aware of the total care plan. To gain this overview, nursing staff may need to take the initiative to institute change in communication patterns. Care conferences between the client's primary nurse and physician could be scheduled.

Change takes time and is sometimes accomplished by small steps. Minimally, a front sheet on the client's chart could be used for the care providers from all professions to record their diagnoses. A perceived need for scheduled joint conferences might evolve from this beginning. If physicians and nurses have separate rounds on all clients, they could be combined. The methods employed to promote change have to be specific to a particular institution.

NURSING DIAGNOSIS AND COMMUNICATION

When more than one person is responsible for health care, communication is necessary. Actually, even in private practice, records of diagnoses and treatments have to be kept. In this section the relevance of nursing diagnoses to various types of written and verbal communication within and among professions will be examined. The problem oriented permanent record and the nursing care plan are important methods of communicating and will be discussed in detail. It will be seen that nursing diagnoses provide a concise and organized means of communication.

Communicating one's diagnoses and interventions, particularly in writing, has benefits. It (1) eases memory strain; (2) encourages one to organize one's data, diagnostic judgments, and treatment decisions; (3) facilitates continuity and coordination of care when two or more people provide care; (4) provides a record in the event of alleged harm to a client; and (5) permits research that can lead to improvement of care. The costs in time and effort are minimal when compared with these benefits.

Verbal Communication

Nurses use verbal communication in shift reports, informal discussions of client's health problems, formal case conferences, nursing rounds, and reports to supervisors. These are examples of nurses' communications with other nurses. During nurse-physician communication, a physician may inquire about a client's sleep pattern or nutritional pattern during hospitalization, or the nurse may initiate a verbal communication about a nursing diagnosis that will have an impact on medical treatment.

In all these kinds of communications, nursing diagnosis provides a succinct and clear mode of communication. Consider the following examples:

1 *Shift report* "Ms. K is ineffectively coping with the threat of impending surgery. I have . . ." [night nurse lists interventions and outcomes] .

2 *Coffee break* "I'm really having trouble coming up with a way of dealing with Mr. G. He has a potential for fluid volume deficit and I can't get him to drink anything. I hate to see him have an I.V. [intravenous infusion] . Can you think of anything?"

3 *Case conference* "I've picked Mr. L because of his major problem that is common to so many of our clients. His diagnosis is self-care deficit due to left-sided neglect. We aren't treating this effectively and so I have done a review of the literature that may suggest some additional possibilities."

4 *Nursing rounds* "Mr. F. is a 45-year old construction worker; his medical problem is myocardial infarct, uncomplicated. Currently he has an independence-dependence conflict. The probable cause is the restriction of his activity and self-care. I am . . ." [states intervention] .

5 *Report to supervisor (service director)* "I have one client with impaired home maintenance management/decreased activity tolerance. I taught her energy conservation techniques but I've decided she also needs a homemaker 2 days a week. Tomorrow I'll orient the homemaker. I also have two clients for whom the referral states altera-

tions in parenting. I'll see them tomorrow. The home health aide is implementing my plan for Ms. S. Her mobility impairment has decreased and. . . ."

6 *Nurse-physician* "I finally found out that Jamie's passive dependence is not due to fear but to parental overprotection. I'm helping the parents develop a plan for allowing independence. When you talk to the parents . . ."

The preceding communications are concise and to the point. Hesitation and confusion over a multiplicity of signs and symptoms are avoided. Data have been organized by use of nursing diagnoses.

Written Communication

In contrast to verbal communication, which relies on human recall and human interaction, written information takes on a quality of permanence. In the developed nations, important observations and decisions are nearly always recorded. One hour, one day, or years later others can read how an event was seen and interpreted.

In health care situations written communications provide a sequential record of the client's health status as well as care provider's diagnostic judgments, treatment plans, and actions. These records provide the means for continuity and coordination of plans across settings, care providers, and time. Written records not only preserve data; certain methods of recording also provide a means for checking thought processes.

Nurses and other care providers use various modes of written communication. Some are permanent records of the client's progress and others are working records that are summarized and discarded at intervals.

A permanent record, commonly referred to as the medical record or client's chart, is used in private, institutional, and community practice. Its main purpose is to provide continuity of care, but it also is used for research and teaching purposes. In addition, this record is used as evidence in legal proceedings. State laws require that a record of care provided to an individual or family be kept for a number of years.

Different chart formats are in use, particularly for nursing recordings. Some institutions separate medical and nursing notes within a chart. Others use one section for all health care providers' histories, examinations, progress notes, and treatment orders.

Historically nurses communicated important observations and actions in long paragraphs. Adding to the record occurred at least three times a day, once on each work shift. Certain of these communications were required: sleeping, eating, comfort, and a doctor's visit.

Sometimes long dissertations were critically important and sometimes not. Little evidence existed that physicians or supervisors read nurses' notes, and after the client's discharge they were discarded. Understandably, this type of nurse's note has become nearly extinct.

In addition, the nurse's judgments were to be carefully worded in the written record. Every student learned the cautious, conservative phrase "appears to be" in the first nursing course. These words were modestly applied to nurses' judgments—"appears to be bleeding," "appears to be uncomfortable," or even "appears to have expired."

In recent years judgment has been emphasized in nursing. Most importantly, *nurses* are beginning to believe their observations, diagnostic judgments, and treatment decisions are important. They diagnose and treat health problems within their scope of practice and communicate these in the permanent record.

In 1969, Lawrence Weed, a physician concerned about the poor quality of records, designed a new format that organizes information around client problems. This format has been implemented in many hospitals, clinics, private practices, and community nursing agencies. Interestingly, it was about this same time that many nurses began to think about their practice in terms of nursing diagnoses. Merging the two ideas permitted nurses to move easily into the new charting system.

Problem Oriented Recording   Realizing that the content of records was usually inadequate and information difficult to find, Weed (1971) introduced the idea of a problem oriented charting system. It is a system designed to facilitate care, teaching, and research.

The problem oriented record (POR) system provides structure and organization for any health professional's written record of care. It has four main parts:

1 A problem list
2 A defined data base
3 Initial and revised plans
4 Progress notes

Plans for care and progress notes are titled and numbered for each problem. As each part is described in the following paragraphs, it will be seen that clear documentation of problem identification (diagnoses) and problem solving (treatment and outcomes) is possible. Another advantage is that this type of recording makes it possible for students to examine and evaluate the logical consistency of their judgments.

The Problem List   Used as a dynamic (continually updated) indexing system, the *problem list* appears on the cover page of notes or the front of the chart. It is a cumulative listing of client problems and potential problems recorded by each health profession independently or through interdisciplinary conferences.

Nursing diagnoses are the problem labels nurses record on the list. Nurses also list potentially important signs and symptoms that cannot be diagnostically categorized at the time. It is important that each diagnosis be well supported by clinical data.

Table 7-3 contains a sample problem list; the nursing diagnoses are listed as numbers 3 and 4. Number 5 is a sign of potential importance and worthy of nursing attention. As soon as the client's condition improves, this sign will be investigated further. Problems that will be deleted from the active list within a short period of time should not be listed.

Because they are concise methods for describing a client's health problem, nursing diagnoses are ideal terms for nurses to use in the problem list. The advantage that results from using concise terminology is that each health team member can see at a glance what problems are being treated by the different professions involved in the client's care.

A Well-Defined Data Base   The need for a well-defined data base obtained by the initial nursing history and examination has been discussed elsewhere. This base-line data are recorded on progress notes or specially designed sheets in the chart.

TABLE 7–3
ADMISSION PROBLEM LIST FOR ONE CLIENT

Problem no.	Active problems	Date entered	Date problem inactive
1.	Diabetes mellitus	5/20	
2.	Hyperglycemia; Acidosis	5/20	
3.	Exogenous obesity/activity–caloric intake imbalance	5/20	
4.	Potential for injury	5/20	
5.	Four-day history of not taking insulin	5/20	

Initial Plans After the nursing history and physical examination are completed, they are recorded in the client's chart. A nursing care plan is written for each problem diagnosed. If applicable, plans include (1) collection of further information, (2) treatments, and (3) patient education.

Goals, or projected outcomes, are also stated. These clarify the degree of function sought or state a reason why treatment is delayed (e.g., patient education delayed until physical condition stabilized).

One example from a problem oriented recording will illustrate the preceding points. The hospitalized client whose problem list is presented in Table 7-3 had decreased sensation in her legs. One bruise and one scratch were evident. Precautionary measures against injury had not been taken in her home because she did not consider them important. The nursing diagnosis, potential for injury, and the initial plan were recorded following the history and examination (*Dx* refers to diagnostic plan, *Tx* to treatment plan, and *Ed* to explanation or educational plan):

4 Potential for injury

Outcome: Absence of leg injuries; states plans for implementing measures in home to prevent injury.

P_{Dx}: Observe degree of caution exercised.

P_{Tx}: Room check for jutting objects, slippery floors; eyeglasses worn during ambulation; adequate lighting at all times when ambulating.

P_{Ed}: Potential for injury with sensory deficit explained. Teach precautions regarding ambulation, adequate vision, lighting, scatter rugs, slippery floors, jutting objects, ill-fitting shoes or boots, nail cutting.

The diagnostic plan (Dx) at admission was to collect further information about the degree of caution exercised by the client when ambulating in the hospital. In addition, plans for further data collection should always be included when the problem list includes uncategorized but potentially important signs, for example, problem 5 in Table 7-3, 4-day history of not taking insulin. Admission data may not be sufficient to specify etiological factors; this situation would also necessitate a plan for data collection.

The treatment plan (Tx) was designed to ensure safety during ambulation in the hospital and attain the stated outcome, absence of leg injury. While these interventions were being implemented, incidental teaching could be done. Yet, to attain the outcome *states plans for implementing measures in home to prevent injury*, an *educational plan* (Ed) was needed.

The three parts of a plan help the nurse to think about possible nursing actions that may be required. Memorizing these three components—diagnostic plan, treatment plan, and educational plan—is useful; they apply to all planning and can be used to check on completeness.

Progress Notes Nursing diagnoses are used in recording progress toward problem resolution. Progress usually is charted on *each* problem every day in hospitals and at each visit in private practice settings, clinics, or community nursing. Theoretically, progress notes are written only when a change is observed in the status of the problem or when there is no response, or an unexpected response, to treatment. In actuality, if treatment is aggressive daily changes are observed.

In the POR system, progress notes are structured. They are headed by the problem and its number from the problem list. Subsections of a note include subjective data (S), objective data (O), assessment (A), and plan (P).

The terms *subjective data* and *objective data* are defined as previously stated in Chapter 4: Briefly, subjective data are those the client reports, and objective data are those the nurse personally observes. *Assessment* in the POR system refers not to data collection but to the care provider's analysis and interpretation of the problem. The etiology is included under assessment (A); so are any factors related to the prognosis of the problem. *Plan* refers to the diagnostic, treatment, and educational plan of care. Not all of these subsections (S, O, A, P) need be included in each periodic progress note. For example, if initial plans have not changed, no entry is made under plan (P).

If the previous example of potential for injury was a *new* diagnosis added to the problem list it would appear in a progress note as follows:

4 Potential for injury
> S: States decreased sensation in legs; cannot recall trauma producing bruise or scratches; states uses scatter rugs without padding, sometimes goes around house without glasses, does not put light on to cross hall to bathroom at night.
> O: Decreased sensitivity to touch (see physician's exam).
> A: No expected improvement in sensory loss.[2]
>
> P_{Dx}: Observe degree of caution exercised.
> P_{Tx}: Room check for jutting objects, slippery floor; eyeglasses during ambulation; adequate lighting at all times when ambulating.
> P_{Ed}: Teach precautions regarding ambulation, adequate vision, lighting, scatter rugs, slippery floors, jutting objects, ill-fitting shoes or boots, nail cutting.

Projected outcomes can also be incorporated into this format.

Table 7-4 has three other examples of recording new diagnoses. Noncompliance with activity prescription was a problem of a 35-year-old construction worker in an intensive care unit for treatment of myocardial infarction (heart attack). In this case the nurse did not have sufficient data to determine etiology. Thus, tentative etiological hypotheses and the etiological factor ruled out (knowledge deficit) were recorded under assessment. An assessment of activity tolerance was included. Potential skin breakdown was diagnosed for another client during a home visit by a community

---

[2] Note that assessment (A) does not include etiology when the condition is a potential problem. As discussed in Chapter 3 potential problems have risk factors such as the (S) and (O) in this example. It would be repetitive to also record risk factors as the etiology although they are the reasons a potential problem exists.

TABLE 7-4
RECORD OF NEW NURSING DIAGNOSES

---

1 Noncompliance with activity prescription

    S: States feels better: "heart OK now," and "able to do my own bath." Told M.D. that he understood need for rest and wanted to "do everything to get it healed."

    O: Out of bed ×3; stays at bedside; heart rate increased 5 beats per minute with no arrhythmias when out of bed; restless when in bed; activity prescription is complete bed rest.

    A: Possible postmyocardial infarction denial or independence-dependence conflict; no knowledge deficit regarding activity limits; heart rate response to being out of bed suggests tolerance.

    P_{Dx}: Etiology of noncompliance: Assess denial or conflict over required dependence.

    P_{Tx}: Anticipate needs; discuss activity orders and patient's tolerance limits with M.D.; may need activity tolerance evaluation.

    P_{Ed}: Problem solve with client regarding activity restriction if prescription is not changed.

2 Potential skin breakdown

    S: States likes to lie on left side to look out bedroom window, has no discomfort at site of redness.

    O: 3-cm reddened area over left greater trochanter; no ulceration; decreased pain perception below L3.

    A: Wife competent and will be able to carry out plan with neighbor's help.

    P_{Ed}: Discuss with wife: (1) relocation of bed, OOB as tolerated when assistance available; (2) 1½-hour position change and functional positioning; (3) signs of impending skin breakdown; (4) care of potential pressure sites; (5) adequate nutritional intake, especially protein.

3 Alterations in socialization

    S: States he doesn't want to sit with or talk to others; they "frighten" him.

    O: Single; no family in this part of country; no group involvement; at times appears to be listening to group conversations from a distance but does not interact.

    A: Inability to trust.

    P: **a** Milieu activities with staff person he relates to.

      b Explore these difficulties with patient when he is observed to be listening to conversations.

      c Assist patient to develop plans for joining activities.

      d Provide support from trusted staff person when he agrees to join in activities.

---

health nurse. The wife was taking care of her husband, who had had a transection of the spinal cord at level of the third lumbar vertebra. The third example was written in a psychiatric setting; the diagnosis was alterations in socialization/inability to trust.

Not all subsections (S, O, A, and P) are used when charting progress of a problem or changes in plans. For example, if only signs and symptoms have changed (as would occur when a problem is resolving) just the S and O subsections would be used.

Adaptations of the POR System The POR system can be modified for use in various nursing settings (Walter, Pardee, and Molbo, 1976). One modification that is encouraged for nurses who are learning to use nursing diagnosis is that the initial plan is written in greater detail than shown in the preceding section entitled *Initial Plans.*

After recording the nursing history and examination, it is helpful to use the complete SOAP format as outlined immediately above instead of listing only the problem and plan. When the nurse has had more experience, the abbreviated system that omits the SOAP list can be used to record the problem and plan.

The reason for this suggestion is that the SOAP format provides immediate feedback on cognitive processes. Contradictions can be seen. For example, one can check to see whether the subjective (S) and objective (O) data are sufficient to support the problem and etiology recorded. A cross-check with a manual of diagnostic category definitions may help. Secondly, the nurse can check to be certain that the plan (P) is relevant to the etiology and problem identified. Finally, seeing the entire plan can enable one to see whether it contains interventions with a high probability for attaining outcomes.

Consider some examples of errors that occurred as nurses were learning to use nursing diagnoses and problem oriented recording. Try to pick out the inconsistencies found in these three charts:

Example 1

1 Self-bathing deficit (level 2)

      S: Fears falling in shower; bathes self at sink daily but has difficulty reaching all body parts due to extreme obesity.

      O: Personal hygiene poor; body odor and urine odor detected; hair unwashed; skin unclean on admission.

      A: Extreme obesity.

      P: 1. Obtain long-handled sponge and tub chair.

          2. Arrange for equipment to be used in shower at home.

          3. Teach 1000 calorie diet.

Example 2

1 Sleep pattern disturbance

      S: "I am unable to fall asleep at least three or four times a week; I awaken easily and have nightmares when I take Valium."

      A: Work and family stress.

   P_{Dx}: Observe and record sleep pattern in hospital.

   P_{Tx}: 1. Back massage at bedtime; check comfort level.

Example 3

1 Impaired verbal communication

      S: States husband died 8 months ago; 4 days ago was told she has extensive cancer of abdominal organs.

      O: Weak, halting speech; uses short sentences; no apparent shortness of breath.

      A: Decreased strength.

P: 1. Facilitate verbalization of feelings.
2. Provide encouragement, support, and motivation.
3. Work with family.

In example 1 a question may be raised about plan number 3: Is "teach 1000 calorie diet" an intervention for self-bathing deficit/extreme obesity? Obesity, especially the exogenous type, due to a caloric intake–energy expenditure imbalance, is a second diagnosis. It should be recorded as problem number 2. Further, the plan is inadequate for the diagnosis of obesity.

Example 2 illustrates a common error of the novice. The data base is inadequate for the diagnosis. The recorded data do not support the etiology stated in A, work and family stress. Actually the nurse had data to support this diagnosis in the role-relationship pattern recorded in the history. In addition, the plan is inadequate for the diagnosis. Palliative treatment is prescribed but no interventions are directed toward the stress factors.

Obviously the nurse who recorded Example 3 did not appreciate how problem oriented recording provides a check on clinical reasoning. The data do not support the diagnosis. It appears that objective data were heavily weighted in the nurse's diagnostic judgment. Look at the subjective data; do they support the diagnosis? Absolutely not. Furthermore there is no data base to support "decreased strength," the etiology recorded under A.

In Example 3, if the nurse had reread and examined the consistency among problem, etiology, and plan, errors would have been obvious. Facilitating verbalization, providing support, and working with a family are not the treatments for impaired verbal communication. Second, the plan, even if appropriate, is too vague. What does support entail? Work with the family toward what objective?

Rather than having to cross-check judgments and decisions in memory, one can use the written SOAP format. Instructors or clinical specialists can provide feedback, but it is important to learn how to pick up contradictions oneself.

Recording Disease-Related Observations and Treatments The emphasis in this chapter has been on nursing diagnosis and treatment. Yet, as pointed out in Chapter 1, nursing practice also includes carrying out aspects of medical therapy that clients cannot manage for themselves. These aspects of nursing care are determined by physicians' orders or established protocols for medical treatment.

Disease-related observations and treatments have to be recorded. Presumably, if a disease or symptom has been identified the physician has recorded it on the problem list. In the sample problem list in Table 7–3 the physician made two entries, diabetes mellitus and hypoglycemia; acidosis. In charting observations or treatments related to the disease process, the nurse can use the SOAP format previously described. The only differences are: (1) plan (P) is not used; the client's physician, not the nurse, determines interventions for disease processes[3] and (2) the medical diagnosis and its number constitute the heading of the nurse's entry. For example, if symptoms of thirst or

---

[3] An exception occurs when a nurse treats a disease under protocols that permit varying the treatment plan.

frequent urination were observed, the nurse would record them under the heading *1. Diabetes mellitus*.

As with nursing diagnoses, one must beware of contradictions in the charting of disease-related information. For example, recording "able to administer own insulin injection effectively" under diabetes mellitus is a contradiction. The client's ability has no *direct* relationship to the pathophysiology of diabetes. This observation may indicate that a nursing diagnosis of knowledge deficit (insulin administration) was present but not diagnosed. Beware of placing observations related to nursing diagnoses under medical problems.

There is no need to create new terms for diseases or pathophysiological processes in order to chart disease-related observations and treatments. The medical diagnoses provide terminology. Use of those terms does not constitute medical diagnosis, provided that the physician has already identified and recorded them in his or her diagnostic judgment. If the medical diagnoses have not been recorded, either the symptoms were overlooked or new problems have occurred. In either case notification of the physician is appropriate.

Kardex Care Plans In addition to recording diagnoses and plans on the client's chart, many nurses use a Kardex, a flip-card tool that has a section for keeping information about each client. Usually the following information is recorded: name; age; room number; religion; admission date; medical diagnoses; scheduled medical tests (e.g., cardiac catheterization) and medical treatments; nursing diagnoses; nursing treatments; and nursing outcomes.

The main advantage of the Kardex is that it provides rapid access to the client's overall plan of care. It is used in shift reports, in planning staff assignments, and as a quick reference about all the clients on the hospital unit. The alternative way to acquire information is to leaf through each client's chart or problem list. Proponents of the Kardex system extol its merits.

Some nurses decry the Kardex's usefulness. They claim the Kardex duplicates information on the chart, is usually not up to date, and is rarely used by the professional staff.

If a Kardex is used, nursing diagnoses provide a method of organizing treatment plans. The diagnoses are stated in the problem/etiology format and the interventions are then listed. The data base for a diagnosis is not included, as may be seen in the following example of one nursing diagnosis of a client who has pneumonia and chronic lung disease:

> Problem: Fear (inability to breathe)/pain on inspiration and cough.
> Intervention: 1. Discuss with M.D. need for a liquefying cough medicine and humidifier.
> 2. Repeatedly reassure (regarding breathing problem) that nurses are present; provide call system that does not require verbalization (client is concerned that he will not be able to speak into intercom if respiratory problems occur).
> 3. Monitor breathing difficulty ever ½ hr.
> 4. Teach relaxation techniques.
> 5. Ensure adequate fluid intake to assist in liquefying secretions.

Outcomes: 1. Verbalizes perception of ability to breathe adequately.
2. Verbalizes comfort on inspiration.

In some institutions a nurse's order sheet specifying interventions is used as a supplement to the client's chart. Orders, for example, "teach relaxation techniques" are transferred directly from the chart to the order book.

Disease-Related Interventions Nurses write nursing orders for treating nursing diagnoses. In addition, they write orders related to a client's disease, possible complications, or adaptations of medical treatments. For example, a client may require observation for heart failure, bleeding, or change in neurological signs. Or observations and adaptations (e.g., "give with orange juice") may be necessary while the nurse is carrying out medical orders for drugs and other aspects of medical treatment.

In ordering or recording nursing interventions related to diseases it is not necessary to label disease-related care with nursing diagnoses. One simply records on the Kardex or in the order book the interventions required. The same format can be used as when recording nursing diagnoses except that the medical diagnosis is listed as the problem. For example:

Problem: Diabetes mellitus.
Intervention: Observe for irritability as sign of impending ketoacidosis. See that daily blood samples are drawn *before* breakfast.
Problem: Right hip fracture.
Intervention: Obtain fracture pan; maintain functional alignment of right leg.

It is not necessary to change a diagnosis of diabetes mellitus to alterations in glucose metabolism in order to write interventions or make observations. Nor is it necessary to change myocardial infarction or congestive heart failure to alterations in cardiac output in order to observe for arrhythmias or pulmonary edema. It is expected that *after* a medical diagnosis is made nurses will make pertinent observations and carry out appropriate treatments. Communications about these conditions are organized under disease labels, not nursing diagnoses.

In summary, nursing diagnoses organize written and verbal communications. They provide a concise label for a health problem and thereby increase the speed and clarity of communication. Use of the problem oriented clinical information system is facilitated by nursing diagnoses. In fact, without diagnostic labels the system is difficult to use. In addition, if a nursing Kardex or nursing order book is employed, diagnoses organize the recording of nursing care plans.

NURSING DIAGNOSIS AND DISCHARGE PLANNING

The high cost of health care requires that needs and resources be correctly matched. Clients should receive a level of care and the technology appropriate to the acuity of their health problems. To match needs and resources may require that clients be transferred through many levels of care within a few months. The following are two rather typical examples:

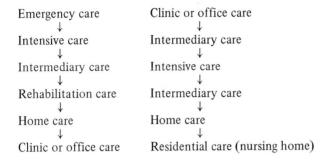

Emergency care	Clinic or office care
↓	↓
Intensive care	Intermediary care
↓	↓
Intermediary care	Intensive care
↓	↓
Rehabilitation care	Intermediary care
↓	↓
Home care	Home care
↓	↓
Clinic or office care	Residential care (nursing home)

These transfers offer the appropriate level of care for different phases of an illness; but from the client's perspective the repeated changes in care providers, routines, and the environment can be additional source of stress. By planning for continuity of care between levels, the nurse can decrease the impact of change.

Ensuring continuity of nursing care between acute care hospitals and the community has been problematic. In response to this difficulty many hospitals have established continuing care programs to assist in coordinating needs and available community resources. Even with these programs, continuity can be jeopardized. If needs are not clearly evaluated and communicated from one care setting to another, fragmented care results.

Requirements for continued medical care as the client moves from one setting to another can be clearly specified. Plans are organized and communicated from physician to physician by using the medical diagnosis. In contrast, nursing has not agreed upon the focus for predischarge evaluation or postdischarge communication of treatment plans. Additionally many times medical and nursing plans for the client's continuing care have not been coordinated.

The set of decisions and activities involved in providing continuity and coordination of care after hospitalization is called *discharge planning*. In many instances it is required by federal or state law (McKeehan, 1979) or by hospital policy.

In the following sections it will be seen that nursing diagnoses provide an excellent focus for discharge planning. Communication of care requirements to nurses in community agencies and coordination of resources for continuing care are also facilitated. In fact, a nurse would not know that a client *needed* continued nursing care unless unresolved nursing diagnoses had been identified. A brief consideration of predischarge planning, referral decisions, and communication of nursing plans will illustrate how diagnoses facilitate these activities.

Predischarge Planning

Discharge planning begins when diagnoses are made. Outcomes that can and should be attained before discharge are projected. These discharge outcomes specify the level of problem resolution and probable time required before a client can (1) undertake independent health management at home or (2) manage with less than 24-hour acute hospital care.

Many currently identified nursing diagnoses can be treated with less expense to the consumer in nursing homes, rehabilitation centers, home care programs, or offices and clinics than in hospitals. Thus a client's discharge is seldom delayed because of nursing diagnoses.

Time of discharge is a combined decision of all health professionals who treat the patient. Sometimes nurses and social workers leave this decision to the physician if it is assumed that the nursing and social work diagnoses (1) will be resolved before the physician is ready to discharge the client or (2) can and should be treated in another setting. In other instances coordinated discharge planning is necessary. No one professional should be expected to make decisions in isolation without information about the client's overall program of care. Too early discharge can result in harm, and delayed discharge adds to financial costs.

Most problems arise because of inadequate communications and delayed planning and intervention. The solution to these problems is (1) early discharge planning, (2) an established structure for multidisciplinary discharge planning, and (3) discharge nursing assessment.

Nursing Activities in Discharge Planning   The structure and implementation of multidisciplinary discharge planning has been described by McKeehan (1979, 1981). In order to participate in multidisciplinary planning, the nurse has to do the following:

1 Assess the level of problem resolution as discharge approaches. Review the status of each current nursing diagnosis. If there is doubt that all nursing problems have been diagnosed, a functional health pattern assessment is done.

2 By reviewing nursing treatment orders, decide what continuing care is needed.

3 Assess the client's capabilities as well as available family and community assistance. The client's (or responsible family member's or guardian's) understanding and plans for personal management of the medically prescribed treatment are also evaluated. (New nursing diagnoses may arise when medical discharge plans are formulated. These may include knowledge or planning deficits in management of symptoms, medication, diet, or activity.)

Discrepancies between the nurse's and the client's (or family member's) assessments of capabilities for managing outside the hospital also need to be identified. For example, if a client does not feel capable of carrying out a health care recommendation, support services will have to be arranged until confidence is developed.

4 Assess the client's need for referral for continued care. When the nurse knows the current diagnoses, the posthospital nursing care that will be required, and the client's capabilities and environmental resources, the next questions are: What care will not be handled adequately by the client, family, or friends? What home or environmental adaptations that are necessary for optimal (or at least acceptable) health promotion cannot be handled by the client, family, or friends? The answers to these questions provide the basis for matching the client's needs for continued nursing care, the available community resources, and the client's preferences about continuing care.

Referral Decisions

The last step in planning for a client's discharge is to determine what type of referral to make. Some options for postacute nursing care are listed in Table 7–5. Clinics, nurses

TABLE 7-5
POSTHOSPITAL RESOURCES AND FACILITIES FOR CONTINUED NURSING CARE

Hospital clinics

Private office practice

Health maintenance organizations

Neighborhood health centers

Rehabilitation centers

Hospital home care programs

Home health care agencies (visiting nurse or public health agencies)

Hospices

Residential centers (long-term care)

Nursing homes

Long-term care hospitals

in private practice, health maintenance organizations, and neighborhood health centers provide periodic nursing care. The emphasis is on health maintenance and promotion. Clients with nursing diagnoses requiring follow-up care on an ambulatory basis would be referred to nursing services such as these.

With certain nursing diagnoses a long period of time and highly skilled nursing care are required to reach optimal outcomes. In these situations plans may be initiated to refer clients to rehabilitation centers or rehabilitation units within acute care hospitals. Specialized services may be considered with diagnoses such as impaired mobility, self-care deficit, perceptual deficit, or chronic pain self-management deficit. Referrals for rehabilitation are appropriate only for clients who have the potential for improvement of their functional pattern.

Both hospital-managed home care programs and community nursing agencies provide family-centered care and help with adaptations from hospital to home. Clients with nursing diagnoses requiring continued home care or supervision are referred to visiting nurses in these agencies. Examples of such diagnoses are potential noncompliance (disease management), self-care deficit due to short-term memory loss, potential for injury, and unresolved grieving. Actual or potential family problems in coping, inter-action, or home maintenance may also require home visits for evaluation and treatment. The availability of professional visiting nurses, homemakers, and home health aides varies from 24 hours a day in some communities to 8 or fewer in others; thus client and family capabilities have to be carefully determined.

Residential and hospice centers provide living environments for clients who cannot manage in their homes. Conditions such as profound mental retardation or severe cerebral palsy may require long-term residential care in a sheltered environment. A hospice is both a living environment and a philosophy of care for terminally ill clients. Residential care and hospice centers, respectively, are options for clients with nursing diagnoses related to permanent cognitive or motor impairments and terminal illness.

Depending on the resources available, a diagnosis such as severe chronic mobility impairment may be treated in the home or may require long-term institutional care. If continuous 24-hour nursing care is required over a period of time, nursing homes or long-term care hospitals may be chosen. The period of care may be weeks, months, or years, depending on the client's progress toward independence in decision making, mobility, and self-care.

The nurse discusses with clients and their families the type of care required and the options available, or clients and their families may attend multidisciplinary planning conferences. These conferences include all health team members involved in the client's care and discharge planning.

Two or more clients may have the same nursing diagnosis but different discharge plans. This is to be expected because interventions are always individualized. Consider the example of two clients with total self-care deficit (level 3) due to sensorimotor loss (spinal cord transection). After rehabilitation, both were able to manage self-care with the assistance of one person and assistive devices. One client was referred to the visiting nurse service for home care. The other was discharged to a long-term care facility. Why the difference? The first client's spouse and neighbors valued home care and were able to adapt the home setting and provide care with the assistance of the visiting nurse. The second client had no family and lived alone although he liked social contact. Twenty-four hour home services were not available; even if they had been they would probably have been too costly and would not have provided sufficient social interaction. A nursing home was chosen where he could be near his friends.

Before discussing the writing of referrals, it is important to examine why discharge planning begins when nursing diagnoses are made and outcomes projected. If referral for continuing care will be necessary, information will be needed for making decisions about the referral. A great deal of information can be collected and charted while daily care is being given. Without this ongoing information gathering, discharge planning appears very time consuming—it is rushed and ineffectively done.

Discharge planning judgments are critically important both for the client's safety and for the quality of the person's life. Diagnoses have to be made accurately. If the capabilities of the client or situation are overestimated, further problems can arise; if they are underestimated, the client is subjected to unwarranted financial expense. The best data available have to be obtained.

Communication of Plans

The communication of plans is as important as planning. Clear and concise treatment orders and the bases for orders have to be communicated to the next care providers. Good communication increases the probability that nursing care will proceed without interruption.

Nursing diagnoses organize communications and clarify the rationale for nursing orders. Problem oriented recording of the diagnoses (SOAP format) further facilitates concise communication of critical information.

Standardized forms are used in most hospitals for client referrals to frequently used community agencies; visiting nurse referral forms are an example. Discharge summaries can also be used by nurses to refer clients with unresolved diagnoses. A discharge summary referral would be sent to nurses in clinics, private practice, and other ambulatory care settings. When particular attention needs to be called to some problem or aspect of follow-up care, a telephone call may be used.

The following two examples of the use of nursing diagnoses in writing referrals demonstrate the clarity and conciseness of communication which results. The first client was a 12-year-old intelligent, sports-loving boy referred for periodic nursing care at a hematology (blood) clinic. His medical diagnosis was hemophilia. The following two nursing diagnoses and SOAP notes were recorded on the nursing section of a referral:

NDx:[4] 1 Potential for injury

    S: Likes sports, especially football; active child; states thinks he can still play on team if plays a different position.

    O: Factor VIII deficiency, 1% plasma factor activity; recent football injury.

    A: Moderately severe risk for hemorrhage; knows about bleeding problem and that he will not be able to play football but can attend games; overheard telling mother he could play.

    P_{Dx}: Assess whether he has resigned from Little League team.

    P_{Ed}: Repeat instructions regarding caution in avoiding trauma. If trauma occurs mother is to bring child to emergency room.

ND_x: 2 Potential parental overprotection

    S: Mother states, "I feel so guilty, but I'll be sure he doesn't get hurt"; father says he will buy books and child can come home and read after school; asking if they should get rid of dog.

    O: Both parents express concern and nervousness whenever child's activity discussed.

    A: Parents understand tendency for overprotection and say they will try to avoid it; plan to contact National Hemophilia Foundation and join parent support group.

    P_{Dx}: Assess for restrictions placed on child by parents; check to see whether they have joined parent support group.

    P_{Tx}: Continue to reassure parents that guilt is normal reaction; assist them in identifying their strengths as parents; to hospital for plasma factor VIII if trauma and bleeding occur.

A second example is that of a referral to a visiting nurse. The client's medical diagnosis was adult onset diabetes mellitus. She was a 65-year-old retired secretary. In the nursing section of the visiting nurse referral the following appeared:

NDx: 1 Dysfunctional grieving

    S: States lost her father 1 year ago; cared for him at home before he died of cancer; verbal expression of distress, sadness; states she has no one now and doesn't know what to do.

    O: Altered sleeping, eating, and dream pattern in hospital; mild inability to concentrate; crying spells.

    A: Loss; possible fear of newly acquired independence. States will try to become involved in community activities after discharge.

    P_{Dx}: Evaluate state of grieving after return home.

    P_{Tx}: Encourage contact with son and his family for support. Encourage joining voluntary community group; client expressed interest in this.

ND_x: 2 Disease management deficit (insulin administration)[5]

---

[4] Abbreviation for nursing diagnosis.
[5] Note: The problem label heads the referral. Etiology is placed under assessment (A).

S: "I don't know if I can do this injection adequately. I could never give my father injections." States knows importance of insulin administration.

O: Has successfully administered morning insulin twice. Hand shakes; dexterity is fair. Client has asked to practice on an orange. Able to draw up dose accurately.

A: Fear (perceived incompetency and error). Motivated but still needs supervision. Supervision and experience increase confidence.

P: Supervise insulin administration in home ×2 (likes to eat breakfast at 9 a.m.) Reevaluate competency.

ND_x: 3 Disease management deficit (compensated)

S: Reassured by plans for nurse's home visit.

O: Verbalizes correct dietary and activity plans. States principles of skin care, urine testing, and signs of complications to be reported; skills demonstrated.

P: Review management during home visit. To be seen in doctor's office in one month.

Nursing referrals about unresolved diagnoses help community agencies to provide continuity of care. Referrals should also be sent from these agencies when their clients are treated in hospitals.

In summary, nursing diagnoses facilitate continuity of care among care settings. Diagnoses provide focus for early evaluation of continuing care needs, and suggested plans can be communicated in a concise, organized manner. Most importantly, individualized interventions can be written and communicated for each problem. Good communication between care providers decreases the client's stress in adjusting to different health care providers, routines, and environments.

NURSING DIAGNOSIS AND THE LAW

From the perspective of many nurses, nursing diagnosis merely recognizes what nurses have always done. This may not be the view of hospital administrators, lawyers, or physicians, for many of whom the term *nursing diagnosis*, when heard for the first time, sets red lights flashing. The lights usually change to green when the concept is explained.

Even nursing colleagues are heard to say, "Legally, you can't do that" or "You'll put your license in jeopardy." Another often-heard comment by nurses is, "Our hospital hasn't accepted nursing diagnosis." The purpose of the discussion in this section is to explore whether the first statements are true or false and to see whether the latter has any relevance. The concepts of duty, cause, and harm, as they relate to negligence, will first be examined in order to provide a basis for judging the truth of the above statements or similar ones encountered in practice. It will be seen that formulating and documenting nursing diagnosis can help nurses and institutions avoid negligence claims.

Negligent conduct on the part of a nurse is a basis for malpractice litigation. The client, relative, or other has to provide evidence about four issues: (1) duty, (2) breach of duty, (3) cause and effect, and (4) personal or economic harm (Mancini, 1979, p. 337).

An example will clarify. A nurse, hospital, and physician were sued by the wife of a client. Her husband fell in the hospital and fractured his femur. She maintained that his care was negligent. The facts of the situation were as follows:

On December 1 the patient, an athletic appearing, sociable, 30-year-old male was admitted to a hospital because of slight muscle weakness. The chart stated that tests for multiple sclerosis were to be done. According to the wife, she told the admitting nurse that her husband had fallen twice at home. The physician's ambulation order was "out of bed as desired." On the morning of December 2, the nurse told the client he could wash in the bathroom and left to care for others. The client fell going to the bathroom. X-rays revealed a fractured femur. The client was unable to reach the call light; the private room door was shut, and it was maintained he lay in pain for one-half hour before the nurse returned.

The Element of Duty

The first element to be established when the possibility of negligence is being assessed is *duty* to the client. Basically, the nurse must protect the client against unreasonable risks by adhering to a certain standard of conduct. How is a nurse to know what the standard of conduct is?

In response to this question, the ANA standards of practice may come to mind, or the ANA code of nursing ethics. These nationally accepted, professional guidelines for the *conduct* of nursing practice can be used by a trial lawyer. The situation would be similar to obtaining a nurse expert witness. A lawyer would ask, "Would this [citing alleged negligence] be common practice by a nurse?"

As previously discussed, the *Standards of Nursing Practice* states that nurses assess and that nursing diagnoses are derived from health status data. There was no indication in the chart that the nurse had assessed mobility or gross muscle strength even though they were the reason for admission.

A nurse expert witness would probably testify that it was reasonable to expect that the risk factors (history of falls, muscle weakness, and possible multiple sclerosis) would suggest the diagnostic judgment of potential for injury. Recognition of potential for injury would be followed by supervision while ambulating and other preventive measures. Although this diagnosis was within the domain of nursing practice (Appendix A), there was no evidence that the diagnosis was made and supervision instituted.

Before resorting to the standards or nursing textbooks, the client's attorney would check the state nurse practice act. The incident occurred in one of the states whose nurse practice law includes the term *diagnosis*.

Lawyers also examine rules and regulations promulgated by state boards of nursing; some states specify the nursing process components as functions of the registered nurse. State practice acts and board of nursing rules and regulations are the legal basis for nursing; standards are professional, not legal, guidelines.

Breach of Duty

The second element that must be present in negligence is breach of duty to a client. The chart, in this man's case, was evidence that the nurse did not conform to the practice act: No diagnostic judgment was on record about the potential for injury. Most importantly, there was no indication that ambulation was being supervised by nurses.

Cause and Effect

A relationship between the nurse's conduct and an alleged injury is the third element necessary for demonstrating negligence. In the case cited, a reasonably close relationship had to be demonstrated between the fracture and the nurse's lack of client supervision. *Why* the nurse did not supervise the client's ambulation is irrelevant from the legal perspective. The court is interested only in the fact that there was negligent supervision. Nurses and hospital administrators ask why in order to prevent future occurrences; for example, why was a nursing history and examination not done at admission?

Nursing diagnosis represents a synthesis of clinical data and a judgment about whether or not a health problem is present. Once this synthesis and problem identification take place, it is difficult to ignore the state of the client. The nurse becomes motivated to act. This is how diagnosis helps prevent a breach of duty that results in harm to the client.

Harm or Injury

The fourth element to be proven in a negligence case is actual injury (physical, psychological, or both) and loss, including economic loss. In the case illustrated, x-ray reports demonstrated a fractured femur. Because of the long period required for healing, economic loss as well as injury was claimed.

The main point to be understood from this discussion is that the law is concerned with diagnosis in only one respect. That is, the court wishes to establish what the state of the client is. Once this is established, the law is primarily concerned with nursing actions appropriate to the client's state. An act that is *committed* or *omitted* in regard to that state *and* results in harm is a basis for a malpractice determination. As Fortin and Rabinow state, "the law is primarily concerned with diagnosis-related action" (1979, p. 553).

Legal Decisions

No cases have been found in which the court cited nursing diagnosis, although "judgment" increasingly appears to be something nurses are expected to exercise.

Can nurses make medical diagnoses? This is not the most fruitful way of framing the question. Rather, ask: What judgments are nurses expected to make? Two cases cited by Fortin and Rabinow (1979) may clarify that judgment is expected beyond the domain of nursing diagnoses.

In the first case, a company nurse was considered negligent for not recognizing a basal cell carcinoma and referring the employee who had developed it. As cited, the court said "a nurse . . . should be able to diagnose . . . sufficiently to know whether it is a condition within her authority to treat as a first aid case or whether it bears danger signs that should warn her to send the patient to a physician" (Fortin and Rabinow,

1979, p. 560). In the second case, nurses judged that a child's fever was not serious. No physician was called. The child died of congestive heart failure after an attack of rheumatic fever (Fortin and Rabinow, 1979, p. 560). In both cases, the courts required tentative medical diagnosis to some degree. In many states the extent of a nurse's responsibility for making medical diagnoses is unclear.

Interpreting signs and symptoms and judging how to treat them (nursing diagnoses) or making referrals (tentative medical diagnoses) are nursing responsibilities. In both instances the nurse has a legal responsibility to use the diagnostic process skillfully. Otherwise, diagnostic judgments may lead to injury and risk of malpractice.

One additional point should be made. There are reasons why some physicians pale when encountering nursing diagnosis. They may believe they are legally responsible for *all* care. What needs to be clarified to such physicians is that a nurse practices under his or her own license, not the physician's. Second, one should clarify that the law requires nurses to make diagnostic judgments; it may be useful to cite the previously mentioned court cases. Third, the nurse can find out whether the state practice acts or rules and regulations specify diagnosis, diagnostic judgments, or merely judgment. If diagnosis is called for, copies of those documents can be obtained for physicians. They may not have had the opportunity to learn the legal scope of nursing. In many medical schools little is taught about nursing practice.

DIAGNOSTIC RESPONSIBILITY

Who should diagnose? The answer sought is usually a classification, such as clinical specialist or professional, technical, or practical nurse. At times the question is abstract; at other times it is highly pragmatic and is asked for legal, administrative, or educational purposes. It also can be reworded: Who *can* diagnose? This wording introduces the idea of ability.

The answer is important when staffing and nursing care delivery are being examined. It is also important in decisions about delegating care to nonprofessionals when the nurse assumes managerial responsibility for groups of clients.

The answer depends on multiple factors. Exploration of these factors and the "state of art" of nursing diagnosis suggests that diagnosing is a professional activity influenced by the situation in which the professional is practicing.

Legal Considerations

Laws regulating nursing practice are not worded consistently from one state to another. In some states, practice acts specify diagnosis as a function of the registered nurse (baccalaureate, associate degree, and diploma graduates). The question is sometimes asked whether initial assessment and diagnosis can be delegated to practical nurses. Practice acts controlling practical nursing usually state that the practical nurse must have the *direction and supervision* of a registered nurse, physician, or dentist. Diagnostic judgment cannot be directed; thus it cannot be delegated. Moreover, supervision during assessment would require presence of the registered nurse as data are being collected; thus there is no point in delegation of assessment.

Direction and supervision usually refers to the activities of observation and treatment. These can be clearly directed *after* diagnoses are made. Noncomplex judgments related to observation and treatment are within practical nurses' scope of practice, but the complex diagnostic judgment is not.

The delegation of nursing diagnosis to practical nurses places a burden on them. If harm occurs, it can easily be established that they are not educated to diagnose and should not have accepted this responsibility. A comparable situation would exist if a physician delegated a liver biopsy to a registered nurse. Both risk malpractice if harm occurs.

This argument does not negate the fact that practical nurses contribute observations of importance to nursing diagnosis. Neither does it detract from their contribution to treatment, once the treatment plan has been specified.

Professional Considerations

Registered nurses consider assessment, diagnosis, care planning, and evaluation to be professional—as well as legal—duties to their clients. Standards of practice, nursing textbooks, and journal articles specify diagnosis as a professional function. In addition, standards of the Joint Commission on Accreditation of Hospitals state that a registered nurse assesses clients and plans their care (Joint Commission on Accreditation of Hospitals, 1981).

Consumers deserve professional nursing care. At a minimum, professional care includes diagnosis and care planning. When care giving is delegated, these two responsibilities must be retained. The basic argument for this statement rests within the educational curricula of nursing programs as will be seen in the next section.

Educational Considerations

Another way of answering the question of who should diagnose is to examine the curricula of nursing programs. Examination reveals that diagnostic judgment is seldom if ever taught in practical nursing programs. In baccalaureate and master's degree programs, nursing diagnoses and the judgment skills used in making diagnoses are usually integrated into nursing courses (McLane, 1981). In diploma and associate degree programs it may be expected that at least an introduction to nursing diagnosis is given when nursing process is taught. Currently diploma and associate degree graduates are preparing for registered nurse functions.

When competency statements for professional and technical practice (and thus, education) are discussed, professional competency includes formulating nursing diagnoses. Technical nurses' competencies are usually viewed as contributing observations to the formulation of diagnoses and understanding relationships between diagnoses and care planning.

Process Considerations

From previous chapters it should be clear that the diagnostic process is not a task to be undertaken by nonprofessional nurses. Diagnosing requires a good clinical knowledge base, training in inferential and analytical skills, and the ability to conceptualize a client's condition for purposes of intervention. Nevertheless it is not uncommon to hear that initial assessment or diagnosis can be delegated to nonprofessionals.

A distinct problem arises if one person collects clinical data, for example, takes the health history, and another tries to formulate diagnoses. A critical step is missed: branching on the basis of clinical knowledge and hypotheses. Discussion in previous chapters pointed out that assessment and diagnosis are not separate activities. The diagnostic process begins after the first few pieces of information signifying a possible problem are collected.

Further, a diagnosis dictates care. It is impossible to separate the components of nursing process into an assembly line activity. The nursing process is just that—a process —not independent steps.

A second major argument for diagnosis as a professional activity is the clinical knowledge base required. If all nurses had equally good diagnostic process *skills*, the successful and unsuccessful diagnosticians could probably be separated on the basis of their theoretical knowledge. This suggests that the best diagnosticians will probably be at the clinical specialist level. These are the nurses who should be used as consultants to the less knowledgeable and experienced.

An example may illustrate. Let us consider what many think is an "easy" diagnosis to make: potential skin breakdown. Anyone can recognize reddened skin if motivated to do so. Yet to make an early diagnosis and institute preventive care, one must weigh a multiplicity of factors in judgment. It is not just that a client is on bed rest; age, nutrition, current pathophysiology, motivation, and emotional state are also factors that determine the risk state. The weight of each factor has to be considered in making the judgment that the client is at risk for skin breakdown.

The diagnoses in the current list (Appendix A) may appear very basic. In fact, from a cognitive perspective, they require more complex judgments than many medical diagnoses.

A third major argument for restricting diagnostic responsibility to professional nurses is the state of the art in nursing diagnosis. Professional nurses at this time are just learning how to formulate clients' actual and potential problems in diagnostic terms. Equally true, the diagnostic nomenclature still needs clinical testing and more explicit definition. When ambiguity exists in diagnosis, professionals are required. This is exemplified in the levels of certainty discussed in Chapter 2, page 49.

In other professions, it takes many years of training to be considered a good diagnostician by one's colleagues. Perhaps in the future, new nursing graduates, like medical interns, will routinely have an opportunity for a year of supervision. The value of postgraduate supervision of diagnosis and treatment is already recognized in psychiatric-mental-health nursing. Most people presumably would agree that clients with other conditions also deserve this quality control.

Situational Considerations

Not all clients who need nursing care have access to professional nurses. This is a reality. In some settings, such as primary care, the shortage of professional nurses can be related to insufficient reimbursement for nursing, a topic to be considered later. The lack of sufficient professional staff in hospital and nursing home settings is very widely recognized.

Why is there a shortage of professional staff? Conditions of employment have been implicated (Wandelt, Pierce, and Widdowson, 1981). Nursing as a profession has not articulated the client problems requiring professional care; in the absence of this information, staffing has been based on the only available data, the medical diagnosis and its acuity. Yet no administrator would be able to refute the need for staff if it is documented that nursing diagnoses are going untreated. Data about staffing needs in relation to the problems nurses treat take time to collect but may prove exceedingly useful in the long run to justify whether professional or nonprofessional staff are needed.

In response to shortages, busy nurses too often delegate the history, examination, diagnosis, or care planning at admission to a nonprofessional person. In actuality, it would be safer to turn over technical or administrative duties. Professional care planning makes a difference. More specifically, diagnosis-based treatment makes a difference. Many will attest to this.

Experiential Considerations

Among professional nurses there are both experienced and inexperienced diagnosticians. Some nurses may not have had the opportunity to learn diagnostic skills in basic or continuing education programs. Inservice programs or self-study groups can remedy this.

As competency is being attained, whether one is a student or graduate, it is important to recognize the need for consultation. No one is an expert on everything. Legal and ethical considerations suggest that assistance should be sought from colleagues or specialists in the problem area. As in medicine, general practitioners in nursing seek specialist consultation for complex diagnostic problems. The practitioner learns and the client receives quality care.

In summary, registered nurses have responsibility for diagnosis. Within this category may be varying levels of expertise. This variety is a result of the nature of educational programs as well as of continuing education opportunities.

Projections about the future indicate that clinical specialists will be the expert diagnosticians of the profession. Baccalaureate graduates will be competent in diagnosis and through experience will build on these competencies. The shorter programs cannot be expected to develop more than an introduction to the concept of diagnosis and diagnostic skills used in referral. Practical nurses will be aware of diagnosis and of the relevant data to be documented. Projections are always tentative, especially when a profession is in the process of change. This is the current state in nursing. Furthermore, projections are not based on research in diagnostic competencies but rather on opinion derived from the legal, educational, and process considerations just discussed.

SUMMARY

The subject of this chapter was how to use nursing diagnoses in direct client care. Nursing process was described as the method nurses use to deliver care and to implement the concepts, values, and standards of nursing.

Two phases of the nursing process were delineated: problem identification (the diagnostic process) and problem solving (care planning and implementation). The link between the two phases is nursing diagnosis; diagnosis is the *end product* of problem identification and the *focus* of problem solving.

Nursing process involves an interrelated set of decisions. The chapter showed how, in the problem-solving phase, a nursing diagnosis, describing the client's present state, is used as a focus for projecting health outcomes to be reached. In combination the diagnosis and desired outcomes are used as a basis for decisions about nursing intervention.

One of the values held by the profession and expressed in its *Standards of Nursing Practice* (American Nurses' Association, 1973) is individualized nursing care. Accordingly, although clients may have the same diagnosis and desired outcomes, their individuality is considered in care planning. Personal factors, the client's perceptions about the problem, level of compensation, acuity, situational effects, and cost-benefit factors were discussed as considerations in care planning decisions that individualize care.

To ensure coordination of care, and for legal reasons, communication of nursing process decisions is necessary. Both written records and verbal communications are enhanced by using nursing diagnoses to organize clinical data. The problem oriented method of recording provides clarity of communication as well as an important crosscheck on cognitive processes.

Using nursing diagnoses increases the clarity and conciseness of verbal and written communications. One result is improved coordination of care. Examples of communication in discharge planning demonstrated how diagnoses could be used to facilitate continuity of care.

In an examination of nursing diagnosis and the law, negligence was defined. In malpractice suits involving negligence one criterion to be demonstrated is duty to the client. According to the professional standards of practice, duty includes diagnostic judgments. Some state nurse practice acts or board of nursing rules and regulations for practice also specify nursing diagnosis as within the scope of generic (general) registered-nurse practice. From a legal perspective, must the nurse diagnose? The law is concerned with whether harm and injury could have been prevented if a diagnostic judgment had been made and whether standards, acts, or rules and regulations were violated.

Nursing diagnosis is a cognitive tool that directs conscious attention to the meaning of a set of cues. Attention to a client's need for care usually results in nursing action. This is how nursing diagnosis, as opposed to isolated and sometimes meaningless cues, protects a nurse against negligence litigation and a client against harm.

Who should diagnose? Standards and laws clearly dictate that this is a professional activity. Nonprofessionals contribute data after initial diagnoses are made. Can diagnosis be delegated to nonprofessionals? Certainly, just as cardiac surgery can be delegated to a registered nurse. No nurse would accept this delegation because none is prepared and licensed to practice medicine. The situation is similar where nursing diagnosis is involved. Delegation is associated with legal risk, both for the person delegating and for the one accepting. Nonprofessional activities, not assessment and diagnosis, are appropriately assigned to nonprofessional personnel. Professional authority cannot be used to subject others to situations they are unprepared to handle.

BIBLIOGRAPHY

American Nurses' Association. *Standards of nursing practice*. Kansas City, Mo.: American Nurses' Association, 1973.

Bloch, D. Criteria, standards, norms: Crucial terms in quality assurance. *Journal of Nursing Administration*, September 1977, 7:20–29.

Combs, A. W., Avila, D. L., & Purkey, W. W. *Helping relationships*. Boston: Allyn and Bacon, 1971.

Fortin, J. D., & Rabinow, J. Legal implications of nursing diagnosis. *Nursing Clinics of North America*, September 1979, *14*, 553–561.

Gordon, W. J. *Synectics: The development of creative capacity*. New York: Collier, 1961.

Joint Commission on Accreditation of Hospitals. *Accreditation manual for hospitals*. Chicago: Joint Commission, 1981.

Mancini, M. Proving negligence in nursing practice. *American Journal of Nursing*, February 1979, *79*, 337–338.

McKeehan, K. M. Nursing diagnosis in a discharge planning program. *Nursing Clinics of North America*, September 1979, *14*, 517–524.

McKeehan, K. M. (Ed.). *Continuing care*. St. Louis: Mosby, 1981.

McLane, A. Nursing diagnosis in baccalaureate and graduate education. In M. J. Kim & D. A. Moritz (Eds.), *Classification of nursing diagnoses: Proceedings of the third and fourth national conferences*. New York: McGraw-Hill, 1981.

Orem, D. E. *Nursing: Concepts of practice*. New York: McGraw-Hill, 1980.

Osborne, A. F. *Applied imagination*. New York: Scribner, 1963.

Walter, J. B., Pardee, G. P., & Molbo, D. M. *Dynamics of problem-oriented approaches: Patient care and documentation*. Philadelphia: Lippincott, 1976.

Wandelt, M. A., Pierce, P. M., & Widdowson, R. R. Why nurses leave nursing and what can be done about it. *American Journal of Nursing*, January 1981, *81*, 72–77.

Weed, L. L. *Medical records, medical education, and patient care*. Cleveland: Case Western Reserve University Press, 1971.

CHAPTER 8

RELEVANCE OF NURSING DIAGNOSIS TO PRACTICE ISSUES

In this chapter the relevance of nursing diagnosis to issues slightly removed from direct care will be considered. The assurance of quality care for populations of clients is one issue. This area will be examined in order to understand how diagnoses can be the focus for nursing quality assurance programs. Ideas in this section will be familiar because quality care review is a review of nursing process components discussed previously. It will be evident that nursing diagnoses have to be recorded during direct care in order for the required review to take place.

One factor that can influence quality care is the client's access to professional nurses. The section on staffing patterns demonstrates that current methods of allocating staff leave much to be desired, in the opinion of institutional administrators. Staffing patterns are unsatisfactory partly because nursing has not sufficiently described client needs from a nursing perspective. Studies are in progress to design staffing patterns that are based on clients' nursing diagnoses. The essential understanding to be gained from the discussion is that each nurse has to record clients' diagnoses and related interventions in order to help institutions plan professional staff allocations.

Access to professional nursing in the community is also problematic. The issue has some similarities to staffing problems in institutional care. In both settings, the rationale for reimbursement for nursing care is either vague or lacking. An understanding of third party payment for the treatment of nursing diagnoses may lead to clearer articulation of what should be reimbursed.

Nursing diagnoses, it will be seen, are relevant to determining the scope of nursing practice. Nurses need to communicate rather specifically to consumers, legislators, and administrators what health conditions they treat. In this chapter it is argued that the scope of practice will become much clearer when nursing diagnoses are identified.

Issues such as how to describe the domain of nursing practice will lead us to consider the development of nursing science. Nursing diagnosis is particularly relevant to this subject. It will be seen that diagnoses may offer a focus for the development of nursing practice theory, which will eventually provide scientific knowledge to be used in direct care activities.

Identifying health conditions that concern practicing nurses will have an impact on the previously discussed issues. Thus, we will come full circle: As nursing diagnoses are identified a focus will be provided for measuring quality client care, for allocation of professional staff, and for third party reimbursement.

NURSING DIAGNOSIS AND QUALITY CARE REVIEW

As costs rise, consumers demand quality goods and services. People have long been concerned about cost and quality of toasters, automobiles, and plumbers' services. Since more public funds have been funneled into government sponsored health programs, demands for assurance of quality care have been heard.

In 1972, the Congress of the United States mandated professional review of health care services, particularly emphasizing medical services. Since that time, care delivered to recipients of Medicare (people over 65 years of age), Medicaid (low-income populations), and maternal and child health programs must be reviewed. A national and statewide system of professional standards review organizations (PSROs) was created. They are responsible for ensuring that all health care reimbursed from federal funds is *necessary*. In addition, care must (1) meet professional standards and (2) be provided economically in an appropriate setting (Public Law 92-603).

The legislation just described was based on the concept of *peer review*. This concept means that members of a profession that delivers a specific type of health care develop the bases for evaluation of that care. They also carry out the evaluation process. Care may be reviewed (evaluated) while it is being given or retrospectively. In the latter case charts are examined after the clients are discharged. The purpose of peer review is to identify less than acceptable care delivery. Once problems are identified, remedial action can be taken. Through educational programs, administrators and practitioners can be helped to bring care to an accepted level.

In addition to the required PSRO review of hospital and long-term care, many institutions voluntarily submit to another type of care review carried out periodically by the national Joint Commission on Accreditation of Hospitals (JCAH). One of their requirements is a well-defined program for identification and correction of problems. The standard to be met in this area is:

> There shall be evidence of a well-defined, organized program designed to enhance patient care through the ongoing, objective assessment of important aspects of patient care and the correction of identified problems. (Joint Commission on Accreditation of Hospitals, 1981)

In the following sections, concepts of quality assurance will be reviewed. This review will provide a basis for understanding how nursing diagnosis can be used in care review, problem identification, and remedial actions. It will also be important to understand the concept of accountability to consumers that underlies quality assurance.

Terms will be introduced that are commonly used in quality assurance literature.

Some will seem familiar because quality assurance deals with nursing process components previously discussed. Large populations of clients will be considered, not individual clients.

Assuring quality care for large groups of clients is sometimes thought of as a responsibility only of administrators. Actually, concepts of quality assurance have to be integrated into every nurse's practice. Irrespective of whether they are directly or indirectly involved in quality assurance, nurses should clearly understand issues, such as this, that affect their professional practice. Understanding is facilitated when each nurse becomes involved in developing standards, reviewing care, or in planning for care improvement. As professionals, all nurses are responsible and accountable for the standards that are set for their practice and the level of care delivered to consumers.

Use of Nursing Diagnosis in Care Review

What are measures of quality nursing care? This is the first question to be answered when a department of nursing begins quality care review. Various options exist. The competency of nurses certainly influences quality care, as do the resources they have available. Also, what nurses do for clients has an impact on care and can be measured. Finally, it is argued that the outcome of care, that is, the health state of the client, is one of the best measures of quality care delivery.

Overview of Care Review Concepts   The assessment areas just named represent the three components of care delivery that can be evaluated: structural, process, and outcome components. In each component standards are developed from research literature and expert opinion. The three types of standards are defined as follows:

Structural standards are statements describing valued characteristics of the care delivery setting that indirectly influence care. Examples would be number and preparation of nurses, physical facilities, equipment, inservice education, policies, and procedures.

Process standards are statements describing valued characteristics of care delivery. They describe what nurses should do for their clients. The American Nurses' Association standards of practice are process standards for assessment, diagnosis, planning, and so forth.

Outcome standards are statements describing health characteristics, behavior, or states of the client. Descriptions of clients' mobility and of clients' knowledge about their medications are examples of the focus of these standards. Outcomes are presumed to result from nursing intervention (although cause and effect relationships are hard to establish).

Theoretically, structural, process, and outcome standards are interrelated as are links in a chain. Structural resources are needed to carry out the processes of care delivery; in turn, processes (interventions) influence client health outcomes. Yet it is recognized that many other factors operating in either the client or the environment can influence outcomes.

Structural, process, and outcome standards are set for populations of clients. A *population* is a classification or grouping of clients that have some characteristic in common. A diagnosis may be a basis for grouping.

The setting of standards of care for client populations is an activity of great importance. Once standards are set, they cannot be ignored. In a sense they are a commitment to certain health care values. Suppose, for example, a standard of care is set in a hospital for clients with potential fluid volume deficit; ethically, the standard should then be met for every patient with that diagnosis. Standards should be based on the best scientific and clinical knowledge available. They have to be realistic and attainable in all situations unless extenuating circumstances can be demonstrated.

When quality assurance was mandated by legislation and accrediting agencies, the health professions had neither relevant research data nor standards with which to proceed. In the last 10 years many debates have occurred about how to measure quality. The major issue involves formulating reliable and valid standards and criteria for measurement. In essence the debate is whether the care (processes), the outcomes of care, or both have to be measured. Block (1975, 1980) in nursing and McAuliffe (1979) in medicine present reviews of the debate.

To experience the issue, imagine for a moment that your colleagues are going to use a set of standards to grade (evaluate) your nursing care or your clients' health outcomes. Imagine further that outsiders are going to know what grade you receive. Are you concerned about *what* is evaluated and *how* the evaluation is done? For example, do you want them to measure *what patient education you provided*? Or, instead, should they evaluate *your clients' health knowledge and skills*? Suppose you taught a client how to take his medications, but when your care was evaluated the client stated incorrect information. Does that mean you gave poor quality care?

There is a second important issue with which nurses must be concerned. Full accountability can be assumed only for health problems nurses diagnose and treat. This statement may seem so logical that it need not be said. As quality assurance began, however, clients were classified according to medical conditions, such as myocardial infarction and appendectomy. This gave the impression that nurses were assuming accountability for quality of care not within their control. Actually, mislabeling of the populations occurred; many of the standards were nevertheless processes and outcomes of unlabeled *nursing* diagnoses.

Focus of Care Review   Nursing diagnoses describe the independent domain of nursing practice. Thus nurses assume accountability for health problems described by these diagnostic labels. It follows logically that nursing diagnoses should be used to define client populations for care review (Gordon, 1980) and that diagnoses provide the ideal tool for writing nursing-specific process and outcome standards, identifying care delivery problems, and planning remedial actions.

Use of nursing diagnoses as a framework for care review brings some uniformity to quality assurance activities in different health care settings. Standards based on diagnoses rather than on unique features of one setting or another can be shared and consequently decrease the cost of implementing review programs. Also, multiple testing of standards in different institutions leads to the improvement of the standards.

Selecting Populations   In a health care setting a small, representative group of nurses usually undertakes the task of developing standards. This task requires a set of decisions. Because of time and costs, it is seldom possible to review all care given to all patients; therefore the first decision is to designate a few diagnostic populations. Later the number of populations can be increased. To decide which patient populations will be studied, high-incidence nursing diagnoses have to be identified by staff familiar with the setting. A listing such as that in Appendix A can facilitate the process.

Tracer methodology is a systematic way of making final decisions about populations. The common nursing diagnoses identified by staff can be narrowed by use of this technique. A tracer is a nursing diagnosis that can reflect the quality of care being delivered. For example, potential skin breakdown may be one good tracer for long-term institutional care. A tracer such as noncompliance may reflect an aspect of ambulatory care quality.

The questions in Table 8-1 can be applied to a list of diagnoses that are common in the particular setting. Those nursing diagnoses having most of the characteristics are probably good tracers, and the clients who have those diagnoses become the tracer populations.

Writing Standards and Criteria   Nursing diagnoses facilitate the writing of standards that are clearly within the realm of nursing accountability. There is now sufficient nursing literature to enable nurses to begin to delineate processes and outcomes for currently accepted diagnoses. As clinical research on these health problems increases, standards will have a more substantial scientific base. Until then theory, the available research, and expert opinion will prevail.

Process standards describe the critical interventions for a diagnosis. When process standards are written both the problem and the etiology have to be considered. Look at the differences in the standards listed in Table 8-2. Although the problem in the two diagnoses is the same, the standards are different because the etiology differs. The cause of a condition directly influences what is done to treat it; thus the acceptable standard for what is done changes with the etiology.

Outcome standards are characteristics of the client that describe a valued health state. They describe only the state of the client, not how it came about. If the health problem disappears or improves, the assumption is made that quality care was delivered.

When outcome standards are being written, the definition and defining character-

TABLE 8-1
USEFUL QUESTIONS FOR IDENTIFYING TRACERS OF QUALITY NURSING CARE

1. Does the tracer diagnosis have a definite functional impact on clients?

2. Is the tracer diagnosis relatively well defined and easy to diagnose?

3. Is the incidence of the tracer diagnosis sufficiently high that adequate data can be collected?

4. Does the quality of nursing care influence progression of the tracer diagnosis?

5. Is the prevention or treatment of the tracer diagnosis sufficiently well defined?

6. Are the effects of nonnursing (environmental) factors on the tracer diagnosis sufficiently understood?

Source: Adapted from Kessner, Kalk, and Singer (1973).

TABLE 8-2
DIAGNOSIS–SPECIFIC PROCESS STANDARDS

Diagnosis:	Impaired home maintenance management/decreased activity tolerance, level 2
Process standards:	1. Energy conservation techniques for cleaning, cooking, lifting, pushing, etc., are taught.
	2. Assistance is given in planning home management activites and rest periods.
Diagnosis:	Impaired home maintenance management/knowledge deficit (hygiene practices)
Process standards:	1. Relationships between lack of hygienic home practices (cleanliness, food storage), spreading of harmful microorganisms, and human infections are explained.
	2. Assistance is given in planning home maintenance responsibiliites with family.
	3. Information is given about methods and resources to prevent vermin.

istics of nursing diagnoses are helpful; for accepted diagnoses these may be found in compilations of national conferences on nursing diagnosis (Kim and Moritz, 1981). When defining characteristics are converted to positive health behaviors, they provide the content for the outcome standards. For example, the standards indicating resolution of impaired home maintenance management could be those listed in Table 8-3. They are the opposite of the critical defining characteristics of the diagnosis. Similarly, converting the characteristics of a diagnosis such as ineffective coping to the signs of effective coping results in measurable outcome standards.

Irrespective of the probable cause (etiology), with quality care the outcome standard should be attained. Therefore, etiological factors are not considered when outcome standards for populations are written. Notice that in Table 8-2 the probable causes of the two diagnoses were decreased activity tolerance and knowledge deficit (hygienic practices). Clients with impaired home maintenance management from *either* cause should reach the same accepted outcome.

Although not influencing the *content* of outcome standards, etiological factors influence the *time* for reaching a standard. Standards must be realistic (attainable); hence the time frame may be different when etiological factors require complex, extended interventions.

In each standard the time by which the outcome has to be reached is specified. For a population with impaired home maintenance management, food stored safely (one week) would be an example. Some outcome standards also require consistency of client behavior across time, for example, food stored safely at three weekly visits (3 weeks). This would mean that the client's behavior would not be evaluated against the standard until after three weeks and three visits.

Process standards also specify a time frame. It indicates the acceptable time(s) that a process of care (intervention) is performed. If the diagnosis is potential fluid volume deficit, for example, fluids offered every 2 hours might be the process standard. The diagnosis potential for violence might have a more frequent time frame, for example, agitation level checked every 10 minutes. One standard for noncompliance with medication therapy/regimen complexity might be: written list of medications,

TABLE 8-3
DIAGNOSIS–SPECIFIC OUTCOME STANDARDS

Diagnosis:	Impaired home maintenance management
Outcome standards*:	1. Food is stored safely.
	2. Wastes are disposed of safely.
	3. Vermin are absent.
	4. Surroundings are generally clean.

*Time and methods of measurement are not specified.

dosage, and time given before discharge. The above examples illustrate that time frames as well as content of the statements are standardized.

In addition to nursing diagnoses, nurses assume accountability for assisting clients in carrying out therapy ordered by physicians. Although no data exist, it may be estimated that nursing judgment is involved in nearly 50 percent of the disease-related acute care clients receive. This percentage includes making and reporting clinical observations and judgments about complications, administering "as necessary" medications, carrying out protocols, and taking other actions. How is this aspect of nursing care reviewed?

The quality assurance review of medical-diagnosis–specific nursing care requires only process standards. Nurses do not assume accountability for medical, or disease-related, outcomes.[1]

Process standards can be developed for complications, actions based on assessments, and actions based on physician orders or hospital protocols. Caution has to be exercised in writing these standards. Expectations cannot go beyond knowledge commonly acquired in professional education, and processes for the treatment of nursing diagnoses must not be mislabeled under medical diagnostic population groups.

Information Retrieval   After standards are written, the quality of care is evaluated. The process is referred to as *auditing*. There are various types of audits. Clients' permanent records are reviewed to see whether (1) admission was necessary (facility utilization review); (2) care being delivered is at an acceptable standard (concurrent review or retrospective review); and (3) outcome standards are reached (retrospective review). The time expenditures and other costs of auditing make it necessary for most audits to be done by reviewing clients' records. Thus it is extremely important that daily recordings be clear, concise, and complete.

There are difficulties, but not unsolvable ones, in grouping clients and writing standards according to nursing diagnoses. In most health care settings clients' records can be retrieved (selected for inclusion in the audit) only on the basis of medical diagnoses. This chart retrieval system exists because hospital statistical reports are based on medical diagnoses. Unless provision has been made also to record nursing diagnoses in the call-up system, record retrieval is difficult. For example, 100 charts of

---

[1] Nurses delivering primary care may have responsibility for treating some common diseases, but in most settings this treatment is given under physician supervision, orders, or protocols.

clients with ineffective coping patterns or impaired home maintenance management cannot be easily retrieved from among 10,000 records.

The mechanical problem of retrieval does not have to dictate the way standards are written. Nurses are working toward the placement of nursing diagnoses on computerized or other information systems. Until this occurs other methods of record retrieval have to be used.

One method is to use medical diagnoses for retrieval and nursing diagnoses as a focus for writing standards and criteria (Gordon, 1980, pp. 85-86). This method

TABLE 8-4
MEDICAL DIAGNOSIS RETRIEVAL MODE AND NURSING DIAGNOSIS AUDIT

Retrieval mode	Audit population	Process standards	Outcome standards
Right cerebrovascular accident*	Potential skin breakdown	1. Assisted to change position at least every 2 hours	1. Skin intact
		2. Special skin care (defined) every 2 hours	
		3. Protein intake monitored for deficits once daily	
		4. Elimination monitored for incontinence every 2 hours	
	Total self-care deficit (level 3)/ uncompensated hemiparesis	1. Assistance required in bathing, dressing, grooming, feeding, and toileting assessed daily	1. Provides own self-care by using equipment or device in bathing, dressing, grooming, feeding, and toileting (level 1)
		2. Use of adaptive equipment taught during bathing, dressing, grooming, feeding, and toileting	
		3. Compensation for deficit assessed daily	
	Ineffective family coping/role changes	1. Assisted in thinking through family management decisions until stated outcome obtained	1. Explains role readjustments made for family management
		2. Assisted in exploring role changes until stated outcome obtained	2. States no more than moderate concern about family role readjustments

*The population can be specified further, for example, as male, 45 to 65 years of age, and married.

requires estimating what high-incidence nursing diagnoses occur with particular medical diagnoses. Table 8-4 presents an example: The medical diagnosis was cerebrovascular accident (stroke) and the predicted nursing diagnoses were potential skin breakdown, ineffective family coping/role changes, and total self-care deficit (level 3)/uncompensated hemiparesis.

A second method of retrieval is to write discharge notes containing both resolved and current (unresolved) nursing diagnoses. This kind of discharge note facilitates record librarians' coding and retrieval of records by nursing diagnoses.

Interdisciplinary Reviews Some institutions combine nursing, medical, and other health professionals' quality care reviews into one program. Again, because of the retrieval process medical diagnosis is usually the main client classification. Nursing diagnoses can be a subset. The nursing standards could be similar to those in the example in Table 8-4.

Interpretation of Care Reviews If standards are not reached by the specified time, two alternative interpretations are possible. One possibility is that quality care *was* delivered but client or situational factors interfered with the expected outcome. If clients with noncompliance/knowledge deficit become disoriented, it is understandable that they may not attain the knowledge level expected. This kind of situation would constitute an exception to the standard, but information about the disorientation would have to be found in the client's chart.

Not reaching an outcome can also mean that treatment of a particular nursing diagnosis was not at an acceptable level. This finding leads to the identification of care delivery problems.

Identifying Problems The use of nursing diagnoses in population audits facilitates identification of care delivery problems. The group of clients receiving less than quality care is clearly specified and reasons for the inadequate care can be determined.

Problems in care delivery are identified by raising questions. For example, Why did 30 percent of the client population with the diagnosis of potential fluid volume deficit develop dehydration? Why did 10 percent of the population with potential skin breakdown develop decubitus ulcers (bedsores)?

Where do auditors find the answers to these questions? The reader who thinks that possible answers lie in the processes of care (nursing interventions) or in the structural resources of the setting has grasped a major concept in quality care assessment. That is exactly where nurses look for the reasons why client outcomes are below standard.

Charts that do not pass the outcome screening standard are examined. Process standards that have been developed for relevant diagnoses (for example, potential fluid volume deficit and potential skin breakdown) are compared to the actual care documented in the chart. It may be found that treatments for these diagnoses were not consistent with accepted standards of treatment. Why?

For answers, structural factors in the setting are examined. Was there sufficient staff competent in the treatment of these diagnoses? Did they have the necessary equipment and materials, such as special mattresses for prevention of pressure ulcerations? Does the method of nursing care delivery or philosophy of care promote individual accountability for treatment of diagnosed problems? These searching questions are asked by both practitioners and administrators.

It is advisable to begin a quality care assurance program with a concurrent audit of all (or a sample of) charts, using the ANA standards of practice (Table 7-1). This preliminary audit can be done while committees are preparing diagnostic population standards. The major elements for this general audit are identified in Table 8-5. Included in the general process audit are assessment, diagnosis, outcomes, interventions, and evaluation of progress toward discharge outcomes. At this early point in the audit just the presence or absence of these elements is the objective of the audit.

An audit of this type will identify gross deficiencies. If nursing diagnoses, plans of care, progress notes, and discharge assessments of care outcomes are not recorded, audits of diagnostic populations cannot be done economically. Thus the first step is to determine whether broad standards are being met. If not, why not? After remedial actions are taken by nurses to correct these charting deficiencies, the previously described tracer population audits can be done from records.

When quality care assurance programs are built on nursing diagnoses, periodic review of the validity of diagnoses may be necessary. Nurses may not be making valid assessments or correct diagnostic judgments; these errors affect audits that are based on recorded diagnoses. Periodic review of items 1 and 2 in Table 8-5 would reveal these diagnostic errors. Actual reassessment of some clients could be done to check diagnostic accuracy, but this procedure involves added time and expense. The same problem occurs in medicine. An elevated blood pressure may have been overlooked, but this lack of diagnosis and treatment would not be revealed in a process or outcome audit of a fractured femur population.

TABLE 8-5
GENERAL PROCESS AUDIT

1. Assessment contains information relevant to the 11 health pattern areas:

Nutritional-metabolic	Cognitive-perceptual
Elimination	Health-perception–health management
Role-relationship	Self-perception–self-concept
Activity-exercise	Sexuality-reproductive
Value-belief	Coping–stress-tolerance
Sleep-rest	

2. Nursing diagnoses are supported by and consistent with history and assessment data.

3. Unstable or potentially unstable physical parameters are identified for observation, for example:

   Blood pressure

   Pulse

   Level of consciousness

4. Outcomes for diagnoses are stated.

5. Diagnosis-specific nursing activities are listed in the plan of care.

6. Progress notes are written about each diagnosis.

7. Information relevant to progress toward outcomes is documented.

Taking Remedial Actions Using nursing diagnoses for developing standards and identifying problems facilitates the next step in quality assurance. That step is the taking of remedial actions by nurses. Let us suppose that both the resources and the care provided are problematic for certain diagnostic populations. As an example, consider the situation in which the incidence of skin breakdown is too high. Nurses and administrators determine that the problem is twofold: inadequate professional staff and inadequate methods of prevention used by current staff.

The ultimate purpose of quality care review is to offer opportunities for institutional administrators and care providers to improve care. In the skin breakdown example reasonable actions would include (1) obtaining more professional staff and (2) increasing staff education programs. The nursing diagnosis and management of potential skin breakdown would be an excellent topic for inservice education programs in this setting. Early diagnosis, judgments about risk factors, and prevention need emphasizing. After a reasonable time a reaudit is done. If the problem was correctly identified and addressed, it should now be found that standards indicating quality care are being reached.

In summary, accountability to the consumer underlies quality assurance programs. Individual nurses of course evaluate the effectiveness of the care they give to individual clients; quality assurance audits evaluate the nursing care delivered to groups of clients. In essence, care review requires that nurses decide in what areas of health care their accountability lies.

Clearly, nurses' accountability, first and foremost, is for the health problems described by nursing diagnoses. Just as physicians assume accountability for quality treatment of diseases described by medical diagnoses, nurses assume accountability for recognizing and intervening in the dysfunctional health patterns described by nursing diagnoses.

Writing standards, identifying problems that exist, and taking remedial actions are made easier when nursing diagnoses are used. Diagnoses impart clear direction to these activities. The result is that nursing assures quality of care within its own domain of practice. When each profession does this, overall health care quality is assured.

Future Directions

Two issues are clearly important as the future of quality assurance is contemplated. One is the need for a scientific base for nursing care evaluation. The second is the identification of care delivery problems and creative solutions that have immediate payoff in terms of quality.

Writing standards of care makes it clear to all involved that "mature knowledge" (replicated studies) in nursing is sparse. When a group of nurses try to state what nurses should do for a particular nursing diagnosis and what health results are expected, diversity of opinion exists. Even setting aside the matter of quality assurance, research is needed to determine effective treatments and related outcomes as a basis for everyday practice.

The second major issue for the next few years is the cost-benefit aspect of quality assurance. In simplest terms, activities have to pay off. This requires that problems in care delivery be prioritized. The highest priority must be given to those care delivery problems that have a significant impact on illness, death rates, and actual financial costs.

Inadequate preventive care is one example of a care delivery problem that when remedied can decrease health care costs. If potential problems were diagnosed and preventive care instituted, many dollars and days of disability could be saved. It is estimated that the treatment of a decubitus ulcer costs thousands of dollars but preventive nursing care of 2 hours daily costs less than twenty dollars a day. As a second example imagine the reduction in cost, disability, and mortality if people were helped to improve their functional health patterns. Merely reducing the speed limit on highways has enormously diminished automobile accidents, one of the leading causes of death and disability.

One hospital, by focusing nurses' attention on the nursing diagnosis potential for injury, substantially reduced clients' falls (McCourt, 1979). Imagine the savings in money and days of disability and discomfort if even 10 fractures of the hip were prevented. This is an example of identifying care delivery problems that have immediate payoff in monetary and human costs. Containing these costs will be the major emphasis in future quality assurance activities.

Others are engaged in demonstration and research projects to develop standards and criteria for measuring care. In one demonstration project nursing diagnosis, quality assurance, and change theory are integrated in a continuing education project for three states, New Hampshire, Vermont, and Maine (Morse, 1980). A research project related to the study of processes (interventions) and related client outcomes is in progress. Nursing diagnoses, as well as medical diagnoses, are providing the focus (Young and Ventura, 1980).

Quality care has a price. The next section will examine economic elements of care delivery and nursing diagnosis.

NURSING DIAGNOSES AND THIRD PARTY PAYMENT

A large proportion of United States citizens pay for nursing care through a third party, commonly an insurance company. In fact, as will be discussed, a fourth party—the physician or hospital—enters into payment for nursing care. A brief overview of the current system of paying for care will demonstrate that some people have minimal access to nursing care and some have little choice. The historical development of the situation is interestingly portrayed by Welch (1975); change in the current situation, as will be described, can be facilitated by nursing diagnosis.

Rather than paying for health services at the time of care delivery, people pay monthly premiums to nonprofit (for example, Blue Cross and Blue Shield) or profit-making (Mutual of Omaha, Aetna, etc.) companies. Also, government funds are available for care of the elderly (Medicare) or medically indigent (Medicaid). Insurance companies and the government are referred to as *third party payers*, and their process of payment is called *reimbursement*.

Treatment of a nursing diagnosis, except in a few instances, is not reimbursed. This means that consumers do not have direct access to nursing unless they are willing to pay the fees themselves. It means, further, that the poor and medically indigent have no choice in the type of care provider they can choose. Yet there are loopholes whereby payment for nursing occurs.

A client who wants nursing care can be admitted to a hospital or clinic; the nursing is included in the reimbursable bed and board charges or clinic fees. But to get into a hospital, the client must have a disease or possible disease. Another route to take is to convince a physician that nursing care is needed. If a physician certifies the need, a client can obtain home nursing, private duty nursing, or community-based care by a nurse in private practice. As Jennings (1979) points out, although consumers are paying high premiums, in the current system a consumer is not entitled to receive any health care unless it is directed or executed by a physician.

Under the current system, many functional health problems are not diagnosed early or are not diagnosed until disease is present. Many cases could be cited: the untreated body image alteration that has to progress to a severe depression, the potential shoulder contracture that when fully developed a year after mastectomy requires surgery, and the ineffective coping pattern that is not diagnosed until child abuse results. As many have said, the current health care system is disease oriented rather than preventive care oriented.

What can be done? Nurses currently are seeking third party payment. This reimbursement will permit an increase in private and group practice. Hospitals are attempting to obtain reimbursement for client health education (Nordberg and King, 1976) and to make a change from the method of including nursing reimbursement in the room rate.

In addition, groups are currently working with legislators and insurance companies to determine reimbursement plans. This, of course, is a threat to the current system. Counteracting proposals, such as reimbursement for health education when ordered by the physician, continue to arise.

Consumers need to be informed about the controls the present system imposes on access to care. Public education requires clear communication about what is to be reimbursed. Communication should be focused on the actual and potential health problems nurses diagnose and treat rather than on tasks nurses do. Competency and quality care can be assured to consumers and third party payers if the reasons (nursing diagnoses) for actions are specified.

In addition to these efforts to obtain reimbursement for community-based care, work is underway to study the use of nursing diagnoses to determine costs of hospital nursing. This work involves the concept of client classification for staff allocation, the subject of the next section.

NURSING DIAGNOSIS AND STAFFING PATTERNS

In the previous section staffing patterns were used as an example of a structural characteristic of the care delivery setting that influences quality of care. *Staffing pattern* refers to the allocation and utilization of nurses. An ideal pattern exists when the number and competency of the nurses who work in a setting match the nursing care requirements of the clients.

The degree of control a nurse has over the number of clients in his or her caseload varies with the institution. Whether or not involved in this determination, each nurse should have some understanding of how staffing is done and how daily assignments are made. If fewer staff are available than are needed, quality care or dedicated nurses suffer; if staffing is excessive, the cost to consumers and taxpayers rises.

This section includes a brief overview of how staffing patterns are determined. The influence of nursing care requirements and budgetary allocations on these decisions will be examined.

Current systems of classifying clients' care requirements receive much criticism. Equally true, the way hospitals are currently reimbursed for care does not allow for variability in nursing care requirements. This in turn has an effect on staffing. Two projects will be reported that involve studies of nursing diagnosis as a basis for determining clients' use of nursing services.

The following pages will emphasize (1) that both internal and external factors influence staffing on a unit, (2) that nurses need to find ways of more accurately describing their practice so that staffing patterns support quality care, and (3) that to study the potential uses of nursing diagnoses requires that every nurse incorporate diagnosis into practice.

Determination of Staffing Patterns

Nurses can set standards of quality care but standards will be difficult to realize if equal consideration is not given to staffing. Many factors influence the number of professional nurses you see on a hospital unit, clinic, or in a visiting nurse district. Two primary factors that we shall consider are client care requirements and budgetary allocations.

Classification of Care Requirements Client care requirements for a nursing unit can be determined by various means. The purpose is to predict the *nursing time* clients on a unit require. Quantifying care in terms of nursing time is the usual basis for allocating nurses.

Global approaches for determining nursing time, such as counting the number of clients, have been used. Such approaches are not too successful in predicting staffing needs because clients differ in their care requirements. Recognition of this has led to client classification as a basis for allocating nursing staff. *Classification* is the process of categorizing clients according to their nursing care requirements.

Classifications can be based on single or multiple indicators of care needs. For example, acuity of illness is one gross predictor of nursing time required. It is assumed that critically ill clients need more nursing care time than convalescent clients. If nurses did only physical care, the assumption might be true.

What if health counseling and teaching were used as indicators of nursing time required by clients? Then it might be found that convalescent clients need more or as much nursing time (and staff) as critically ill clients. Clearly, the indicator used for classifying clients ultimately influences decisions about staffing.

Most current systems of classification are based on task oriented, "doing for" views of nursing. Clients' needs for bathing, feeding, ambulation, and medication are not always valid predictors of professional nursing time required. These indicators do not take into account the scope of client problems and current standards of nursing care. By maintaining the status quo, classification systems of this type restrict developments in professional practice. In turn, clients are deprived of new developments in practice. A comparable situation would exist if a faculty-student ratio did not permit instructors to institute new methods of teaching or a physician-client ratio did not permit clients to benefit from new medical developments.

If professional staffing is based on poor predictors or poor use of predictors, shortages become the rule, not the exception. Understaffing readily limits the implementation of current practice standards, including nursing diagnosis. Yet, if instituted, nursing diagnoses may provide a more valid measure of staffing needs.

Simmons (1980) has recognized the utility of diagnosis as a basis for staffing specifically in relation to community health nursing. Her comments about the use of nursing diagnoses (nursing problems) apply to other levels of care also:

> Problem labels and their signs and symptoms, stated clearly and concisely, can be useful in interpreting community health nursing services to others. A clear interpretation of services can be especially crucial when the agency must compete for funding and justify the need for existing or new programs.
>
> Cost analysis and cost effectiveness can be enhanced by using the problem classification scheme. Nursing activities can be related to specific client problems resulting in cost centers for different client needs. Proficient use of the problem classification scheme will demand less time in recording and allow more nursing time for direct client care. (Simmons, 1980, p. 5)

Giovanetti (1978) notes that classifications are consistent with current ways of thinking about practice and with the nomenclature of the time. When nursing was conceptualized as tasks and procedures, the presently used classification systems developed. She states:

> As the nomenclature changes, so will the basis for classification. Two relatively new nomenclatures to describe nursing process are now beginning to emerge: (1) patient problems and (2) nursing diagnoses. It seems reasonable to expect that as the validity of these descriptions becomes more evident, one or both may well lead to new patient classification systems, which, in turn, may be more responsive to the true nature of the patients' care requirements. (Giovanetti, 1978, p. 92)

Budgetary Allocations A second important factor influences the number and competency of the nurses with which a unit is staffed. This factor is the budget for nurses' salaries in the institution. The nursing department budget for salaries is usually about one-third of a total hospital budget. To a great extent the hospital budget, and thus the salary budget, is controlled by outside forces.

Hospital income is based on direct client payments and reimbursement by insurance companies and public funds. The external control of reimbursement rates (by state agencies) directly influences nursing department budgets. State rate-setting commissions determine the reimbursement hospitals receive per client.

It must be recognized that in the majority of institutions the cost of nursing care *is included in the basic daily room charge*. This charge is a flat rate for all clients at particular levels of care (acute, intensive, long term). As an example, reimbursement is not provided for clinical specialist consultation. When nursing provided glorified maid service or apprenticeship training, inclusion in the "hotel rate" may have been appropriate.

Today many nurses argue that nursing should be a separate charge as are physical therapy, radiology, and other hospital services. Would this increase consumers' bills? Perhaps not; rather, there might be more equitable distribution. Those clients requiring minimal care would probably pay less than they now pay. Charging separately for nursing would also pressure the profession to determine the basis for fee-for-service charges. Actual and potential problems diagnosed and treated by nurses may be an answer. Two important studies that relate to this idea are in progress.

Staffing and Reimbursement Based on Diagnosis

Around the midseventies two studies were initiated to test the idea of using nursing diagnoses in staffing pattern and reimbursement decisions. Underlying both studies was the need to find valid measures of nursing care requirements of hospitalized clients. Both studies incorporated the concept of nursing diagnosis; the nomenclature employed was based on that developed by participants at the first and second national conferences on classification of nursing diagnoses, 1973 and 1975.

Process Oriented Nursing Staffing   Halloran (1980) has begun to study nursing diagnoses as a basis for staffing decisions. Rather than studying only the tasks nurses do, researchers are examining the influence of diagnoses on time allocation by nurses. Thirty-seven diagnoses from the 1975 accepted list of the national conference group are being used.[2] The sample of approximately 2560 clients' medical diagnostic groupings, nursing diagnoses, and nursing care time allocations should provide useful conclusions. Progress reports indicate that nursing diagnoses are much better predictors of nursing time than are medical diagnoses.

Reimbursement Based on Diagnosis   Currently hospitals are reimbursed for the number of days a client stays. A new concept developed by Yale University and a computer firm proposed set fees for disease treatment. Medical diseases have been classified into 383 diagnostically related groups (DRGs). Groupings are based on clinical characteristics and resources used. The question is asked whether nursing services can be related to DRGs and, further, whether standard rates for various types of hospitals and DRGs can be set (Thompson, 1981). Interest in the DRG concept of reimbursement by the U.S. Department of Health and Human Services resulted in funding the New Jersey Department of Health for a study of the cost of resources used by clients in the various DRGs.

Within this ongoing project nursing diagnoses are being used as a focus for measuring nursing service resources used. Twenty-seven nursing diagnoses are included in the study; many are similar to the currently accepted listing ("News and Reports,"

---

[2] In a longitudinal study of this type nomenclature cannot be changed, although revisions were made by the conference group in 1978 and 1980.

1980). Others, such as G.I. function/activity, possibly imply disease-related nursing observations rather than nursing diagnoses.

Both the staffing research and the reimbursement study address practice issues that can be explored using nursing diagnoses. For the practitioner, research may lead to better predictions about clients' needs for care, more valid staffing patterns, and, finally, equitable daily caseloads of clients. Yet until nursing diagnosis is implemented in practice settings, the research will proceed slowly and exploration of the potentialities of nursing diagnosis will be delayed.

In summary, hospital staffing patterns are controlled both from within an institution and by external forces. In institutions, clients are categorized (usually by medical diagnosis and acuity of illness) and their care requirements are estimated and translated into the nursing time that will be needed to give that care. This process is the basis for staffing patterns. More accurate predictions of nursing time requirements may result from using nursing diagnoses to estimate the care that will be needed.

Externally, the regulation of reimbursement rates by state agencies influences hospital budgets and, thereby, staffing patterns. Charges for nursing care are included in the daily room rate along with the cost of laundry, meals, and housekeeping. Other ways of establishing charges for nursing care are being studied; hospitalized clients of the future may pay a direct fee for nursing services.

As professionals, nurses have an obligation to clients to see that current standards of quality care are not compromised. The responsibility also exists to see that excess costs are not imposed by overstaffing. As employees, nurses seldom have much direct control over caseloads; as professionals, they are responsible for communicating clients' care requirements to enhance staffing pattern decisions.

NURSING DIAGNOSIS AND THE SCOPE OF PRACTICE

What is nursing practice? That question is asked by career-seeking high school students, by legislators who pass laws that regulate practice, and by hard pressed financial vice presidents of agencies delivering nursing care. It is asked by educators designing curricula, by third party payers, and by research funding agencies.

Nursing is caring for the whole person. Yet that statement is too vague for those who have to decide how many nurses to hire or what courses should be in a curriculum.

In recent years gigantic steps have been taken to define and describe the scope of nursing practice. Conceptual frameworks have been proposed to clarify the focus, and nurses now lament the proliferation of views. They forget that not long ago nursing was conceptualized only as being a handmaiden to other health care providers, who made all the decisions. The nursing process, requiring actions based on judgment, was "kept in the closet."

Theory and nursing process have led to even clearer articulation of the scope of nursing practice. In 1980 the Congress for Nursing Practice of the American Nurses' Association defined 11 actual or potential health problem areas that are the essence of nursing practice (American Nurses' Association, 1980, p. 12). Within these areas, theoretical knowledge guides diagnosis and treatment.

Still clearer definition of the scope of practice will occur as nursing diagnoses are identified, standardized, and classified. Then nurses could, if they chose, point to a list of actual and potential problems and say nurses assume responsibility and accountability for the diagnosis and treatment of these. At a very specific, concrete level it can be said that nursing diagnoses are the focus of caring because they represent human health-related responses.

Both the ANA *Social Policy Statement* (1980) and the classification of problems in the domain of practice will increase nursing's future scope. If true responsibility is taken for a problem area such as knowledge deficit (health maintenance), imagine the opportunities for practice that will be open. Clinical research can be done about the quality and quantity of knowledge that correlates with health maintenance behavior. Nurses will be able to lobby for health education and learning centers; the media can be used to reach target populations, and third party payers can be pressured to reimburse clients for preventive health education. These are only a few examples of what can occur as the domain of practice is clearly defined by nursing diagnoses.

NURSING DIAGNOSIS AND NURSING THEORY

The current effort to identify and classify nursing diagnoses has been described as theory development (Bircher, 1975; Kritek, 1978, 1979; Henderson, 1978). Interestingly, this position can produce various responses. One reaction is "If the work on diagnosis is theory development, then it's the *first* useful thing about theory I've seen." People with this point of view usually become involved in diagnostic category identification *even though* it could be theory development! The reaction that rarely leads to involvement is "Oh, another theory; probably too abstract for practice." Lacking appreciation of the use of theory in practice, nurses who hold this second view devalue diagnosis because it sounds theoretical.

Probably the most meaningful way for the learner to think about the issue is in the context of practice theory, as defined by Dickoff, James, and Wiedenbach (1968). They define four distinctive levels of theory. These levels will structure our discussion of the relationship between nursing diagnosis and theory. We shall see, as these authors propose, that theory begins and ends in practice.

Factor-Isolating Theory

Identifying and formally labeling phenomena is the first step in the development of theory in a science. This step is referred to as the factor-isolating level of theory development.

Phenomena of concern are isolated and categorized. Then the categories are given names. As previously described, categorization is a method humans use to deal with the otherwise overwhelming complexities of even their simplest environments. Things judged to be similar are given the same name. The names represent concepts or ideas that are the basic building blocks for other levels of theory.

Nursing practice has been commonly represented as a set of tasks related to clients' therapeutic needs. Categorization has been done in terms of needs for nursing such as "needs suctioning" or "needs emotional support." Grouping clients into a category like "needs emotional support" ignores the diverse health problems that may be present. These could be fear, anxiety, role conflict, and so forth. It also ignores the different interventions that may be required.

This type of categorization bears a striking resemblance to task oriented categories in which *things are described by the actions performed in regard to them* (Bruner, Goodnow, and Austin, 1956, pp. 5-6). The formal categories of a science are established in quite a different way. Rather than describing phenomena by the response to them, *formal categories specify the intrinsic characteristics of phenomena*. In the case of nursing, intrinsic characteristics would be clusters of client characteristics such as the critical defining signs and symptoms previously discussed in chapters 5 and 6. Formal categories such as nursing diagnoses provide a better cognitive focus for determining nursing intervention than do task oriented categories with their prespecified interventions.

Currently, nursing diagnoses describing clients' actual or potential problems are being defined. Thinking of these as formal categories or concepts in a clinical science emphasizes the need for a scientific approach to their development. This approach will be discussed in Chapter 9 in a section on diagnostic classification systems. At that time, current identification and classification efforts will also be reviewed.

Having seen that the basic building blocks of nursing practice theories are diagnostic concepts, we can now consider other levels of theory. As will be seen, each level of theory presupposes development at lower levels (Dickoff, James, and Wiedenbach, 1968, pp. 415-435).

Higher Levels of Theory

The reader may have recognized that factor-isolating theories are the basis for concepts taught in courses such as physiology and chemistry. These disciplines isolate phenomena and create concepts such as chemical, atom, organ, and system. They then proceed to describe these and predict causal relations. This approach requires three levels of theory development: isolation, description, and prediction.

Nursing requires higher levels of theory development. As will be described, nursing extends beyond description and causal relations to the prescriptive theory level.

After actual and potential health problems are identified, their natural history can be described. This type of theory is called *descriptive theory*. It results in the depiction of relationships among factors in a client and situation. This description of relationships permits the study and development of third-level theories that are *predictive*. An example would be prediction of the effect A has on B. Situation A may be a nursing intervention and B a problematic health situation. Or A may be some causal factor in the development of B, a health problem.

Predictive theories are indispensable for the fourth level of theory. This is *prescriptive theory*, which assists in producing desired health outcomes.

> Prescriptive theories are situation-producing or goal-incorporating theories. They are not satisfied to conceptualize factors, factor relationships, or situation relationships, but go on to attempt conceptualization of desired situations as well as conceptualizing the prescription under which an agent or practitioner must act in order to bring about situations of the kind conceived as desired in the conception of goal (Dickoff, James, and Wiedenbach, 1968, p. 420).

In summary, identification and naming of health problems described by nursing diagnoses is the first level of theory development. Building on these diagnostic concepts, higher levels of theory can be developed that will be a basis for treatment. In essence, the identification and classification of nursing diagnoses is the first step in developing a clinical science that can be used by all nursing clinicians. Theory development begins and ends in practice.

SUMMARY

Selected issues of practice have been examined to clarify the relevance of nursing diagnoses. It was argued that because the focus of nursing care is the client's diagnoses, it follows logically that diagnoses can provide a focus for programs designed to assure quality care.

Perhaps an even more basic issue is availability of and access to professional nursing care in institutions and communities. The suggestion was made that staffing of institutions may be improved if nursing diagnoses were considered in planning nursing staff allocations. In community practice as well as in institutions, financial reimbursement for care is an issue. As nursing moves toward third party payment for services, nursing diagnoses will be a mechanism upon which to base reimbursement.

For many years it has been difficult to define the scope of nursing practice. Nursing diagnosis may make it possible to arrive at a clearer definition of nursing's domain of responsibility. Once the domain is defined, research and the development of practice theory can be focused on the health problems that are relevant to nursing.

Throughout this and the preceeding chapter the reader may have thought that everything is being tied to nursing diagnosis! This observation is true. It suggests that perhaps clients' health problems are the basis for thinking about all nursing issues.

In essence, nursing's main social responsibility is to ensure that nursing services are available, accessible, and of a quality that promotes or maintains health. This is a huge undertaking unless the effort is narrowed to those conditions nurses are best able to prevent and treat. The next chapter deals with the ways those conditions can be identified.

BIBLIOGRAPHY

American Nurses' Association Congress on Nursing Practice. *A social policy statement.* Kansas City, Mo.: American Nurses' Association, 1980.

Bircher, A. V. On the development and classification of diagnoses. *Nursing Forum,* 1975, *14,* 20–29.

Bloch, D. Evaluation of nursing care in terms of process and outcome. *Nursing Research,* July-August 1975, *24,* 256–263.

Bloch, D. Interrelated issues in evaluation and evaluation research. *Nursing Research,* 1980, *29,* 69–73.

Bruner, J. S., Goodnow, J. J., & Austin, G. A. *Study of thinking.* New York: Wiley, 1956.

Dickoff, J., James, P., & Wiedenbach, E. Theory in a practice discipline: Part I. Practice oriented theory. *Nursing Research,* September-October 1968, *17,* 415–435.

Giovanetti, P. *Patient classification systems in nursing: A description and analysis.* (Publication No. HRA 78-22). Washington, D.C.: U.S. Department of Health, Education and Welfare, 1978.

Gordon, M. Determining study topics. *Nursing Research*, March-April 1980, *29*, 83–87.

Halloran, E. J. Analysis of variation in nursing workload by patient medical and nursing condition. Chicago: University of Illinois, 1980 (Doctoral Dissertation #8106567).

Henderson, B. Nursing diagnosis: Theory and practice. *Advances in Nursing Science*, October 1978, *1*, 75–83.

Jennings, C. P. Nursing's case for third party reimbursement. *American Journal of Nursing*, January 1979, *79*, 110–114.

Joint Commission on the Accreditation of Hospitals. *Accreditation manual for hospitals, 1981 edition.* Chicago: 1981.

Kessner, D. M., Kalk, C. E., & Singer, J. Assessing health quality: The case for tracers. *New England Journal of Medicine*, January 25, 1973, *288*, 189–194.

Kim, M. J., & Mortiz, D. A. (Eds.) *Classification of nursing diagnoses: Proceedings of the third and fourth national conferences.* New York: McGraw-Hill, 1981.

Kritek, P. B. Generation and classification of nursing diagnoses: Toward a theory of nursing. *Image*, June 1978, *10*, 33–40.

Kritek, P. B. Commentary: The development of nursing diagnosis and theory. *Advances in Nursing Science*, October 1979, *2*, 73–79.

McAuliffe, W. E. Measuring the quality of medical care: Process versus outcome. *Millbank Memorial Fund Quarterly*, 1979, *37*, 118–152.

McCourt, A. Personal communication, 1979.

Morse, S. *Trice tablet.* Tri-State Continuing Education Project, 48 West Street, Concord, New Hampshire, 03301. 1980.

News and reports: New Jersey works toward new reimbursement model. *Nursing Outlook*, November 1980, *28*, 652–655.

Nordberg, B., & King, L. Third-party payment for patient education. *American Journal of Nursing*, August 1976, *76*, 1269–1271.

Simmons, D. A. *A classification scheme for client problems in community health nursing.* Hyattsville, Md.: U.S. Department of Health and Human Services (Publication No. HRA 80-16), June 1980.

Thompson, J. D. Prediction of nurse resource use in treatment of diagnosis-related groups. In H. H. Werley & M. R. Grier (Eds.), *Nursing information systems.* New York: Springer, 1981. pp. 60–81.

Welch, C. A. Health care distribution and third-party payment for nurses' services. *American Journal of Nursing*, October 1975, *75*, 1844–1848.

Young, D. E., & Ventura, M. R. Application of nursing diagnoses in quality assessment research. In A. McCourt (Ed.), *American Nurses' Association Quality Assurance Update*, December 1980, *4*, 1–4.

CHAPTER 9

NURSING DIAGNOSIS: ACCEPTANCE, IMPLEMENTATION, AND CLASSIFICATION

What is the status of nursing diagnosis in the profession, and what work is ahead? This chapter will attempt to answer these questions. Many of the realities have been saved until last in order to allow the reader to focus on the diagnostic process and its application. It will be evident in the first section of this final chapter that some nurses have difficulty with the term *diagnosis* but that the diagnostic process, or clinical judgment, are accepted as nursing functions.

The second section will review implementation in clinical units, including some suggestions for helping nurses acquire diagnostic skills. The novice in diagnosis may not have the responsibility of helping others learn to diagnose but when curiosity is expressed, suggestions can be offered.

A classification system for nursing diagnoses cannot be developed by armchair theorizing. Clinicians practicing nursing are the ones identifying client conditions and testing diagnoses in their daily care. For these reasons, even the beginner should appreciate how classification systems are developed, why they are developed, and how each nurse can contribute. The last section of the chapter describes classification systems and the current national effort to classify nursing diagnoses. Let us begin by reviewing comments and criticisms of nursing diagnosis.

ACCEPTANCE IN THE PROFESSION

The idea of identifying a client's condition as a basis for planning nursing care is well accepted. That this condition should be conceptualized at a level beyond a set of observables (phenomena that can be directly perceived by use of the senses) is also accepted. What produces difficulty for a small minority is the name applied to the process. The issue seems to be the word *diagnosis*. Levine (1966) reacted to the term for reasons having to do with its legal implications and suggested *trophicognosis* as a substitute. Her concern was justified, since she conceived of nursing diagnosis as diagnosis of "disease and its manifestations . . . without using the formal language of medical diagnosis" (1966, p. 58).

A few current diagnoses *do* fit her definition and increase the potential for harming clients if they are treated inadequately. These include fluid volume deficit, ineffective breathing patterns, impaired gas exchange, alteration in tissue perfusion, and alteration in cardiac output (decreased). If placed in the position of consumer, this writer would request a physician rather than a nurse to treat these problems as they are currently defined (see Kim and Moritz, 1981). The current defining signs and symptoms represent diagnoses for purposes of referral, not nursing diagnoses for purposes of nursing intervention.

The existence of conditions usually requiring medical evaluation among the conference-approved diagnoses points to inconsistencies in defining a nursing diagnosis. Some nurses in intensive care settings would support the use of these labels (fluid volume deficit, ineffective breathing patterns, and so forth) and broaden the concept of diagnosis to include pathophysiological conditions traditionally within the domain of medicine. They appear to use the above terms to cluster a set of nursing diagnoses and physician-directed activities. It is not clear whether clustering of problems under these labels is a habitual focus in disease-related care (the objective of intensive care units) or whether it facilitates some cognitive activity.

A second reaction to nursing diagnosis is that it pigeonholes clients. This concept of care has a negative emotional connotation in nursing. People who see diagnosis as pigeonholing fail to appreciate the fact that humans are disposed to organize and categorize experiences in order to choose appropriate behavior in a situation. The need to categorize in order to understand is found in simple societies and even in cultures with a more holistic philosophy of humankind than our own. The categories of ying and yang, used by people in certain eastern cultures, are examples.

Nurses categorize clients; this activity did not originate with nursing diagnosis. In fact, various professions, including nursing, use categories of various sorts to classify clients. Among categories sometimes used are uncooperative, turkey, crock, and vegetable. A recently published article specified etiological factors and treatment for one of these "diagnostic" classifications (Whitney, 1981). Such categories are nonproductive for determining therapy. Certainly most nurses would prefer the current nursing diagnoses, for both ethical and practical reasons.

A variation on the pigeonholing argument against nursing diagnosis is: "If nurses diagnose, they *will* pigeonhole or stereotype clients." Admittedly, this could happen. An inadequate data base for diagnosis and too early closure are errors that can occur. Shall we blame the nurses or the concept? Perhaps recognizing this possibility will lead to an emphasis on avoidance of these errors.

Some say that nursing diagnosis does not permit individualized care. Correct; neither do any other concepts nurses use to describe a client's condition or behavior. Care is individualized by treatment planning, not problem identification. If every client had a unique problem and required a totally unique care plan, learning would be useless. Perhaps complaints should be directed at the standard care plan rather than at diagnosis.

One occasionally hears that use of the term *diagnosis* is a status-seeking behavior (presumably by a low-status profession). Rather, use of the word diagnosis avoids the confusion inherent in inventing a new label for an accepted process. As King (a physician) has pointed out (1967), although traditionally associated with medicine, diagnosis is a process used by many. One can even take one's car to a diagnostic clinic.

Hesitancy to use the word *diagnosis* is seconded by others who predict physicians will be upset by nurses' use of the word. Some will; others, with explanation and examples, say nursing becomes so much clearer. One hears of physicians' having asked directors of nursing why nursing diagnosis is not used in their institutions or agencies. In other situations comments are heard that a physician wants his or her client assigned to "the nurse that does nursing diagnosis" or wants the client admitted to one unit instead of another because "the care is better" (diagnosis is used). These examples are not the crux of the counterargument. Nurses have to resolve for themselves the conflict between upset doctors and professional nursing standards.

The current list of nursing diagnoses has been criticized as containing "euphemisms" (unoffensive terms substituted for explicitly offensive terms) (Gamer, 1979). Since medical terms that do the same thing have not been criticized by nurses, perhaps the intended word was *euphuism* (affectation of elegance). The accusations that the accepted nursing diagnoses contain imperfectly defined words and imprecise expressions are justified. But one can argue with the complaints that diagnoses dealing with tying shoelaces and brushing teeth (presumably self-care deficits) are too detailed; these activities are critically important client concerns after a stroke or spinal cord injury.

Gast (1979, p. 2) describes the status of diagnostic nomenclature development realistically: "Nursing diagnoses are still largely ambiguous in regards to parameters, disordered in regards to classification, and isolated in regards to theories which might serve as a basis for deduction." This also was the state of biological classification in the eighteenth century before Linnaeus. Recognizing the state of the art in nursing diagnosis, let us turn to clinical testing through implementation, a process that is of critical importance in addressing the problems Gast lists.

IMPLEMENTATION

In this book, clinical judgment has been viewed as predominantly a logical process. Those who take this perspective believe that known components of the diagnostic process can be described in words, learned, and applied in practice to the extent one's intelligence allows. Some people, on the other hand, view judgment as an intuitive act; under this model, learning to make clinical judgments requires a description of the subjective, "aha" experiences of great nursing clinicians. This intuition model would seem to suggest imitation and apprenticeship training for the student of diagnosis.

By pulling together what is known about how humans reason, one can formulate a base for clinical teaching and learning of diagnosis. Helping others to implement nursing diagnosis may be done informally in conversation or formally through conferences. In either case, being aware of current practice and steps in implementation will be useful.

Implementation in Practice

Not all professional developments in the health fields spread across the nation as fast as some people would desire. In medicine the application of new knowledge and techniques is sometimes delayed 5 or more years; the situation is no different in nursing.

One indicator of interest in a topic is the frequency of its appearance in journals and textbooks. Since the beginning of the national effort to identify nursing diagnoses in 1973, more than 60 articles have appeared in leading journals, and all recent textbooks in nursing process deal with the subject. Interest is high.

Interest does not help improve care, at least not until motivation leads to implementation. No data exist and thus no estimate can be made about how many nurses use nursing diagnosis to organize their clients' care.

The personal experience of the author suggests that many are implementing the concept in practice. Yet this impression is biased by association and contact mostly with those so motivated. In some regions the question of implementation has long passed. Nurses are discussing the application of diagnosis to quality assurance programs and the implications for clinical research. When a hospital requires that students know and use nursing diagnosis before affiliating for clincial experience, and when another advertises for a clinical specialist knowledgeable in nursing diagnosis, it is clear that diagnosis is established in those places.

Within the same or other regions situations are encountered in which even nursing process is not a familiar concept. Although different levels of competency are currently encountered, those interested in nursing practice are generally enthusiastic about learning nursing diagnosis. It is sometimes said that ideas arise from the academic ivory tower. This was not the case with nursing diagnosis. Clinicians seemed to appreciate its importance more than educators did in the early years.

Implementation in Education

Although interest has increased, diagnostic skills do not always appear "in bold type" in curricula of all professional programs (McLean, 1981). Looking to the future, educators will have to assure that all students develop beginning competency in diagnosis and treatment of common nursing diagnoses (Fredette and O'Connor, 1979). Otherwise, new graduates will not be prepared to practice at a level consistent with national standards of practice (see Table 7-1). State board examinations will begin to reflect this requirement as these standards are implemented.

Competency in diagnosis is something graduates will use, as clinicians, the remainder of their professional lives. This usefulness criterion alone places nursing diagnosis into the category of essential content in educational programs.

Clinical experiences in disease-related judgment may not transfer to nursing diagnostic judgments. There are indications that beyond the general diagnostic process, knowledge is a significant factor in success as a diagnostician (Elstein, Schulman, and Sprafka, 1978). Clinical knowledge and nursing process have to be synthesized. Dealing with uncertainties and variability among clients requires repetitive experience in the diagnosis of common problems amenable to nursing care.

Clearly, the most economical way to acquire diagnostic skill is under the guidance of faculty. Feedback in early stages of training and guided clinical experiences offered in the educational setting are critical in developing this competency.

Currently, both remedial education and expertise in diagnosis have to be built into masters' degree and clinical doctoral programs. Graduation as a clinical specialist or teacher should guarantee to society that a nurse has the ability to diagnose and treat high-incidence nursing diagnoses in his or her specialty. Master's-prepared nurses are the ones who will act as consultants in differential diagnosis and provide feedback to generalists on the development of their competencies. They are also the more sophisticated clinical experts who have the responsibility for studying new or unlabeled diagnoses.

Inservice educators continually remind us that they have to fill in the gaps that result not only from deficiencies in educational programs but also from new developments in practice or nurses' lack of continuing education. Orientation programs, workshops, and even classes in the identification and treatment of specific diagnoses are useful. Many inservice educators find, as Aspinall (1976) remarked, that nursing diagnosis and diagnostic judgment are the "weak link" in nursing process competencies.

Clinicians are eager to learn. They find organizing their care around nursing diagnoses makes practice interesting and challenging and care planning more focused.

Assisting with Implementation

The usual roles of student and graduate may be reversed where nursing diagnosis is concerned. It is not uncommon to find students helping graduates learn about nursing diagnosis. This section will review the implementation process. It will be useful to be acquainted with methods and resources when opportunities to help are encountered. One should always use others' curiosity to advantage.

Nursing care settings will be encountered where the idea of nursing diagnosis is unheard of, controversial, seen as student activity, or considered interesting but unclear. In such settings it is appropriate for a student to present a brief description and examples of nursing diagnosis, if questioned. Follow this by suggesting some reading or a conference to discuss the idea. The staff may not be ready to think about diagnosis; a "back door" approach could include helping staff plan a conference on any of the following:

1 Are we implementing our institution's philosophy and objectives of nursing on this unit? (Each person at the meeting has a copy of the philosophy and objectives to examine.) Usually objectives specify identification of clients' health problems.

2 Is our practice on this unit consistent with national standards? (Each person has a copy of the generic or specialty ANA standards of practice to examine and perhaps also an article about legal aspects, such as the Fortin and Rabinow article listed in this chapter's bibliography.) Standard 2 specifies nursing diagnosis.

3 Is our scope of practice consistent with the scope defined nationally? (Each person has a copy of the American Nurses' Association's *A Social Policy Statement* to examine.) Diagnosis is included within the scope of practice.

4 Is our practice consistent with the law? (Each person has copies of the state practice act and board of nursing rules and regulations; this approach is useful if diagnosis or judgment is specified in those documents.)

The topics provide a basis for thinking about current practice. The objective is to examine personal role concepts relative to outside criteria. This comparison, combined with one selected reading on the concept of nursing diagnosis, should lead nurses to consider the idea of using diagnoses, which is step one. Conversations and questions about diagnosis suggest readiness for step two.

The second step in implementation is to provide information. One or more of the following may be helpful:

1 Provide a small bibliography of two or three articles about nursing diagnosis, especially articles that are relevant to the type of clients the present staff serves.

2 Secure a speaker who is expert in nursing diagnosis, either a member of the staff or someone from elsewhere in the town or city.

3 Some staff members may be able to attend a continuing education offering about nursing diagnosis and report to the others.

If interest in trying nursing diagnosis as a means of organizaing nursing care is present, inform physicians before recording on charts. They may not understand the new way of recording. Think about (1) their level of knowledge and attitudes and (2) how nursing diagnosis may positively influence client care, and be ready with examples relevant to the particular physician's interest. Have the support within nursing before informing other professionals.

The group is ready for step three when even a few staff want to learn more. Step three begins the staff's educational process. The first learning objective is application of the definition of nursing diagnosis.

Diagnostic recognition exercises, such as those on page 7 and in Appendix H, Section A, are useful. These exercises require knowledge and application of the definition of a nursing diagnosis. Recognition of what is and what is not a diagnosis is present when discriminations can be made and reasons stated for choosing, and not choosing, items.

The group is then ready to move to *diagnostic selection exercises*; an example is provided in Appendix H, Section B. It is useful to prepare exercises at various levels of difficulty. For example, in vignettes the cues can range from obvious, critical defining signs and symptoms to cues which are ambiguous or conflicting. Also, a higher level of difficulty is attained if no diagnoses are provided at the end of the vignette and diagnostic hypotheses have to be generated during the reading of the vignette. A list of diagnoses and defining characteristics, such as those provided in a manual (Gordon, 1982) or book (Kim and Moritz, 1981) are used to assist in problem-identification. An example of this second type of diagnostic selection exercise is contained in Appendix H, Section C. Early diagnostic concept learning is facilitated if (1) a language is provided (diagnostic labels) and (2) vignettes are constructed directly from defining characteristics of diagnoses. Ambiguities and uncertainties can be introduced *after* the basic concepts are acquired.

The next level of learning, problem formulation, utilizes total case data rather than vignettes. Learning can be facilitated by *diagnostic formulation exercises*. Examples are contained in Appendix G. This exercise is the most difficult but also the most meaningful. It simulates the process used in actual client care. Answers to exercises in Appendix G and H are provided in Appendix I.

Repetition of diagnostic formulation exercises increases the group's skill in analyzing and integrating clinical data. When expertise is developed in formulating nursing diagnoses from simulated case data, each participant can be asked to bring to the group admission data and diagnoses from one of his or her own clients. Deficiencies in assessment, hypothesis generation, and testing, and in problem formulation can be discussed; this discussion can benefit both the individual and the group. After one or two experiences, diagnostic process (the hypothesis-testing model) should be discussed. This will focus attention on the *process* being used as well as on diagnostic labeling of health problems.

Step four involves using the diagnostic process with clients. One of the factors that facilitates formulating nursing diagnoses is collecting a *nursing* data base. Difficulties arise if the collected information is more appropriate to medical than nursing diagnoses.

As implementation of the diagnostic process begins, nurses may become aware of needs to improve their interviewing and assessment skills. In addition, branching, hypothesis testing, and problem formulation usually need to be discussed.

Some may wish not to record their first efforts in the client's chart. Provide opportunities for review by the group, a colleague, or whoever is guiding their learning. This helps alleviate anxiety about mistakes in labeling and charting.

Step five in implementation may last for a year. This is the questioning and doubting phase. Topics usually needing discussion include doctors' reactions, ways to treat diagnoses, the need for further work on terminology, and the creation of new terms to describe client conditions. The most common basis for discouragement in the novice is the time diagnosis and care planning take.

One or more of the following may help the staff get through the phase of feeling that "nursing diagnosis takes too much time":

1 Can I help? In what aspect are you having difficulty?

2 How many times have you gone through the diagnostic process (systematic health status assessments, problem identification, and care planning)? Oh, just once?

3 Do you remember how long it took you to give your first bath and make a client's bed?

4 Have you noticed how long it takes a medical student to do a history and exam? [Or] When you go to a physician for the *first* time, I imagine the history and examination take at least 30 minutes, and the doctor is probably experienced; I guess most of us would not refuse this much attention.

5 Oh, do you think there are areas in the functional patterns assessment that are not important? [This induces conflict.]

6 Could you be intervening as well as assessing? Oh, that's why it takes so long.

7 What nursing diagnoses did your client have? Oh, you wouldn't have wanted to miss *these.*

8 Yes, but now you have a base; daily assessments can be done from this base, and look how many problems you can prevent that would otherwise take nursing time to treat.

9 I promise that if you keep practicing, the *most complex* assessment, diagnosis, and care planning can be done in 30 minutes. For most clients this whole process may take 15 minutes.

10 Don't clients deserve the time functional health assessment takes? [This is the ethical-moral-legal appeal.]

Systematically assessing functional health patterns and identifying and labeling problems, if there are any, takes time. This is why in other professions the skills are developed during the educational program. Those not having this opportunity to learn while in school will have to spend the time it takes, just as the others have had to do. There is nothing magical that will produce overnight the competency needed in current practice. The consolation is that diagnostic skills have lasting value, in contrast to learning how to use the latest machine that may be outdated in a year.

Resources Available   The literature contains a number of articles useful in implementing nursing diagnosis in practice settings. Sharing even one of these may stimulate interest.

Feild's (1979) excellent description of her experience with the change process for implementing diagnosis is a good resource for staff, head nurses, and administrators. Dalton (1979) and Weber (1979) provide many insights about establishing diagnosis-based care in a community setting and private practice, respectively. Bruce (1979) describes a program of implementation stimulated by nursing administration.

As implementation proceeds, resource information from articles listed in the bibliographies of chapters and the Annoted Bibliography at the end of the book may be helpful. The Clearinghouse for Nursing Diagnosis, discussed in the next section, provides a newsletter, *NR DX*, containing national, regional, and state activities. Continually updated bibliographies about specific nursing diagnoses, prepared by the Massachusetts Conference Group on Classification of Nursing Diagnoses, are also available from the Clearinghouse.

Clearly, the best way to exchange ideas about implementation is to hold local meetings. In Massachusetts, three groups meet in different parts of the state to share ideas and experiences. All participants in the monthly meetings comment on the learning that has occurred as a result of discussions with nursing colleagues. The local groups that have been formed in a few states can provide leadership through its members' practice and through conferences held in conjunction with state nurses' associations. Most importantly, having a local group offers a forum for nurses to extol or criticize the latest developments in nursing diagnosis.

In summary, one should not expect to find outstanding diagnostic competencies in all clinical settings. Change takes time. Yet the time can be reduced. Professional education can be designed to enable students to learn beginning diagnostic and therapeutic skills before graduation.

The complexity of diagnostic judgment probably lies more in the environment than in the process. Clients and their situations vary widely, so that a broad knowledge base is required. Repeated practice and feedback are critically important. This kind of learning environment is provided most economically in educational settings.

When students or staff members begin to use nursing diagnoses in obvious places, such as care plans and charts, other nurses ask questions. In order to prepare the reader for these questoins, a brief overview of stages of implementation and available resources has been provided. Introducing the staff to a professional role concept compatible with using nursing diagnosis is a basic step in implementing diagnosis; this leads them to examine the concept. The next steps in implementation center on the use of diagnostic nomenclature and process skills. No one has become an expert in diagnosis overnight, but once skills are developed they last a lifetime.

Diagnostic judgment is a process that requires a "language" for describing conclusions. In the next section, current developments in naming client conditions encountered in practice will be described.

DEVELOPMENT OF THE CLASSIFICATION SYSTEM

Some identifiable group has to develop a diagnostic classification system. The following discussion begins with the national group that has assumed responsibility for this activity. As in other professions, it is a voluntary group not aligned with any nursing organization. There is no outside financial funding. Liaisons with nursing organizations exist and representatives from medical classification groups and medical record librarians have participated in national conferences.

The purposes and methods for developing the classification system are described in this section, as well as current problems and issues. It will be seen that there is need for a clear concept of what is and what is not a nursing diagnosis. The multiplicity of conceptual frameworks complicate this decision. Experts are currently working on developing the conceptual categories for organizing the system and guiding further development.

As each of these separate topics is discussed it will be seen that no decisions have been finalized. Even the currently listed accepted diagnoses are accepted only for clinical testing. This means that every registered nurse can, and should, participate and influence the course of development.

The National Conference Group

The National Conference Group for Classification of Nursing Diagnoses (NCG) is the main group coordinating the national effort to develop a diagnostic classification system. It was formed at the First National Conference on Classification of Nursing Diagnoses in 1973 by the enthusiastic participants in that meeting. At that time nursing diagnosis was a vague entity to most nurses. Today 42 diagnoses have been classified.

The NCG is highly committed, as evidenced by the group's sustained effort for approximately a decade. The NCG membership includes broad representation from practice, education, research, nursing specialties, and geographic areas of North America. The NCG is open to all nurses' participation.

Participants attending the first and subsequent conferences are the designated national group. They represent nearly every state in the United States and also a few provinces of Canada. Among the group are staff nurses, clinical specialists, directors of nursing, deans, faculty, theorists, and researchers. Some are recent graduates; others have many years of education and experience in nursing. All are committed to the development of nursing diagnoses, some because of everyday practical reasons and others because of abstract theoretical interests in this nursing concept. Probably at no other conference is such interest, enthusiasm, and working together demonstrated by nurses from diverse positions, backgrounds, clinical specialties, and geographic areas. It is truly a unique group committed to the development of nursing. (Gordon, 1981)

To sustain developmental activities between biennial conferences, the NCG appointed a task force in 1973. This voluntary group represents all regions of the United States. Its members are from practice, education, and research. Task force responsibilities include information dissemination and exchange, educational and research activities, and planning of national conferences.

To help nurses throughout the country acquire and exchange information, a central Clearinghouse for Nursing Diagnosis was established in 1973 at St. Louis University.[1] This center was made possible through the support of Sr. T. Noth, Dean of the School of Nursing; today the Clearinghouse is nearly self-supporting. Its first coordinator, Kristine Gebbie, initiated a publication, *Nursing Diagnosis Newsletter* (NR DX), which through the years has had 1500 subscribers. The readers ask questions, critique activities, and submit abstracts of their work on diagnosis.

The task force maintains a liaison with the Congress on Nursing Practice of the American Nurses' Association. One individual is a member of both this group and the task force. The liaison between the two groups facilitates the exchange of information about national practice issues and classification system development. The Congress is concerned with the implementation of standards of practice, nursing process, quality assurance, and credentialing. All of these, as previously discussed, depend on the development of diagnostic nomenclature.

Less formal, but effective, communications have been established with other national nursing groups and specialty organizations. It is expected that in the next few years these relationships within nursing and between nursing and medical classification system developers will be more formalized.

Educational activities of the task force are directed toward implementation of nursing diagnosis in practice and education. The position was taken that educational efforts should be made primarily at the state or local level; conference groups have been started in a few states to reach this goal. Regional conferences, which occur between national meetings, are held for the purpose of stimulating diagnostic category identification and reviewing regional activities.

State and regional educational efforts permit conferences at the national level to serve other purposes. The primary role of biennial national meetings is to add, revise, or delete diagnostic nomenclature. Review of developments in practice, education, and research is an additional feature of national meetings.

The stimulation of research activities is also within the scope of responsibilities the task force assumes. Although it is clear that diagnostic categories have to be clinically validated, ongoing research is minimal relative to the need that exists. Both methodological and conceptual issues have contributed to this dearth of research (Gordon and

---

[1] The current Clearinghouse coordinator is Ann Becker, R.N., M.S., of St. Louis University, School of Nursing, 3525 Caroline St., St. Louis, Missouri 63104.

Sweeney, 1979). During the relatively short time period of the NCG's existence, diagnostic classification has moved from an idea in the minds of the two coordinators of the first conference, Kristine Gebbie and Mary Ann Lavin, to a national priority in professional practice. The next decade will probably be equally exciting.

Before this discussion turns to development of the diagnostic classification system, general characteristics of a system will be described. It will be seen that a system has a purpose, a focus, and an organizing principle. Structurally, there is a vertical hierarchy of categories proceeding upward from the least to the most abstract level. Horizontally each level has a set, or class, of concepts at a similar level of abstraction. Nursing diagnoses and their definitions would be placed in a horizontal class on the lowest level of the hierarchy. They are the least abstract concepts in the system.

Characteristics of a Classification System

Whenever the term *nursing diagnosis* is heard, the words *diagnostic classification system* usually follow closely. In general, a *classification system* is the ordering of phenomena in a systematic way for some purpose. One familiar example of a useful system is student classification in colleges and universities—freshman, sophomore, junior, and senior—the purpose of which is to classify students' progress in the educational system. In some instances classification is tied to privileges, expectations, and requirements.

Classification is also used in a science to sort and code the phenomena of interest. Concepts are identified, defined, and classified in the factor-isolating, or naming, stage of theory development discussed previously. Biology is an example; it orders classes of living things. Chemistry classifies elements, and medical science classifies diseases. The purpose of classification systems is to describe, explain, and develop theories about how to influence relevant phenomena.

In nursing, clusters of signs and symptoms representing health problems are being identified and labeled. When the process is completed a nomenclature system will be available. A *nomenclature* is defined as a compilation of approved terms for describing phenomena; in this case the terms describe clusters of signs and symptoms. The diagnoses listed in Appendix A represent a beginning nomenclature for nursing, which can be used as basic categories in a classification system.

Taxonomy is another term that will be heard in discussions of nursing diagnosis. It refers both to the theoretical study of classification and to the classification system that results. The term originally applied to theory and principles of biological classification; it is now used in other contexts: disease taxonomy, taxonomy of educational objectives, nursing taxonomy, and so forth.

Each classification system has a *purpose* and an underlying concept and *principle of organization*. The conceptual organization of the system dictates the vertical arrangement of classes within the system. Furthermore, the conceptual organization that pervades a discipline before classification is begun influences the way phenomena are conceived and classified.

Purpose, focus, and ordering principle are three decisions to be made in the development of any classification system. Hangartner (1975) clarifies these ideas by using an analogy to the common telephone book. By enlarging his example, the idea of purpose, focus, and ordering principle can be illustrated.

The *Bell System Yellow Pages, Boston Area* includes a passage entitled "How to Use the Yellow Pages" that describes a system for classifying large and small businesses that provide a product or a service. Underlying the structure of this system is the everyday "theory" of classifying businesses according to their services. Purpose, focus, ordering principle, and description are evident. *Purpose:* "Telephone directories are provided as an aid to good telephone service." *Focus:* "Exclusively business related heading, 'Product or service.'" *Ordering principle:* "Headings are always alphabetical. Think of the heading most likely to carry what you want. Flip to it and you'll find names, addresses and phone numbers of business people ready to serve you. Forgotten the name? Again, turn to the heading best describing the firm's type of business. Glancing down the list [alphabetical] will usually bring the name back to mind" ("Bell System," 1980, p. 8). Under "employment" one finds employment agencies, employment contractors–temporary help, and employment training service. Under each is an alphabetical listing of names. This constitutes a three-level ordering hierarchy.

A classification system of nursing diagnoses might have a similar format: broad categories, diagnostic categories, and etiological subcategories. This kind of system would provide a dictionary type of reference to the health problems within the scope of nursing practice. Nursing diagnoses would be arranged at one horizontal level with similar problems separate from dissimilar ones. The basis for separating diagnoses under broad categories is found in the conceptual framework of the classification system.

Functional health patterns would be examples of second-level vertical classes. Role-relationship pattern, one class at this level, would serve to classify related diagnoses. At a third level, broader concepts would classify the patterns. Appendix B illustrates two levels; diagnoses are at the basic level and patterns at the second level.

It is important that all horizontal elements at a particular level are at the same level of abstraction. For example, in a classification of living things, which of the following would not be at the same level: dogs, cats, animals, spaniels, and cows?

If you picked animals and spaniels, you have grasped the idea that concepts exist at different levels of abstraction. *Animals* is a *higher* level of classification of living things. The category includes dogs, cats, and cows. *Spaniels*, on the other hand, is a *lower* level of classification because spaniel is included in the class *dog; red spaniels* would be at an even lower class level as red spaniels are included in the class *spaniel*. The level of abstraction in a classification system relates to the level of inclusiveness.

We shall pursue this example further for both practical and theoretical reasons. When caring for a client, a nurse may have to create a diagnostic label to have a focus for intervention; this will occur until the accepted diagnosis list is more complete. To create a label to describe a cluster of signs and symptoms, one has to know the "right" level of abstraction.

Think of the difficulties that could result if one classified observations as animal when in fact the thing one began to hug (action) was a subclass of animal called a wolf. Similarly, if the diagnoses created in nursing practice and in a classification system are not at a useful level for determining action, intervention can be unsafe or ineffective.

Consider an example in the nutritional-metabolic pattern area. "Nutritional alteration" is not a useful diagnosis; neither is "nutritional alteration: less than minimum daily requirements," a subclass of the former. Protein deficit, a subclass of nutritional deficit, points toward nursing action. Is it adequate for determining intervention? Not really. A nurse would intervene differently for the problem of protein deficit/lack of finances than for protein deficit/inadequate knowledge of daily requirement.

The most useful level of abstraction in classifying (or identifying) client conditions is the level that permits one then to determine what intervention to use. Diagnoses have to be *basic level* categories in the system. This is a "level of abstraction that is appropriate for using, thinking about, or naming" a client condition in situations where the condition occurs (Rosch, 1976, p. 43).

The first task in classification is to identify basic level categories in light of present knowledge. A few generations ago, *dropsy* was a diagnostic category in medicine. Using this concept clinically and studying the phenomenon in many clients demonstrated that the level of abstraction was too high. Discrimination among various forms of dropsy has led to the identification of more useful categories to guide treatment.

Examination of the *changes* occurring in nursing diagnostic nomenclature between 1973 and today does not reveal what the NCG views as a useful level of abstraction for the diagnoses to be classified (Appendix F). Some nursing diagnoses listed today are more inclusive, thus at a higher level of abstraction, than in 1973. Others have become more specific. Two factors appear to have influenced these developments: (1) changes have not been based on systematic clinical testing, (2) no position has been taken by the NCG on the level of abstraction of basic categories and how the level is defined. Does this discussion hint of a previously discussed issue? Exactly; these ideas bring us back to the recognized need for an operational definition of a nursing diagnosis.

Before proceeding to examine the current process of classification, let us explore the assumption that the purpose of diagnostic classification is to facilitate practice. The purpose must be clearly established before classification efforts are begun.

Purpose of Classification

Why does nursing desire a classification system? What purpose will it serve other than filling the pages of a manual? These are critically important questions that have to be answered before beginning development. What is classified—that is, the focus of classification—and how the classes are ordered depend on the purpose of the system.

Classification systems designed for one purpose are more desirable than multipurpose schemes that have to accommodate to many types of operations (Giovanetti, 1978, p. 8). The initial purpose of developing a classification system in nursing was to facilitate practice. Diagnostic nomenclature did not exist; it was not a situation in which basic level diagnoses had been identified and standardized and were awaiting a system of classification that would be relevant to practice. It was necessary to start "from scratch." The task was to begin to develop a way of naming the client conditions that generated therapeutic concern. In essence, nurses had to sort and code their world of practice.

In their foresight, Gebbie and Lavin, coordinators of the first conference, set the focus for classification system development: nursing diagnoses. A few articles had appeared in the literature (Durand and Prince, 1966; Komorita, 1963; Fry, 1953), but in the early 1970s most nurses still described their practice in terms of nursing objectives and tasks. The client conditions necessitating care were not articulated. In fact, the first classification system relevant to practice focused on therapeutic objectives as can be seen in the 21 problems listed in Table 2-1 (Abdellah, 1959, p. 26).

When a diagnostic classification system is developed, nurses in practice will be able to consult a manual that contains the entire diagnostic nomenclature. This will enable them to label client conditions consistently. When a diagnostic label is used, it will have a standard definition. This uniformity decreases the probability of communication errors.

A diagnostic classification system can be used to construct other systems with other purposes. There may be systems for computerizing nursing information; one such system of interest to nursing administrators would relate diagnoses to nursing care time. Classifying clients' diagnoses and the time required for intervention would assist in determining staffing patterns and hospital reimbursement. In addition, the development of a clinical science would be facilitated by classification of the client conditions amenable to nursing therapy.

In summary, current efforts in classification are directed toward establishing a system to facilitate practice. Yet this system can be used to design others. Let us now examine what progress has been made and the methodology used. Identification, definition, and ordering of diagnostic categories will organize the discussion.

Methods and Progress in Classification

Development of a diagnostic classification system entails identification, definition, ordering, and numerical coding. Gebbie and Lavin (1974) outlined these activities to guide the work of the national conference group. In the following sections each of these activities will be defined and the progress to date will be reviewed. An appreciation of issues and current work will provide knowledge for the reader's future participation in classification system development.

Identification of Nursing Diagnoses   In a previous section on nursing diagnosis and nursing theory, it was seen that naming and defining concepts was the first step in developing practice theories. When concepts are organized in hierarchical sets in a classification system, they are referred to as classes or categories. In a diagnostic classification system, nursing diagnoses are the basic class or category. More specifically, what has been referred to as the problem in the problem/etiology format is a class in the classification system; etiologies are subclassifications.

The first conceptual issue encountered in identification is how to define diagnoses. The definition is critical. The "world" of practice must be divided into two domains, client conditions that are classifiable as nursing diagnoses and client conditions that are not.

Let us try, step by step, to narrow down the whole of practice. Nurses are concerned with individuals, families, and communities that (1) feel a therapeutic concern, that is, a need for care, and/or (2) arouse a therapeutic concern in physicians or nurses (Taylor, 1971). Underlying the concerns, we shall assume, is a problematic or potentially problematic condition. The task will be to isolate and name the specific conditions that clients or others bring to a nurse's attention *or* that arouse concern in the nurse.

Conceptual Focus for Identification The domain *therapeutic concern* is too large to provide guidelines for identification of nursing diagnoses. Many conditions encountered in nursing practice generate therapeutic concern. Some are already labeled by other professions.

Logically, the actual or potential problems *amenable to nursing therapy* should be the focus in identification and classification. Or, as defined by the NCG:

> . . . those patient problems or concerns most frequently identified by nurses, problems which are usually identified by nurses before they are recognized by other health care workers, and problems which are amenable to some intervention which is available in the present or potential scope of nursing practice. (Gebbie and Lavin, 1974, p. 250)

After we have come this far in delineating the domain, the next step is to specify a concept of health problem. One way of conceptualizing problems amenable to nursing therapy is as dysfunctional or potentially dysfunctional health patterns. This approach would lead to identifying problematic patterns in the 11 pattern areas:

Health-perception-health-management pattern
Nutritional-metabolic pattern
Elimination pattern
Sleep-rest pattern
Activity-exercise pattern

Cognitive-perceptual pattern
Self-perception–self-concept pattern
Role-relationship pattern
Sexual-reproductive pattern
Coping–stress-tolerance pattern
Value-belief pattern

Some actual and potential problems have already been identified in the pattern areas (Appendix B). For further identification, a sample question would be: Are there any other dysfunctional role-relationship patterns that respond primarily to nursing treatment? The patterns are the areas nurses say they assess; thus they provide a structure for the basic level of category identification and classification.

Bircher (1975) has also proposed a way of identifying diagnostic concepts. Following the human needs classification developed by Maslow (1970), problems in mastery or competence in fulfilling needs are proposed as broad categories for classifying diagnoses. The needs framework is a theory explaining motivation; some question the use of a nonnursing theory as a basis for a nursing classification. Yet the idea of behavioral competence in meeting needs could be fruitfully applied to the pattern areas. Models of the client that were discussed in Chapter 3, such as Roy's adaptation model, Orem's self-care deficit framework, and Johnson's behavioral systems, have also been proposed as guidelines for identifying diagnostic concepts.

These various views again remind us that in nursing there is no unified model of the client and no agreed upon way of describing the domain of client problems. In the biased view of this author, the functional health pattern areas employed in assessment could be used in basic-level classification of nursing diagnoses resulting from assessment. Higher-order syntheses of patterns into more abstract categories may ultimately reveal relationships among them and, thus, among the diagnoses. Identification should begin at the most concrete level, the functional health pattern areas that nurses assess.

Before examining current work in classification, it is well to note that the problem oriented approach is a source of controversy. On one side of the controversy is the argument that nursing is health oriented, not only problem oriented. Clinical examples are offered as follows:

1 Client family with *no* actual or potential parenting (or nutritional or other) problem but with a curiosity, interest, or desire to further enhance its knowledge, alternatives, and status

2 Well, grieving client who is further interested in exploring his grief reaction and/ or the grieving process

It is expected that nurses who are particularly interested in the development of diagnoses in this area will continue to submit categories. One was accepted in 1980— family coping: potential for growth.

On the other side of the controversy it is argued that there is a large population of clients who do have health problems or are at risk for problems. Highest priority, it is said, should go toward identifying and classifying these conditions. This classification would enable nurses to identify to third party payers and administrators the *professional* services clients require.

Finally, the argument is heard that (1) practice is being eroded by a proliferation of health care workers who treat parts of the client, (2) if nurses do not establish a domain of practice *soon*, the client will be exposed to a multitude of care providers daily, (3) the health care systems that employ nurses value problem oriented care, and thus (4) initial efforts should concentrate on *problems*. As may be seen, many other issues interact. These influence decisions about problem oriented or wellness oriented diagnoses and priorities in identification activities.

Practice-Based Identification of Diagnoses Since classification activities began in 1973, the constant theme has been that all nurses should be involved in the development of diagnostic nomenclature. In this section, some ideas will be explored for practice-based identification of diagnoses. As one's skill increases in the use of diagnoses and the diagnostic process, one becomes able to contribute to the development of diagnosis. The following discussion includes information about how to identify and test nursing diagnoses and how to submit a nursing diagnosis to the national conference group.

Suppose, as mentioned in Chapter 6, a nurse observes a cluster of signs and symptoms that cannot be labeled with current terminology (Appendix A). The cluster may represent an entirely new diagnostic area or may be in an area already identified but not sufficiently labeled. Second, a nurse may notice in clinical practice that a current diagnostic label is too broad. Alteration in parenting is an example. For purposes of treatment, discrimination among various forms of the identified condition may be necessary. Inability to plan treatment for a stated diagnosis is a signal that a current diagnostic category is too broad.

Third, in clinical practice it may be noticed that a particular cluster of signs and symptoms is associated with the development of the client's problem. An etiological factor may not be currently named or may be too broad to guide treatment. To summarize, in clinical situations a category label should be created if an observed cluster of signs and symptoms:

1 is not described by any current diagnostic label

2 represents a distinguishable form of a currently labeled problem (needs a more specific label)

3 is an etiological subcategory (of a diagnosis) that either has not been named or has been named too broadly

In any of these situations, the immediate need is to create a label. Eventually, as will be seen, the label can be shared with others.

The importance of having a clear concept of nursing diagnosis cannot be overstressed. Before one creates labels and calls them nursing diagnoses, one must have a definition upon which the labeling is based. If the definition of nursing diagnosis employed in this book is used, the cluster of signs and symptoms manifested by the client (1) must represent a dysfunctional or potentially dysfunctional health pattern *and* (2) can be predicted to respond primarily to *nursing* treatment.

These guidelines are intended to help nurses avoid labeling conditions they cannot treat. Such labeling is a waste of time and intellectual ability. Admittedly, these guidelines can be supplemented and improved. Articulating *exactly* how a nursing diagnosis is defined and discriminated from client problems referred to other care providers requires further thought by the profession.

At times there is a tendency to label pathophysiological conditions that are not actually amenable to nursing treatment. A check of the *International Classification of Disease—Hospital Adaptation* (Commission on Professional and Hospital Activities, 1978)[2] may provide further help in excluding medical diagnoses. If one is tempted to label single symptoms, it is helpful to remember that a diagnosis describes a *cluster* of signs or symptoms.

The boundaries of psychiatric–mental-health nursing, psychiatric social work, psychiatry, and clinical psychology sometimes seem to overlap. Thus the above guideline *responds to nursing treatment* may not sufficiently discriminate nursing from those other domains. The *Diagnostic and Statistical Manual III (DSM III)* (American Psychiatric Association, 1980) is considered by some nurses in this specialty to contain labels for client problems they treat. Others contend that the scope of conditions listed in DMS III is too limited for nursing practice and that the diagnoses do not represent a nursing perspective. This issue will no doubt get further attention in the coming years.

Nurses who identify and label new (or revise current) nursing diagnoses need to keep a record of the cluster of signs and symptoms observed. Small file cards may be useful. As cases accumulate, the *common* signs and symptoms occuring among clients become apparent. The nurse should be sure also to record probable etiological factors for the problem; clients with the same problem can be expected to have different etiological factors.

New or revised diagnoses should be reviewed by colleagues in the practice setting. Feedback may lead to improvement and encourage further testing in practice. Some have found it beneficial to hold conferences in their unit, hospital, or city to review new diagnoses.

When a category is clearly identified according to guidelines (Appendix D), it

---

[2] Readers who are unable to locate this manual of medical diagnoses are referred to a medical records department.

should be submitted to the national conference group.[3] A review by nurses from across the country will follow and may result in acceptance of the diagnosis. Publication in the accepted listing permits widespread clinical testing of the diagnosis. Another avenue that may encourage testing of new or revised diagnoses is publication as an article in a nursing journal.

Many nurses are heard to complain that the accepted list is not complete, that diagnoses are too broad, or that definitions of diagnoses are vague. Recognition of deficiencies is an excellent motivator for generating new terminology or revising current diagnoses.

When nursing diagnosis and the diagnostic process are implemented, interesting questions can be raised and projects started. For example:

1 Do our clients exhibit the nursing diagnoses (clusters of signs and symptoms) in the accepted list?

2 What are the common nursing diagnoses our clients exhibit?

Gordon and Sweeney (1979), Brown (1974), and Gebbie and Lavin (1974) provide some direction for finding answers to questions such as these. Practice in looking at one's own clients in a unit may lead to larger studies, as will be described later. Yet one's own clients may number 500 or more in a year. Imagine how great a contribution could be made to identification of diagnoses if the diagnostic labels and observed signs and symptoms were collected.

In summary, the process of clinical identification of nursing diagnoses has been linked to actual practice. The immediate need in practice, to conceptualize a client's condition for determining treatment, can be used to contribute to diagnostic category identification. The process is not complex, and the payoff is great. Nurses providing direct care are the ones that will use diagnostic terminology; therefore they are encouraged to contribute to its development.

Progress in Classification   Currently 42 diagnoses have been identified and accepted by the NCG for clinical testing. Each is defined by a set of signs and symptoms. The diagnoses have been classified alphabetically (Appendix A). The NCG, recognizing the diversity of conceptual views, in 1973 decided upon a primarily inductive approach to diagnostic category identification. Recall that induction proceeds from specific cases to a generalization. Conference participants utilized their accumulated nursing experience stored in memory to proceed from observed cases to generalizations. During small group work sessions, 100 to 200 participants at each conference described and labeled problems of clients treated in their practices.

In order for a diagnosis to be accepted, (1) definition and other specifications have been required (Appendix D) and (2) the majority of the group had to recommend acceptance. Additionally, in 1980 a committee reviewed the diagnoses for consistency in format and naming procedures. Diagnoses have been submitted to the NCG by individuals, state or regional conference groups, and by participants. It may be expected that data from clinical studies will be the basis for refining diagnostic categories in future years. Data describing the common, critical diagnostic cluster of signs and

[3] See Appendix D for address.

symptoms are the only reasonable basis for changes in categories. Studies will have to be carried out, replicated, and reported to the NCG.

All methods of identifying actual and potential conditions nurses treat rely on both inductive generalization and deductive processes. The retrospective review of clinical experience used by the NCG has been primarily inductive, utilizing participants' experiences with numerous clients. Deductive generation of diagnoses from a conceptual framework was initially advocated by some conference participants. They suggested that a framework assumed to represent the real world of practice be used to deduce diagnostic categories. This would ensure that client conditions described by nursing diagnoses would share common general features.

A conceptual framework identifies the domain of nursing and thus the diagnoses within that domain. A variety of frameworks exist in nursing so it may be expected that nurses within the NCG generated diagnoses from various conceptual viewpoints. It is advantageous to represent the diversity in nursing. The disadvantage is that diagnoses (Appendix A) are at various levels of abstraction and disparate in conceptual focus.

As the accepted diagnosis list grew longer, there was reconsideration of the need for adopting one conceptual framework and an organizing principle of classification. As may be seen in Appendix A, alphabetization has been the basis for organizing diagnoses. A member of the task force, Sr. Callista Roy, was asked to convene a group of nursing theorists in 1977. Since that time, a group consisting of those who have published theories or frameworks and others who are experts in theory construction has met once or twice yearly (Appendix E). This group was invited to generate a framework from currently accepted diagnoses; this clearly was an inductive task.

The theorists, separately, analyzed the accepted diagnoses of 1975 (see Appendix F) as to level, conceptual derivation, and nature of the problem implied. These analyses were discussed at the theorist group's first meeting at the third national conference. Incidentally, this was the first time major theorists in nursing had met together to discuss theoretical concepts. Their spirited discussion and scholarly exchange was evidence of interest in the development of a framework for guiding the further development of nursing diagnosis. A preliminary report of their deliberations was presented at the third national conference, in 1978.

The interaction between theorists and clinicians at the work sessions of the third and fourth conferences fostered exchange of abstractions and practical realities. A joint presentation in 1980 of a progress report, case examples, and critique was most stimulating.

The theorists have emphasized a holistic view of the client which is a traditional focus of nursing. Consistent with the holistic view is their conceptual model of the client, unitary man (referring to human beings in mutual interaction with their environment). Considerable attention was given, initially, to generating a model of the client evident in the diagnoses already developed. Added to this was a synthesis of their personal views.[4]

The model the theorists have created has a set of assumptions about the client. These are: unitary man (1) is growing and developing, (2) is a four-dimensional energy

---

[4] Kim and Moritz (1981) present a complete report of the work of the theorist group.

field, (3) has patterning of energy and (4) is goal seeking. Both the conference group and the theorists recognize that further definition of terms is required to communicate these assumptions.

The theorists' concept of the goal of nursing is to promote a rhythmic pattern of energy exchange between client and environment that is mutually enhancing and supports full life potential. Nurses accomplish this goal by the use of self and a body of nursing knowledge. The concept of nursing intervention and the concept of goal have not as yet been fully developed; most attention has been given to identifying broad categories for classifying nursing diagnoses.

At the most abstract level of diagnostic classification three factors have been identified: interaction, action, and awareness. These characterize unitary man. At a lower level of classification, the following characteristics are in the process of being defined more fully (Kim and Moritz, 1981, pp. 244-245):

A Interaction
  1 Exchanging: interchange of matter and energy between man and environment
  2 Communicating: interchange of information between man and environment
  3 Relating: connecting with other persons or objects
B Action
  1 Valueing: the assigning of worth
  2 Choosing: the selection of one or more alternatives
  3 Moving: activity within the environment
C Awareness
  1 Waking: refers to levels of arousal
  2 Feeling: refers to quality of sensation and mood
  3 Knowing: refers to meaning associated with a world view

Continued development of the assumptions, categories, and definitions is planned. This will permit evaluation of the conceptual model and its categories relative to the purpose of classification previously outlined.

The proposed characteristics listed under interaction, action, and awareness should serve as categories for classifying nursing diagnoses. At present, accepted diagnoses are not easily classified under these characteristics. (Firlit, Glass, and Nolan, 1980). A bridge is needed between the abstract and concrete. Precise definitions of the characteristics of unitary man are currently being developed. Definitions will help to determine whether a bridge can be constructed between the concrete diagnoses (Appendix A) and the abstract characteristics describing unitary man.

As well as providing a basis for organizing and classifying nursing diagnoses, characteristics of the client contained in a conceptual framework provide a focus for assessment. Behavioral manifestations of each characteristic of unitary man have to be identified in order to permit data collection. The functional health patterns discussed in this book may serve as the behavioral manifestations of characteristics. Functional patterns could then serve as the guide for client assessment within the unitary man conceptual framework.

In a previous discussion it was suggested that a cluster of nursing diagnoses may point to an overriding life pattern of the client. Perhaps a thread exists that seems to tie together all of the current health problems or risk states. For example, a person's discernible behavior may indicate self-concept alterations, role conflicts, violence potential, and other problems. A synthesis of these may reveal that there is a larger problem with relationships in general. If intervention deals with the client's pattern of relating, the more concrete problems may all improve.

The question arises: Can clinical observations of a client's coexisting dysfunctional *patterns* (nursing diagnoses) be synthesized at a higher and more holistic level? If so, is this holistic level useful for organizing clinical data and for planning care? Ultimately the question, which level of conceptualization (dysfunctional patterns or some synthesis of them) leads to better health outcomes, will have to be addressed. Perhaps both levels are necessary from a cognitive perspective and perhaps parallel levels of intervention are required.

In order to identify diagnostic categories at the higher level of synthesis, many clients would have to be studied and patterns of relating, exchanging, and so forth identified and labeled. Higher levels of synthesis impose two requirements: (1) the clear definition of less abstract categories (current nursing diagnoses) and (2) clear definition of categories in the theorist's framework previously described. These definitions are necessary if the first level of abstraction is used in the process of conceptualizing the second.

It is expected that the inductive and deductive approaches to classification will run parallel for a time. Diagnoses will continue to be developed and refined. As the NCG becomes more sophisticated in this process, the basic-level categories will be more alike in form and level. Secondly, the interest of the theorist group suggests that current work on developing a framework for classification will proceed. The NCG will continue to provide a forum for discussion of all approaches. As McKay (1977) has said, the usefulness of any approach is discovered only by testing it in the marketplace.

Definition and Standardization Diagnostic labels will someday be standardized. This means there will be an established usage and meaning for each diagnostic label. All those who have been educated in the profession will know the proper usage and employ it. Yet standardization does not imply that the labels will be written in stone. As with dictionaries, periodic revisions will occur.

Why standardize? Before answering this question directly, let us try something important. Please turn to the back of the pamphlet.

If you are confused, that is expected. The *standard usage* of the word pamphlet was not employed; I described what you are reading as a pamphlet instead of a book. This resulted in poor communication between us. The situation is similar in nursing practice. Phenomena have to be called by the same name or communication suffers; different labels generate different meanings.

Whether or not to standardize is not the question. The issue is what word labels describe the clusters of signs and symptoms that are of concern to nursing. Are the to-be-named clusters human processes or patterns, or are they states?

Many of the labels in the current list of diagnoses (Appendix A) describe *states*: constipation, pain, fluid volume deficit, knowledge deficit. Others describe behavioral *processes* or *patterns*: impaired mobility, self-care deficit, sleep pattern disturbance. From a treatment perspective, one removes a state or at least modifies it. A state closely borders on an entity or static condition. Medicine also describes states; cancer, diabetes. Current nursing diagnoses are not as rigid; no *client* could be called a constipatic or a grievic, as in the use of diabetic, schizophrenic, cardiac, or asthmatic.

Standard average European (English), as our language is called, leads to defining client conditions as if they were concrete, material objects. The idea of change, which certainly we recognize, is not readily expressed in English (Warner, 1976).

Although diagnoses describe the state of the client at the time of encounter, is that the state of a pattern or process or a state-as-entity? For example, do we treat "pain" as an entity? Or do we treat "pain self-management deficit" as a subclass of comfort management and a human functional pattern? Do we treat constipation-as-entity or an intermittent constipation pattern?

Functional patterns or processes are close to the concept of "human responses" in the ANA statement on scope of practice (American Nurses' Association, 1980). Patterns and processes also approach a more holistic (total person) philosophy, especially when the defining signs and symptoms are biopsychosocial. But can all therapeutic concerns be expressed in one naming format? Will this prove useful for treatment decisions? We do not know.

This discussion illustrates that questions arise as each aspect of identification, standardization, and classification is considered. The answers refer back to the conceptual framework and forward in time to the projected use of diagnoses in practice. Nursing may be likened to "the new kid on the block." Rules for "good form" in taxonomy development have been set and they need to be considered.

Coding for Information Systems   One of the purposes of identifying nursing diagnoses is to specify the basic data sets for computerized information systems. In addition to naming, standardization, and classification, numerical coding of diagnoses is planned. Incorporation of nursing diagnoses into the information processing systems of health care facilities requires this. Computerization is the only feasible way to retrieve large numbers of data for studies related to practice, education, or nursing research. A number of care delivery settings are currently requesting nurses to specify what they wish to incorporate into the information processing system. Others already use computerized storage systems and have incorporated nursing diagnoses or other information of interest to nurses (Cook and Mayers, 1981, pp. 149-161; Hanchett, 1981, pp. 235-242).

Coding for use in an institution may merely require that every diagnosis be given a number. As an example, anticipatory grieving could be 3.018. The first digit might be a nursing code and the next three might refer to the specific diagnosis in a manual. More useful coding would include various levels, such as:

1.000 Nutritional metabolic patterns
1.100 Nutritional deficit
1.110 Total nutritional deficit
1.120 Protein deficit
1.130 Calorie deficit
2.000 Role relationship patterns
2.100 Role conflict
2.110 Marital role conflict
2.120 Parent-child role conflict

For record searches all charts of clients with various nutritional deficits could be retrieved by the call up code 1.100; if 1.120 was used only the protein deficit subset would be retrieved. A diagnosis might be entered as 1.121; the last digit specifying etiology.

These examples are just possibilities selected at random; the coding depends on the system for entering and retrieving data. The major point is that information systems require numerical coding. In turn, coding requires classification at various levels.

Grier (1981) has identified six categories of data that would be included in a nursing information system. Although all of the following categories are importrant, she views identification of nursing diagnoses and their defining characteristics as basic to developing an information system:

1 Selected observations of patient situations (assessment data)
2 Characteristics defining nursing diagnoses
3 Criteria of desired health states
4 Sets of alternative nursing actions
5 Potential outcomes of nursing actions
6 Observations of patient outcomes (Grier, 1981, p. 25)

Werley and Grier (1981) and Spotts (1981, pp. 76–84) argue that nurses must first identify data sets and then work with others to devise means for incorporating data into computerized systems used in health care. Nursing data are important for health care, education, and research. Communicating this fact would dispel notions that nurses' notes are only messages to the physician and can be discarded at client discharge (Huffman, 1972).

Articulation of Classification Systems   A major consideration in developing nomenclature and classification systems is that they articulate with other relevant classification systems. "Classification systems must provide for communication not only with users but also with other systems" (Hangartner, 1975, p. 11). The national conference group has explored the articulation of a nursing classification system with medical systems in current use, but no concentrated effort has been applied to work with the developers of the *International Classification of Disease American Adaptation*, or others.

Why does nursing have to design a totally new classification system instead of using the current ones? Nurses *can* use the current medical systems when they talk about or chart medical problems. Obviously, if nurses do not treat diseases and if the systems are disease oriented and medically labeled, then those systems cannot be used for nursing diagnoses. Newer client record systems, specifically the problem oriented record system, accommodate the health problems described by all care providers. This versatility should also characterize computerized information systems used in health care facilities.

Thinking idealistically, the *health professions* should have a classification system for use in health care delivery. Instead we have a classification oriented to pathology and surgical procedures. Perhaps if nurses label, develop, and standardize the nomenclature of nursing this could be incorporated into an international classification of health problems. One could surmise that each health profession would contribute its nomenclature to the overall system and the system would be capable of retrieving statistical data of interest to each profession.

Issues in Current Systems   Developers of classification systems are aware of the methodological problems encountered in identifying diagnostic categories from assessment data or from retrospective recall (Gordon and Sweeney, 1979). The following are the most common:

1 There is need for a conceptual focus and for categories to guide the collection of assessment data or recall of client conditions from memory, so that, for example, *apples* and *chairs* will not be put into the same class.

2 The level of abstraction to be used in naming must be established in order to avoid classifying *red apples, fruit,* and *food* at the same level.

3 A method of defining labels must be established that prevents unreliability in the use of the name for a client condition. This standardized definition avoids errors of recognition when one encounters an "apple" or an "orange."

4 The type of concept definition has to be determined. Is a diagnostic concept defined by the joint presence of a set of client attributes and their values—a conjunction ($a + b + c = Dx$)? Or is the concept defined by a disjunction of attributes ($a + b + c$ *or* $a + d + e = Dx$)?

5 The diagnostic competencies required of assessors or developers must be explicated. Otherwise cues could be missed and diagnoses formulated incorrectly during clinical identification studies. These errors could lead to a situation analogous to missing the pineapples when fruit is assessed or retrospectively recalled from a memory search.

The national conference group list of nursing diagnoses that have been accepted for clinical testing can be criticized in the above five areas. The group is aware of some inconsistencies and is relying on clinical testing and the theorists' work to bring forth others. It may be important also to consult experts in language development.

Perhaps a review of a recently published classification scheme will illustrate how any proposed system can be examined. The scheme selected is one recommended for use in practice. It reveals the many methodological problems encountered in classification system development.

Simmons (1980) and her colleagues developed a classification scheme for 45 *client and family health problems* addressed by nurses in community health practice. Examination of the list of problems suggests that the total practice of the nurses was studied, not just the aspect organized by nursing diagnoses. Conditions "addressed by nurses" appear to refer to actual or potential health problems in the four categories identified on pages 23–24 in this book:

1. Problems in health management (e.g., sanitation: deficit)

2. Problems secondary to disease, developmental, or situational factors (e.g., role change: impairment)

3. Problems for referral (e.g., circulation: impairment)

4. Possibly problems identified and treated under medical orders (e.g., urinary function: impairment–burning/painful urination)

The classification scheme is the first effort to describe and code for computerization the problem areas nurses address in the community health specialty. Those employing the scheme as a nomenclature system for planning care may have difficulties with the lack of a uniform labeling system. In some instances the "signs and symptoms" reported are problems in themselves and are clustered under too broad a category for planning intervention. Examples are *demonstrates inappropriate suspicion* and *demonstrates inappropriate manipulation*, which appear under the problem label *behavioral pattern: impairment*. Others might wish to delete the term *inappropriate*.

Nurses in the study must have used the "client problem" for purposes other than planning nursing intervention. Most problems classified are too broad to direct therapy and lack any etiological specification. With continued use of the terms, more useful discriminations will probably occur. Publication of this classification system permits others to help in its refinement.

Some of the health problems identified in this clinical study are similar to items on the national conference list or lie in the same problem area. This fact suggests that there is some degree of consensus among nurses. It would have been helpful to the national effort if, in the Simmons study, health problems amenable to nursing therapy had been distinguished from health problems within the domain of medical treatment.

Interestingly, no evidence of problems in family coping or family dynamics were evident in the categories identified in Simmons' classification. Although a focus on the family and community is a stated philosophy of community health nursing, the majority of diagnoses nurses identified pertain to individuals. Perhaps most interventions are directed toward individuals in a family context rather than toward families per se.

The Simmons classification system was designed for incorporation into a computer system. Each domain, diagnosis, and sign or symptom has a numerical code. The second phase of Simmons' project is to identify expected outcomes of nursing care. Difficulties may be encountered. For example, what is the expected outcome of *nutrition: impairment*? Is it weight gain, loss, or other changes? Before one can write outcomes for a health problem, the problem has to be more specifically described.

The five methodological issues identified above are unresolved in this system. This difficulty in no way negates its importance. Having this scheme available in the nursing literature will allow others to take on the task of further refinement.

Simmons' classification; the NCG accepted list; and the Jones (1981, pp. 138-145; 1981, pp. 196-203), Gottlieb (1981), and Minnesota group (1976) lists share diagnoses in common. In the near future it will be advantageous for these groups to consolidate findings in the common areas. To hasten the development of a classification system for the profession, efforts should be coordinated; individual initiative and creativity would not be hampered by this interchange.

SUMMARY

In this final chapter are three issues critical to future development of nursing diagnosis: acceptance of diagnosis, current status of implementation, and problems and prospects of classification. For various reasons not everyone accepts the term *diagnosis*. At this point the reader will have sufficient background in the subject to take a position.

Should nurses use this term to describe the judgments they make? Or must we create a new word? That nurses make clinical judgments of the type described by nursing diagnoses is not the issue.

Implementation of nursing diagnosis and the diagnostic process is not seen in every clinical setting. Yet when outside accreditors cite the organized approach to care resulting from diagnosis, nurses may consider the concept. When nurses become bored with a routine approach to every "gallbladder patient," they may consider using the diagnostic process. Diagnosis-based care planning may become so habitual during educational programs that new graduates will be unable to consider any other way of determining nursing interventions.

Classification of nursing diagnoses has been reviewed. The problems and prospects are evident. The development of nomenclature and a classification system for nursing practice will not be done by an elitist group. Students, clinicians, and clinical specialists will have to be involved. It is hoped that this review will stimulate more nurses to become enthusiastic about contributing to the future direction of nursing diagnosis.

FUTURE DIRECTIONS

Many forces within and external to nursing will influence the future direction of nursing diagnosis. Nurses using diagnosis and those with whom they communicate in practice settings will encourage clearer definition of the concept. Shoemaker's (1981) forthcoming report of a study on the "critical, defining characteristics" of a nursing diagnosis will contribute to clarification. It may be expected that potential problems, requiring preventive nursing intervention, will continue to be defined as nursing diagnoses. As primary care specialists become more involved in identifying these high-risk health patterns, additional nomenclature will be added. Research will follow to identify methods of helping clients decrease health risks. When risk reduction can be demonstrated and related to cost and quality-of-life, the public may be persuaded to finance preventive care.

Financing of nursing care will be a major factor influencing development of a diagnostic classification system. Hidden within the costs of room and board or medical care, nursing is not clearly perceived by the public. What nurses do and why they do it will become obvious when direct reimbursement is a reality. At that point in time it will be important to articulate what actual or potential problems are treated, what outcomes result, and how these health outcomes contribute to goals society values.

In acute-care settings nursing's concern with the quality of life will encourage assessment of functional patterns. Recognition of actual or potentially dysfunctional patterns will stimulate experimental studies of nursing intervention. Intervention-outcome links will be established which enhance decision making in care planning.

If current predictions are correct, the aged will comprise a high percentage of clients in acute-care settings. Ways will have to be found to sustain their optimal function. Otherwise, the dire predictions for the year 2000 made by some analysts of health care—financial collapse of the health care system and euthanasia—may come true. Nurses focus on optimal patterns of functioning; this focus is especially useful in health care of the elderly. If nursing's domain of practice is established as the detection of potential problems and restoration of integrated function after dysfunctional patterns occur, nurses may need to assume coordinating responsibilities in hospitals and long-term care settings. Beliefs and values traditionally held by nurses may influence society to recognize the aged for their wisdom, rather than their disabilities.

The validity of long-range prediction rests on attainment of short-term goals. One immediate goal is to assess the diagnostic reliability of currently identified signs and symptoms for each diagnostic category. If diagnostic category labels generally represent client problems encountered by nurses, reliability studies are worthwhile.

What would reliability studies accomplish? If a sign or symptom can be demonstrated to occur in 95 out of 100 clients, it is a reliable predictor of a condition. Nurses caring for clients need clusters of highly reliable cues to diagnose actual or potential problems. Without these predictors, diagnostic errors occur. Diagnostic errors lead to inadequate care plans and interventions. In turn, inadequate interventions rarely permit health outcomes to be attained and can result in harm and suffering. Clinical studies of diagnostic categories will provide nurses with clusters of critical, defining signs and symptoms (criteria for a diagnosis). Steps in this direction have been taken by Guzzetta and Forsyth (1979), Martin (1979), Nicoletti, Reitz, and Gordon (1981), and Burgess (1974).

Establishing the level of reliability of current lists of defining characteristics (Kim and Moritz, 1981), would greatly facilitate education. Students could learn the few critical cues that reliably predict the presence of a diagnosis. Other cues currently listed may be useful to support a judgment but not critical. Noncritical cues can be learned later, as clinical experience in diagnosing a condition accumulates.

Future graduates of professional nursing programs will demonstrate competence in using diagnostic categories to organize client data and plan care. This will occur only if both diagnostic process and diagnostic categories are learned in educational programs.

Clinical studies of the diagnostic process used by health care providers will increase. The search for knowledge to increase diagnostic efficiency and validity of diagnosis will be influenced by a continued emphasis on cost and quality control. Expanding knowledge of the diagnostic process will facilitate teaching of the process in nursing. Studies similar to those done by Tanner (1981, pp. 145-152), Grier (1981), Kim (1981, pp. 158-167), Gordon (1980), and Aspinall (1976) will test the application of knowledge about cognitive processes to specific diagnostic situations in nursing. As faculty appreciate the need for training in uncertainty-based judgment, methods of controlling uncertainties will become part of the educational preparation of nursing practitioners (Light, 1979).

Perhaps the future will reveal a unified perspective on what information is included in a nursing data base. A unified perspective on assessment would mean concensus had been reached regarding nursing's conceptual view of the client. (It may be expected that multiple models of intervention and nursing goals will continue to be used.) Classification would be greatly influenced if a unified perspective was reached because diagnostic categories would have to be logically consistent with the agreed upon conceptual model. Some are concerned that professional nurses will divorce themselves from ill clients leaving this area of nursing to the technically prepared. This is unlikely. It is especially unlikely if studies demonstrate complex *nursing* diagnoses occur in intensive and acute care, as well as in primary care, settings.

A few of the issues that will influence the future direction of nursing diagnosis have been briefly reviewed. To those who have the sensitivity to see beyond the mere obvious, the curiosity to wonder why, and the intellect to reason how, is left the future of nursing and nursing diagnosis.

BIBLIOGRAPHY

Abdellah, F. G. Improving the teaching of nursing through research in patient care. In L. E. Heidgerken (Ed.), *Improvement of nursing through research*. Washington, D.C.: Catholic University of America, 1959.

American Nurses' Association, Congress on Nursing Practice. *A social policy statement*. Kansas City, Mo.: American Nurses' Association, 1980.

American Psychiatric Association. *Diagnostic and statistical manual of mental disorders*. Washington, D.C.: American Psychiatric Association, 1980.

Aspinall, M. J. Nursing diagnosis: The weak link. *Nursing Outlook,* July 1976, *24,* 433–437.

Bell system yellow pages, Boston area. New England Telephone and Telegraph Co., Boston, 1980.

Bircher, A. B. On the development and classification of diagnoses. *Nursing Forum*, 1975, *14*, 20–29.

Brown, M. M. The epidemiological approach to the study of clinical nursing diagnoses. *Nursing Forum*, 1974, *13*, 346–359.

Bruce, J. A. Implementation of nursing diagnosis: A nursing administrator's perspective. *Nursing Clinics of North America*, September 1979, *14*, 509–516.

Burgess, A. W. Rape trauma syndrome, *American Journal of Psychiatry,* September 1974, *131,* 981–986.

Commission on Professional and Hospital Activities. *International Classification of Diseases: Clinical Modification*, ICD-9-CM. Volume 1–3, 9th revision. Ann Arbor: Commission on Professional and Hospital Activities, 1978.

Cook, M., & Mayers, M. Computer-assisted data base for nursing research. In H. H. Werley & M. R. Grier (Eds.), *Nursing information systems*. New York: Springer, 1981.

Dalton, J. M. Nursing diagnosis in a community health setting. *Nursing Clinics of North America*, September 1979, *14*, 525–532.

Durand, M., & Prince, P. Nursing diagnosis: Process and decision. *Nursing Forum*, 1966, *5*, 50–64.

Elstein, A. S., Schulman, L. S., & Sprafka, S. A. *Medical problem solving: An analysis of clinical reasoning*. Cambridge, Mass.: Harvard University Press, 1978.

Feild, L. The implementation of nursing diagnosis in clinical practice. *Nursing Clinics of North America*, September 1979, *14*, 497–508.

Firlit, S. L., Glass, L. K., & Nolan, J. W. A response to classification of nursing diagnoses. Unpublished paper. University of Illinois, College of Nursing, Department of Public Health Nursing, 1980.

Fortin, J., & Rabinow, J. Legal implications of nursing diagnosis. *Nursing Clinics of North America*, September 1979, *14*, 553–562.

Fredette, S. & O'Connor, K. Nursing diagnosis in teaching and curriculum planning. *Nursing Clinics of North America*, September 1979, *14*, 541–552.

Fry, V. The creative approach to nursing. *American Journal of Nursing*, March 1953, *53*, 301–302.

Gamer, M. Ideology of professionalism. *Nursing Outlook*, February 1979, *27*, 108–111.

Gast, H. L. Review of some recent studies of nursing diagnosis. In *Monograph on nursing diagnosis, fall 1979*. Denton, Tex.: College of Nursing, Texas Woman's University, 1979.

Gebbie, K., & Lavin, M. A. Classifying nursing diagnoses. *American Journal of Nursing*, February 1974, *74*, 250–253.

Giovanetti, P. *Patient classification systems in nursing: A description and analysis.* (Publication No. HRA 78-22). Washington, D.C.: U.S. Department of Health, Education and Welfare, 1978.

Gordon, M. *Manual of nursing diagnoses.* New York: McGraw-Hill, 1982.

Gordon, M. Nursing diagnosis: The state of the art. In N. Chaska (Ed.), *The nursing profession: A time to speak.* New York: McGraw-Hill, 1982.

Gordon, M. Predictive strategies in diagnostic tasks. *Nursing Research*, January-February 1980, *29*, 39–45.

Gordon, M., & Sweeney, M. A. Methodological problems and issues in identifying and standardizing nursing diagnoses. *Advances in Nursing Science*, October 1979, *2*, 1–15.

Gottlieb, L. N. Small steps toward the development of a health classification system for nursing. In M. J. Kim & D. A. Moritz (Eds.), *Classification of nursing diagnoses: Proceedings of the third and fourth national conferences.* New York: McGraw-Hill, 1981, pp. 203–213.

Grier, M. R. The need for data in making nursing decisions. In H. H. Werley & M. R. Grier (Eds.), *Nursing information systems.* New York: Springer, 1981.

Guzzetta, C. E., & Forsythe, G. L. Nursing diagnosis pilot study: Psychophysiological stress. *Advances in Nursing Science*, October 1979, *2*, 27–44.

Hangartner, C. Principles of classification. In K. M. Gebbie & M. A. Lavin (Eds.), *Classification of nursing diagnoses: Proceedings of the first national conference on classification of nursing diagnoses.* St. Louis: Mosby, 1975.

Huffman, E. K. *Medical record management* (6th Edition). Berwyn, Ill.: Physician's Record Co., 1972.

Hanchett, E. S. Appropriateness of nursing care. In H. H. Werley & M. R. Grier (Eds.), *Nursing information systems.* New York: Springer, 1981.

Jones, P. E. Developing terminology: A University of Toronto experience. In M. J. Kim & D. A. Moritz (Eds.), *Classification of nursing diagnoses: Proceedings of the third and fourth national conferences.* New York, McGraw-Hill, 1981, pp. 138–145.

Jones, P. E. The revision of diagnostic terms. In M. J. Kim & D. A. Moritz (Eds.), *Classification of nursing diagnoses: Proceedings of the third and fourth national conferences.* New York, McGraw-Hill, 1981, pp. 196–203.

Jones, P. E. A terminology for nursing diagnoses. *Advances in Nursing Science*, October 1979, *2*, 65–72.

Kim, M. J., & Moritz, D. A. (Eds.) *Classification of nursing diagnoses: Proceedings of the third and fourth national conferences.* New York: McGraw-Hill, 1981.

Kim, M. J., Suhayda, R., Waters, L., Yocum, C. Effect of using nursing diagnosis in nursing care planning. In M. J. Kim & D. A. Moritz. *Classification of nursing diagnoses: Proceedings of the third and fourth national conferences.* New York: McGraw-Hill, 1981, pp. 158–167.

King, L. S. What is a diagnosis? *Journal of the American Medical Association*, November 20, 1967, *202*, 154–167.

Komorita, N. Nursing diagnosis. *American Journal of Nursing*, December 1963, *63*, 83–86.

Levine, M. E. Trophicognosis: An alternative to nursing diagnosis. *Exploring progress in medical-surgical nursing practice* (Vol. 2). American Nurses' Association, 1965. Kansas City, Mo.: American Nurses' Association, 1966.

Light, D. Uncertainty and control in professional training. *Journal of Health and Social Behavior,* 1979, *20,* 310–322.

Martin, K. S. Variables in the nursing diagnosis of impaired parenting relative to the preschool child: A pilot exploration. In *Monograph series 79: Clinical nursing research: Proceedings of the sixth annual research conference.* Indianapolis: Sigma Theta Tau, 1979, pp. 208–220.

Maslow, A. *Motivation and personality.* New York: Harper & Row, 1954 (rev. ed., 1970).

McKay, R. P. What is the relationship between the development and utilization of a taxonomy and nursing theory? *Nursing Research,* May–June 1977, *26,* 222–224.

McKeehan, J. M. Nursing diagnosis in a discharge planning program. *Nursing Clinics of North America,* September 1979, *14,* 517–524.

McLean, A. Nursing diagnosis in baccalaureate and graduate education. In M. J. Kim & D. A. Moritz (Eds.), *Classification of nursing diagnoses: Proceedings of the third and fourth national conferences, April 9–13, 1980.* New York: McGraw-Hill, 1981.

Minnesota Systems Research, Inc. *Nursing problem classification for children and youth.* Rockville, Md.: U.S. Public Health Service, 1976.

Nicoletti, A. M., Reitz, S. E., & Gordon, M. Descriptive study of the parenting diagnosis. In M. J. Kim & D. A. Moritz (Eds.), *Classification of nursing diagnoses: Proceedings of the third and fourth national conferences.* New York: McGraw-Hill, 1981, pp. 176–183.

Rosch, E. Principles of categorization. In E. Rosch & B. B. Lloyd (Eds.), *Cognition and categorization.* Hillsdale, N.J.: Lawrence Erlbaum Associates, 1976.

Shoemaker, J. Personal communication. 1981.

Simmons, D. A. *A classification scheme for client problems in community health nursing.* (Publication No. HRA 80-16). Hyattsville, Md.: U.S. Department of Health and Human Services, June 1980.

Spotts, S. J. Nursing information systems. In M. J. Kim & D. A. Moritz (Eds.), *Classification of nursing diagnoses: Proceedings of the third and fourth national conferences.* New York: McGraw-Hill, 1981.

Tanner, C. A. Instruction on the diagnostic process: An experimental study. In M. J. Kim & D. A. Moritz (Eds.), *Classification of nursing diagnoses: Proceedings of the third and fourth national conferences.* New York: McGraw-Hill, 1981, pp. 145–152.

Taylor, F. K. A logical analysis of the medico-psychologic concept of disease (Part I). *Psychological Medicine,* 1971, *1,* 356–364.

Warner, R. Relationship between language and disease concepts. *International Journal of Psychiatry in Medicine,* 1976, *7,* 57–68.

Weber, S. Nursing diagnosis in private practice. *Nursing Clinics of North America,* September 1979, *14,* 533–540.

Werley, H. H., and Grier, M. R. Research directions. In H. H. Werley & M. R. Grier. (Eds.) *Nursing Information Systems.* New York: Springer, 1981.

Whitney, F. W. How to work with a crock. *American Journal of Nursing,* 1981, *81,* 86–91.

World Health Organization. *International classification of diseases.* Geneva: World Health Organization, 1977.

LIST OF DIAGNOSES ACCEPTED[1] AT THE FOURTH NATIONAL CONFERENCE, 1980

Airway clearance, ineffective
Bowel elimination, alterations in: constipation
Bowel elimination, alterations in: diarrhea
Bowel elimination, alterations in: incontinence
Breathing Pattern, ineffective
Cardiac output, alterations in: decreased
Comfort, alterations in: pain
Communication, impaired verbal
Coping, ineffective individual
Coping, ineffective family: compromised
Coping, ineffective family: disabling
Coping, family: potential for growth
Diversional activity, deficit
Fear (specify)
Fluid volume deficit, actual
Fluid volume deficit, potential
Gas exchange, impaired
Grieving, anticipatory
Grieving, dysfunctional
Home maintenance management, impaired
Injury, potential for (poisoning, potential for; suffocation, potential for; trauma, potential for)
Knowledge deficit (specify)
Mobility, impaired physical

[1] Accepted by the National Conference Group for Classification of Nursing Diagnoses and published in M. J. Kim and D. A. Moritz, *Proceedings of the Fourth National Conference on Classification of Nursing Diagnoses,* New York, McGraw-Hill, 1981.

Noncompliance (specify)

Nutrition, alterations in: less than body requirements

Nutrition, alterations in: more than body requirements

Nutrition, alterations in: potential for more than body requirements

Parenting. alterations in: actual

Parenting, alterations in: potential

Rape-trauma syndrome (compound reaction, silent reaction)

Self-care deficit (specify level): feeding, bathing/hygiene, toileting, dressing/grooming

Self-concept, disturbance in (body image disturbance, self-esteem disturbance, role performance disturbance, disturbance in personal identity)

Sensory perceptual alterations (specify visual, auditory, kinesthetic, gustatory, tactile, or olfactory perception)

Sexual dysfunction

Skin integrity, impairment of: actual

Skin integrity, impairment of: potential

Sleep pattern disturbance

Spiritual distress (distress of the human spirit)

Thought processes, alterations in

Tissue perfusion, alteration in (specify cerebral, cardiopulmonary, renal, gastrointestinal, peripheral)

Urinary elimination, alteration in patterns

Violence, potential for

GROUPING OF CURRENTLY ACCEPTED DIAGNOSES UNDER FUNCTIONAL HEALTH PATTERN AREAS

1 Health-perception–health-management pattern
   Noncompliance (specify)
   Injury, potential for
   Poisoning, potential for
   Suffocation, potential for
   Trauma, potential for
2 Nutritional-metabolic pattern
   Skin integrity, impairment of: actual
   Skin integrity, impairment of: potential
   Nutrition, alterations in: less than body requirements
   Nutrition, alterations in: more than body requirements
   Nutrition, alterations in: potential for more than body requirements
   Fluid volume deficit: actual
   Fluid volume deficit: potential
3 Elimination pattern
   Urinary elimination, alterations in patterns of
   Bowel elimination, alterations in: constipation
   Bowel elimination, alterations in: diarrhea
   Bowel elimination, alterations in: incontinence
4 Activity-exercise pattern
   Home maintenance management, impaired
   Mobility, impaired physical
   Self-care deficit (specify level): total
   Self-care deficit (specify level): feeding
   Self-care deficit (specify level): bathing/hygiene
   Self-care deficit (specify level): dressing/grooming
   Self-care deficit (specify level): toileting

Airway clearance, ineffective
Gas exchange, impaired
Breathing pattern, ineffective
Diversional activity, deficit
Tissue perfusion, alteration in (cerebral, cardiopulmonary, renal, gastrointestinal, peripheral)
Cardiac output, alterations in: decreased

5 Sleep-rest pattern
Sleep pattern disturbance

6 Cognitive-perceptual pattern
Knowledge deficit (specify)
Sensory perceptual alterations (visual, auditory, kinesthetic, gustatory, tactile, olfactory)
Comfort, alterations in: pain
Thought processes: alterations in

7 Self-perception–self-concept pattern
Fear (specify)
Self-concept, disturbance in (body image, self-esteem, role performance, personal identity)

8 Role-relationship pattern
Grieving, anticipatory
Grieving, dysfunctional
Parenting, alterations in: actual
Parenting, alterations in: potential
Communication, impaired verbal
Violence, potential for

9 Sexuality-reproductive pattern
Sexual dysfunction
Rape-trauma syndrome
Rape-trauma: compound reaction
Rape-trauma: silent reaction

10 Coping–stress-tolerance pattern
Coping, ineffective individual
Coping, ineffective family: compromised
Coping, ineffective family: disabling
Coping, family: potential for growth

11 Value-belief pattern
Spiritual distress (Distress of the human spirit)

ASSESSMENT OF FUNCTIONAL HEALTH PATTERNS

Functional health patterns provide both a format for the admission assessment and a data base for nursing diagnosis. There are two phases in assessment: history taking and examination. The format given here for assessment is a screening format. Further questions and observations are necessary if data or the client's situation suggest that problems (dysfunctional patterns) are present. A sample data recording sheet is also presented here.

NURSING HISTORY

A nursing history provides a description of a client's functional health patterns. The description is from the client's (or parent's or guardian's) perspective and provides data in the form of verbal reports. Information is elicited by questions. The nursing history format that follows is designed to collect information in a systematic manner and to facilitate nursing diagnosis. In the manual that accompanies this book[1], diagnoses are grouped under the pattern areas and can be used to label health problems in a pattern area.

1 Health-perception–health-management pattern
   a How has general health been?
   b Any colds in past year?
   c Most important things done to keep healthy? Think these things make a difference to health? (Include family folk remedies, if appropriate.) Use of cigarettes, alcohol, other drugs? Breast self-exam?
   d In the past, has it been easy to find ways to do things doctors or nurses suggest?
   e If appropriate: Concerns about illness? Hospitalization?

---

[1] Gordon, M. *Manual of Nursing Diagnoses*. New York: McGraw-Hill, 1982.

    f If appropriate: What do you think caused this illness? Actions taken when symptoms perceived? Results of action?

    g If appropriate: Things important to you while you're here? How can we be most helpful?

2 Nutritional-metabolic pattern

    a Typical daily food intake (describe)? Supplements?

    b Typical daily fluid intake (describe)?

    c Weight loss or gain (amount)?

    d Appetite?

    e Food or eating: discomfort? diet restrictions?

    f Heal well or poorly?

    g Skin problems: lesions, dryness?

    h Dental problems?

3 Elimination pattern

    a Bowel elimination pattern (describe). Frequency? Character? Discomfort?

    b Urinary elimination pattern (describe). Frequency? Problems with control?

    c Excess perspiration? Odor problem?

4 Activity-exercise pattern

    a Sufficient energy for desired and required activities?

    b Exercise pattern? Type? Regularity?

    c Spare time (leisure) activities? Child: play activities?

    d Perceived ability for: (code for level—see Functional Levels Code below)

        Feeding_____ Dressing_____ Home maintenance_____ Bathing_____
        Grooming_____ Shopping_____ Toileting_____ General mobility_____
        Bed mobility_____ Cooking_____

    Functional Levels Code

      Level O: Full self-care

      Level I: Requires use of equipment or device

      Level II: Requires assistance or supervision from another person

      Level III: Requires assistance or supervision from another person and equipment or device

      Level IV: Is dependent and does not participate

5 Sleep-rest pattern

    a Generally rested and ready for daily activities after sleep?

    b Sleep onset problems? Aids? Dreams (nightmares)? Early awakening?

6 Cognitive-perceptual pattern

    a Hearing difficulty? Aid?

    b Vision? Wear glasses? Last checked?

    c Any change in memory lately?

    d Easiest way for you to learn things? Any difficulty learning?

    e Any discomfort? Pain? How do you manage it?

7 Self-perception–self-concept pattern

    a How would you describe yourself? Most of the time, do you feel good or not so good about yourself?

    b Changes in your body or the things you can do? Problem to you?

    c Changes in way you feel about yourself or your body (since illness started)?

    d Do things frequently make you angry? Annoyed? Fearful? Anxious? Depressed? What helps?

8 Role-relationship pattern
   a Live alone? Family? Family structure (diagram)?
   b Any family problems you have difficulty handling?
   c How does family usually handle problems?
   d Does family depend on you for things? How are they managing?
   e If appropriate: How do family and others feel about your illness and hospitalization?
   f If appropriate: Problems with children? Difficulty handling these problems?
   g Belong to social groups? Close friends? Feel lonely (frequency)?
   h Do things generally go well for you at work (school)? If appropriate: Income sufficient for your needs?
   i Feel part of (or isolated in) the neighborhood where you live?
9 Sexuality-reproductive pattern
   a If appropriate: Any changes or problems in sexual relations?
   b If appropriate: Use of contraceptives? Problems?
   c Female: Age when menstruation started? Last menstrual period? Menstrual problems? Para? Gravida?
10 Coping–stress-tolerance pattern
   a Tense a lot of the time? What helps? Use any medicines, drugs, alcohol?
   b Who's most helpful in talking things over? Available to you now?
   c Any big changes in your life in the last year or two?
   d When (if) you have big problems (or any problems) in your life, how do you handle them? Most of the time, is this way successful?
11 Value-belief pattern
   a Do you generally get things you want out of life?
   b Is religion important in your life? If appropriate: Does this help when difficulties arise?
   c If appropriate: Will being here interfere with any religious practices?
12 Other
   a Any other things that we haven't talked about that you'd like to mention?
   b Questions?

CLIENT EXAMINATION

Some functional patterns have indicators that can be observed during the examination phase of the admission assessment. Data about these indicators support or negate health problems suggested by the history. It is also possible that observations will reveal unreported problems or potential problems. The functional pattern indicators listed below provide data for nursing diagnoses. Further examination is necessary if data or the client's situation suggest that problems are present. (If presence of disease is to be assessed, the traditional areas of physical assessment should be added.)

In Section A, below, a sequence for conducting the examination and summarizing the observations is presented. This sequence illustrates how data can be *collected*. For example, temperature (T) is the last measurement taken. While body temperature is measured, the remaining indicators can be summarized from observations made during the history and examination.

In Section B the pattern indicators are grouped. Section B shows the relevance of data to pattern description and demonstrates how examination data are *used* in identifying dysfunctional patterns and diagnoses.

Section A. Screening Examination Format

General appearance, grooming, hygiene_____

Oral mucous membranes (color, moistness, lesions)_____

Teeth: dentures_____ Cavities_____ Missing_____

Hears whisper?_____

Reads newsprint?_____ Glasses?_____

Pulse (rate)_____ (rhythm)_____

Respirations_____ (depth)_____ (rhythm)_____ Breath sounds_____

Blood pressure_____

Hand grip_____ Can pick up pencil?_____

Range of motion (joints)_____ Muscle firmness_____

Skin: bony prominences_____ Lesions_____ Color changes_____

Gait_____ Posture_____ Absent body part_____

Intravenous, drainage, suction, etc. (specify)_____

Actual weight_____ Reported weight_____

Height_____

Temperature_____

During history and examination:

Orientation_____ Grasp ideas and questions (abstract, concrete)?_____

Language spoken_____ Voice and speech pattern_____Vocabulary_____

Eye contact_____ Attention span (distraction)_____

1└──────┘5
Nervous or relaxed (rate from 1 to 5)_____

1└──────┘5
Assertive or passive (rate from 1 to 5)_____

Interaction with family member, guardian, other (if present)

_____

Section B. Grouping of Indicators, Demonstrating Relevance of Data to Pattern Description

Nutritional-Metabolic Pattern

Weight	Skin (bony prominences, lesions)
Height	Oral mucous membranes
Temperature	(color, moistness, lesions)
(intravenous, drainage, suction)	Teeth (dentures, cavities, missing)

Activity-Exercise Pattern

Gait	Prostheses
Posture	Assistive equipment
Absent body part	Pulse rate, rhythm
Hand grip	Respiratory rate, depth, rhythm
Coordination	Breath sounds
Range of motion (joints)	Blood pressure
Muscle firmness	

Cognitive-Perceptual Pattern

Grasp of Ideas, questions	Vocabulary
Language spoken	Attention span
Hearing	Vision
Orientation	

Self-Perception–Self-Concept Pattern

Body posture	Eye contact
Attention span	Nervous or relaxed
Voice and speech pattern	

Role-Relationship Pattern

Interactions with family member, guardian, other (if present)   Assertive or passive

DATA RECORDING SHEET

The admission assessment data recording sheet is placed in the client's chart. It becomes part of the permanent health care record. The following format with sufficient space for recording can be imprinted on a permanent record sheet.

Nursing History:

General description of client (age, general appearance, chief concerns, etc.) ⎯⎯⎯⎯

Health-perception–health-management pattern ⎯⎯⎯⎯⎯⎯⎯⎯⎯⎯

Nutritional-metabolic pattern ⎯⎯⎯⎯ ⎯⎯⎯⎯⎯⎯⎯⎯⎯⎯

Elimination pattern ⎯⎯⎯⎯⎯⎯⎯⎯⎯⎯⎯⎯⎯⎯

Activity-exercise pattern ⎯⎯⎯⎯⎯⎯⎯⎯⎯⎯⎯⎯

Sleep-rest pattern ⎯⎯⎯⎯⎯⎯⎯⎯⎯⎯⎯⎯⎯⎯

Cognitive-perceptual pattern ⎯⎯⎯⎯⎯⎯⎯⎯⎯⎯⎯

Self-perception–self-concept pattern ⎯⎯⎯⎯⎯⎯⎯⎯⎯

Role-relationship pattern ⎯⎯⎯⎯⎯⎯⎯⎯⎯⎯⎯⎯

Sexuality-reproductive pattern ⎯⎯⎯⎯⎯⎯⎯⎯⎯⎯

Coping–stress tolerance pattern ⎯⎯⎯⎯⎯⎯⎯⎯⎯⎯

Value-belief pattern ⎯⎯⎯⎯⎯⎯⎯⎯⎯⎯⎯⎯⎯

Examination: (See Section A, p. 332)

GUIDELINES FOR REVIEWING AND PREPARING DIAGNOSTIC CATEGORIES TO BE PRESENTED FOR CONSIDERATION BY THE NATIONAL CONFERENCE GROUP[1]

In making a nursing diagnosis, a nurse places a client in a diagnostic category for purposes of determining therapy. Diagnostic categories can have different levels of abstraction. Diagnoses that are clinically useful are sufficiently specific to provide the basis for the plan of therapy.

A diagnostic category has three parts: (1) the term describing the problem or the category label, (2) the probable cause of the problem (the etiological subcategory), and (3) the defining characteristics. The following are characteristics of each part of a diagnostic category. Please use these as criteria for preparing diagnoses for the conference group.

A The category label
  1 The label is a term that describes a health problem of client (individual, family, or community).
  2 The label refers to an identifiable clinical entity (health problem) that nurses can identify and treat.
  3 The label is clear and concise (two or three words).
  4 The label is sufficiently specific to be clinically useful.
B Common etiological factors: the etiological subcategory (if probable cause can be identified)
  1 An etiological subcategory is a term describing one probable cause of the health problem.
  2 The etiological subcategory, when combined with the category label, suggests a treatment plan.
  3 The term describing the etiological subcategory is clear and concise (two or three words).

---

[1] Guidelines were prepared by Marjory Gordon.

    4 The term describing the etiological subcategory is sufficiently specific to be clinically useful.

C The defining characteristics of the diagnostic category

    1 The defining characteristics are *observable* signs and symptoms that are present when the health problem is present.

    2 The critical defining characteristics are included. (Please star those signs and symptoms that *must* be present for the category to be used clinically. These are the signs and symptoms that permit discriminations or differentiations between categories. Other signs and symptoms that *may* be present, and contribute to identifying the problem may be included but are not starred.)

    3 The characteristics that are related to development (age) are indicated.

D Supporting materials

    1 Literature to support category label (if available).

    2 Literature to support etiological categories (if available).

    3 Literature or clinical data to support defining characteristics (if available).

E Degree of nursing independence in treating the health problem

    1 Diagnoses vary in the degree of independent nursing therapy involved in preventing or treating the health problems they describe. For example, nurses are considerably more independent in treating skin breakdown or anxiety than altered states of consciousness or altered body fluid composition.

    a Rate the diagnostic category as to degree of independent nursing therapy *commonly* involved in preventing or treating the health problem: *high, medium*, or *low*.

Submit diagnoses to Marjory Gordon, R.N., Ph.D., F.A.A.N.; Chairperson, Task Force of the National Group for Classification of Nursing Diagnoses; Boston College School of Nursing; Chestnut Hill, MA 02167.

MEMBERS OF THEORIST GROUP

Andrea Bircher, R.N., Ph.D.
University of Oklahoma
College of Nursing

Rosemary Ellis, R.N., Ph.D.
Case Western Reserve University
School of Nursing

Joyce Fitzpatrick, R.N., Ph.D.
Wayne State University
School of Nursing

Marjory Gordon, R.N., Ph.D.
Boston College
Graduate Medical-Surgical Nursing

Margaret Hardy, R.N., Ph.D.
Boston University
School of Nursing

Imogene King, R.N., Ph.D.
University of South Florida

Rose McKay, R.N., Ph.D.
University of Colorado
School of Nursing

Margaret A. Newman, R.N., Ph.D.
The Pennsylvania State University
College of Human Development

Dorothea Orem, R.N., Ph.D.
Consultant

Rose Marie Parse, R.N., Ph.D.
Duquesne University
School of Nursing

Martha Rogers, R.N., Sc.D.
New York University
Department of Nursing

Sr. Callista Roy, R.N., Ph.D.
Mount St. Mary's College
Department of Nursing

M. J. Smith, R.N., Ph.D.
Duquesne University
School of Nursing

Gertrude Torres, R.N., Ed.D.
Consultant

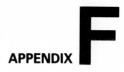

NOMENCLATURE DEVELOPMENT, 1973–1980

The following chart depicts diagnostic nomenclature development from 1973–1980. Reading horizontally provides information on how diagnoses (1) were added (blank spaces in previous years), (2) changed, or (3) deleted (blank spaces subsequent years). Vertical reading of the columns for each year provides the list of accepted diagnoses in 1973 (first national conference), 1975 (second national conference), 1978 (third national conference), and 1980 (fourth national conference).

1973	1975	1978	1980
Anxiety, mild	Anxiety, mild	Anxiety, mild	
Anxiety, moderate	Anxiety, moderate	Anxiety, moderate	
Anxiety, severe	Anxiety, severe	Anxiety, severe	
Panic	Panic	Panic	
Body fluids, depletion of	Body fluids, depletion of		
		Fluid volume deficit	Fluid volume deficit
		Fluid volume deficit, potential	Fluid volume deficit, potential
	Body fluids, excess	Body fluids, excess	
Bowel function, irregular: constipation	Bowel elimination, alteration in: constipation	Bowel elimination, alteration in: constipation	Bowel elimination, alteration in: constipation
Bowel function, irregular: diarrhea	Bowel elimination, alteration in: diarrhea	Bowel elimination, alteration in: diarrhea	Bowel elimination, alteration in: diarrhea

1973	1975	1978	1980
	Bowel elimination, alteration in: impaction	Bowel elimination, alteration in: impaction	
	Bowel elimination, alteration in: incontinence	Bowel elimination, alteration in: incontinence	Bowel elimination, alteration in: incontinence
	Cardiac output, alteration in: decreased	Cardiac output, alteration in: decreased	Cardiac output, alteration in: decreased
	Circulation, interruption of	Circulation, interruption of	
		Tissue perfusion, chronic abnormal	Tissue perfusion, alteration in subcategories (see Appendix A)
Cognitive functioning alteration in level of			
Distractibility			
Hypovigilance			
Hypervigilance			
		Consciousness, altered levels of	
Cognitive dissonance			
Inappropriate and unrealistic based thinking			
Decreased capacity for abstract conceptualization			
Inaccurate interpretation of environment			
Increased egocentricity			
Thought processes impaired	Thought processes impaired	Thought processes impaired	Thought processes, alterations in
Impaired perception			
Impaired retention			

1973	1975	1978	1980
Impaired reflection			
Impaired decision making			
Impaired judgment			
Confusion	Confusion		
Comfort level, alterations in	Alterations in comfort: discomfort	Comfort, alterations in: pain	Comfort, alterations in: pain
Physiological comfort level, alterations in			
Psychological comfort level, alterations in			
Environmental comfort level, alterations in			
Spiritual comfort level, alterations in			
Verbal communication, impairment of		Communication, impaired verbal	Communication, impaired verbal
Nonverbal communication, impairment of			
		Coping patterns, maladaptive (individual)	Coping, ineffective (individual)
		Coping patterns, ineffective family	Coping, ineffective family: disabling
			Coping, ineffective family: compromised
			Coping, family: potential for growth
Adjustment to illness, impairment of significant others	Adjustment to illness, impairment of significant others	Adjustment to illness, impairment of significant others	
Adjustment to illness, impairment of all significant others			

1973	1975	1978	1980
Adjustment to illness, impairment of spouse's			
Adjustment to illness, impairment of child's			
Adjustment to illness, impairment of non-family's			
Digestion, impairment of (impaired digestion)			
			Diversional activity deficit
Faith, alterations in			
Faith in self, alterations in			
Faith in others, alterations in			
		Spirituality: spiritual concern	
		Spirituality: spiritual distress	Spiritual distress (distress of the human spirit)
		Spirituality: spiritual despair	
Fear			Fear (specify)
Functional fear, mild			
Functional fear, moderate			
Functional fear, severe			
Functional fear, panic			
Nonfunctional fear, mild			
Nonfunctional fear, moderate			

1973	1975	1978	1980
Nonfunctional fear, severe			
Nonfunctional fear, panic			
		Functional performance, variations in *or* Self-care activities, alterations in ability to perform	
		Home maintenance management, impaired	Home maintenance management, impaired
Self-care activities, altered ability to perform	Self-care activities alteration in ability to perform		
Self-care in all spheres, altered ability to perform		Total self-care deficit	Self-care deficit (specify level)
Impairment in performance of established hygiene activities	Self-care activities, alteration in ability to perform: hygiene		Self-bathing/hygiene deficit (specify level)
			Self-dressing/grooming deficit (specify level)
		Self-feeding deficit	Self-feeding deficit (specify level)
		Self-toileting deficit	Self-toileting deficit (specify level)
Grieving	Acute grieving	Grieving	
Normal grieving			
Normal grieving, potential			
	Grieving, anticipatory		Grieving, anticipatory
Arrested grieving	Delayed grieving		Grieving, dysfunctional

1973	1975	1978	1980
Arrested grieving, potential			
Delayed onset of grieving			
Delayed onset of grieving, potential			
Injury, potential for		Injury, potential for	Injury, potential for (see subcategories Appendix A)
		Accidental falling, potential for	
		Knowledge, lack of (specify area)	Knowledge deficit (specify)
Understanding of state of health, lack of			
Understanding of etiology of state of health, lack of			
Understanding of preventive health measures, lack of			
Understanding of therapy, lack of			
Manipulation, verbal	Manipulation		
Manipulation, non-verbal			
Mobility, impaired	Mobility, impairment of	Mobility, impairment of	
Mobility, impaired physical			Mobility, impaired physical
Mobility, impaired social			
Mobility, impaired emotional			
Mobility, impaired intellectual			

1973	1975	1978	1980
Mobility, impaired developmental			
Motor incoordination Motor incoordination, gross Motor incoordination, fine			
Noncompliance	Noncompliance	Noncompliance	Noncompliance (specify)
Noncompliance with diet Noncompliance with drug therapy Noncompliance with environmental therapy Noncompliance with activity regimen			
Nutrition, alterations in: undernutrition Nutrition, alterations in: obesity	Nutritional alteration: less than required (MDR) Nutrional alteration: more than required Nutritional alteration: potential	Nutritional alteration: less than body requirements Nutritional alteration: more than body requirements Nutritional alteration: related to changes in body requirements	Nutrition, alteration in: less than body requirements Nutrition, alteration in: more than body requirements Nutrition, alteration in: potential for more than body requirements
		Parenting, alterations in: actual Parenting, alterations in: potential	Parenting, alterations in: actual Parenting, alterations in: potential

1973	1975	1978	1980
Respiration, impairment of	Respiratory dysfunction	Respiratory dysfunction	Airway clearance, ineffective
			Breathing pattern, ineffective
Respiratory distress			Gas exchange, impaired
Family process, inadequate			
Group relations, noneffective			
Social isolation			
Self-esteem or self-actualization, impairment of			
Self-concept, altered		Self-concept, alterations in: (self esteem, role performance	Self-concept, disturbance in (see subcategories Appendix A)
Altered body image	Self-concept: alterations in body image	personal identity, body image)	
Depersonalization			
Identity conflict			
Role disturbance			
			Rape trauma syndrome
			Rape trauma, compound reaction
			Rape trauma, silent reaction
Sensory disturbance			
Sensory deprivation			
Sensory overload			
Sensory impairment	Sensory-perceptual alterations	Sensory-perceptual alterations	Sensory-perceptual alterations (see subcategories Appendix A)

1973	1975	1978	1980
Disturbances in visual perception			
Disturbances in auditory perception			
Disturbances in kinesis			
Disturbances in gustatory perceptions			
Disturbances in tactile perception			
		Sexuality, alterations in patterns of	Sexual dysfunction
Skin integrity, impairment of	Skin integrity, impairment of: actual	Skin integrity, impairment of: actual	Skin integrity, impairment of: actual
	Skin integrity, impairment of: potential	Skin integrity, impairment of: potential	Skin integrity, impairment of: potential
Skin, impairment of regulatory function of			
Altered internal regulatory function			
Altered relationships with self and others			
Susceptibility to hazards			
Altered external regulatory functions			
Sleep-rest patterns, ineffective	Sleep-rest activity, dysrhythm of	Sleep-rest activity, dysrhythm of	Sleep pattern disturbance
		Susceptibility to hazard (specify) (accidental burn, poisoning, suffocation)	

1973	1975	1978	1980
Urinary elimination, impairment of	Urinary elimination, impairment of: alterations in patterns	Urinary elimination, impairment of: alterations in patterns	Urinary elimination, alterations in pattern
Inability to control initiation of urine flow	Urinary elimination, impairment of: incontinence	Urinary elimination, impairment of: incontinence	Urinary elimination, alteration in patterns
Inability to control cessation of urine flow			
Inability to generate urine flow	Urinary elimination, impairment of: retention	Urinary elimination, impairment of: retention	
			Violence, potential for

The books containing lists from which this was prepared are:

Gebbie, K. M., & Lavin, M. A. (Eds.) *Proceedings of the First National Conference on Classification of Nursing Diagnoses.* St. Louis: C. V. Mosby, 1975

Gebbie, K. M. (Ed.) *Summary of the Second National Conference on Classification of Nursing Diagnoses.* Clearinghouse for The National Group for Classification of Nursing Diagnoses, 1310 South Grand Blvd., St. Louis, Mo. 63104, 1976.

Kim, M. J., & Moritz, D. A. *Classification of Nursing Diagnoses: Proceedings of the Third & Fourth Conferences.* New York: McGraw-Hill, 1981.

DIAGNOSTIC
FORMULATION
EXERCISES

The following three cases illustrate a basic data base collected at admission when the clients were added to a nurse's caseload. To simulate the way data were collected and hypotheses generated, stop at the end of each pattern area assessment (e.g., Health Perception–Health Management, Nutritional-Metabolic, etc.) to formulate any tentative nursing diagnoses that may be indicated by cues. Discard, revise, or reformulate diagnoses as you continue reading. At the end of each case, state nursing diagnoses and the data that support your admission diagnoses. A list of accepted diagnoses appears in Appendix A; diagnostic terms should be generated if the list is inadequate. Defining signs and symptoms are found in the manual accompanying this book (Gordon, 1982) or in the compilation of national conference proceedings (Kim and Moritz, 1981). Answers (suggested diagnoses) appear in Appendix I.

CASE 1

Nursing History and Examination

First prenatal clinic visit of 24-year-old, married, former secretary with no history of chronic disease. Last menstrual period, February; expected date of confinement November 15; 5 weeks pregnant. Husband is 25-year-old machine operator who receives health care at company clinic and is in "good health."

Health-Perception-Health-Management Pattern: Sees self as healthy and pleased about pregnancy. Usual childhood diseases, including chicken pox, measles, mumps. No recent colds or other illnesses. Keeps healthy by "eating right" and "supporting each other." Sees this making a difference when compared to other families she knows. No use of cigarettes or drugs; one glass wine per week, socially. No pattern of breast self-exam; doesn't know how. No delay in coming to clinic when missed first period; came to clinic because parents use this hospital clinic for care.

Nutritional-Metabolic Pattern: Typical diet: *Breakfast*: orange juice, cereal with fruit, coffee, toast and butter; *Lunch*: alternate lunchmeat or cheese sandwich and salads, soft drink (no-cal) or coffee; *Dinner*: two vegetables, meat, rolls and butter, coffee, dessert or fruit; *Snacks*: 1 cookie or fruit, coffee, or soft drink. No vitamin supplements. Fluids: 1–2 glasses water, 3–4 c. coffee. Appetite good; tries to restrict calories; states has gained about 1 pound. No nausea, dental problems, skin dryness. Some tingling and fullness of breasts; lotions helpful.

Elimination Pattern: Regular bowel movements qd. No changes or discomfort. Knows that has to maintain roughage and fluid intake. Slight increase in urinary frequency; realized this is due to enlarging uterus; no problems in control. No excess perspiration or odor.

Activity-Exercise Pattern: Resigned secretarial job because of pregnancy and time pressures in job. Worked for busy executive who wanted her to stay another 4–6 months. Does housework; has restricted other exercise; drives car instead of walking; stopped playing tennis; wants to be "careful and sure nothing happens to baby." States too much activity could cause miscarriage, but doesn't know exactly how. Leisure activities: T.V., movies with husband, and visiting friends. Has felt more fatigue since stopped working; attributes this to pregnancy.

REPORTED FUNCTIONAL LEVEL

Feeding	0	Dressing	0	Home Maintenance 0
Bathing	0	Grooming	0	Shopping 0
Toileting	0	General Mobility	0	
		Bed Mobility	0	Cooking 0

FUNCTIONAL LEVEL CODE

Level O: Full self care
Level I: Requires use of equipment or device
Level II: Requires assistance or supervision from another person
Level III: Requires assistance or supervision from another person *and* equipment or device
Level IV: Is dependent and does not participate

Sleep-Rest Pattern: Feels rested in A.M. Tires by afternoon and takes 2-hour nap. Sleep onset delayed since stopped work; states due to excitement of being pregnant and starts thinking about plans; can't get to sleep. No history of sleep disturbances.

Cognitive-Perceptual Pattern: No perceived hearing or vision problems, discomfort, memory changes. Learns "easily"; likes to read and then discuss questions.

Self-Perception–Self-Concept Pattern: Feels she is "easy to get along with," "bright" and "reasonably good-looking." Thinks she will be a "good, careful" mother. "Excited about changes" in her body and has been looking at maternity clothes; doesn't want to wait until dresses or slacks get tight and press on baby. No feelings of anger, depression. States "every new mother is a little fearful and anxious in case something happens to baby." Has stopped work; will devote time to "getting things ready," but friends and neighbors all work and few to talk to; day "seems long."

Role-Relationship Pattern: Lives with husband; 25-year-old machine operator; married 3 years; "he is excited about baby." Both hope it is a boy. Perceives no family problems. Handle problems by "attacking them"; discusses things. Social activities at tennis club; have close friends, couples same age. Moved into neighborhood 3 years ago, people friendly and help each other. No perceived financial problems. Parents and in-laws live in same town. She and husband are only children so this will be first grandchild. Client's mother had two miscarriages and client does not want this to happen to her. Parents available to help after baby born. Gets on well with parents and in-laws.

Sexuality-Reproductive Pattern: Sexual relations decreased so "nothing happens to baby." Told husband this was important and he agrees. Previous sexual pattern: no perceived problems. Stopped contraceptives 6 months ago; wants three children. Menses started age 13, regular cycle 30 days; length 4 days. Last menstrual period 5 weeks. Para O, Gravida O. Plans to breast feed.

Coping-Stress Tolerance Pattern: Feels "a little tense about a miscarriage," Hasn't talked to anyone about this. Usually talks over problems with husband; very supportive; but doesn't want to worry him. States they "deal with problems, not shove them under the table." Perceives this as successful but has had no big problems. No other life changes in last few years.

Value-Belief Pattern: Thinks "do what you can in this life; we've no aspirations to be rich." Comes from close family and learned "family important." Methodist; practices religion and finds it supportive.

Examination

General appearance, grooming, hygiene___Good_____
Oral mucous membranes (color, moistness, lesions)___Normal_____
Teeth: dentures___0___ Cavities___0___ Missing___0___
Hears whisper? _Yes____
Reads newsprint? ___Yes_____ Glasses ___No___
Pulse (rate) ___84____ (rhythm) _____Reg_____
Respirations ___18___ (depth) _Normal__ (rhythm)_Reg__
Breath sounds_Normal_____
Blood pressure___118/70___ Hand grip___Strong___ Can pick up pencil?_Yes_
Range of motion (joints)_Full_ Muscle firmness_Firm___
Skin: bony prominence:___0___ Lesions___0___ Color changes___0___
Breasts___Firm, developed, areolas darkened, no tenderness_____
Pelvis:___gynecoid (see medical exam)_____
Gait_Reg_ Posture_Good___ Absent body part_____0_____
Intravenous, drainage, suction, etc. (specify)_____0_____
Actual weight___120___ Reported weight__Pregravida 119_____
Height___5'6"_____
Temperature____98.6°_____
During history and examination:
Orientation_Yes_ Grasp ideas and questions? (Abstract, concrete)_Both___

Language spoken___Eng___ Voice and speech pattern___Normal___
Vocabulary___Good___
Eye contact___Yes___ Attention span (distraction)___Good span___
1   5
Nervous or relaxed____3____
1   5
Assertive or passive____3____
Interaction with family member, guardian, other (if present)
_____Husband not present; at work_____

Nursing Diagnoses (See Appendix I for answers.)

CASE 2

Nursing History and Examination

First admission of unconscious 5-year-old boy, with facial lacerations and linear skull fracture. To Emergency Room by ambulance after car accident; accompanied by anxious, distraught father who was not injured and provided history. Mother out of town visiting sister. (Screening assessment because of father's anxiety.)

Health-Perception–Health-Management Pattern: Previously alert, healthy child. Has had usual childhood diseases and immunizations, including tetanus; no colds this winter. States hasn't insisted son use seat belts when riding in front seat.

Nutritional-Metabolic Pattern: Appetite has been good; no vitamin supplements, no weight loss; seen by pediatrician 2 weeks ago; told developing normally.

Elimination Patterns: Bowel movements regular; no nighttime incontinence.

Activity-Exercise Pattern: Energetic 6 year old; plays actively with children in neighborhood; baseball favorite sport.

REPORTED FUNCTIONAL LEVEL

Pre-trauma:

Feeding	0	Dressing	0	Home Maintenance —
Bathing	2	Grooming	2	Shopping —
Toileting	0	General Mobility	0	
		Bed Mobility	—	Cooking —

FUNCTIONAL LEVEL CODE

Level O: Full self care
Level I: Requires use of equipment or device
Level II: Requires assistance or supervision from another person
Level III: Requires assistance or supervision from another person *and* equipment or device
Level IV: Is dependent and does not participate

Sleep-Rest Pattern: No sleep problems; stopped naps at 4 years.

Cognitive-Perceptual Pattern: Comatose since accident; no convulsions. No previous hearing, vision, or learning problems. Speech has been clear.

Self-Perception–Self Concept Pattern: Described as generally outgoing and friendly with strangers. Recently calls self "bad boy" when things go wrong. Made "big fuss" last week over skinned knee and whether "would get better."

Role-Relationship Pattern: Looking forward to school in fall. Has three good friends in neighborhood. At times takes older brother's clothes to try on but relationship perceived as good. Family structure: 2 brothers 14 and 16, mother, father; paternal grandmother lives next door; other grandparents deceased. Family relationships good; no perceived problems. Father states he feels "guilty," about accident; "although not my fault"; hit from rear by another car; "Why couldn't I be the one to die"; relates unconsciousness to approaching death of child. Father pacing in room.

Sexuality-Reproductive Pattern: Deferred.

Coping–Stress Tolerance Pattern: Seeks parents for security when situations stressful. Father states he and wife are supportive to each other. He'll "feel better when she gets here."

Value-Belief Pattern: Religion: Episcopal. Assessment deferred.

Examination

General appearance, grooming, hygiene _____ ― _____
Oral mucous membranes (color, moistness, lesions) _Normal color; no lesions_
Teeth: Dentures __0__ Cavities __0__ Missing _2 upper front_
Hears whisper? __No__ Reads newsprint: _Comatose_ Glasses? _No_
Pulse (rate) _100_ (rhythm) _Reg_
Respirations _20_ (depth) _Deep_ (rhythm) _Reg_
Breath sounds _clear_ Blood pressure _98/58_ PO$_2$ _78mm_
Hand grip _Absent_ Can pick up pencil? _No_
Voluntary movement _Absent LL, LA, RL, RA_ Functional Level _4_
Range of motion (joints) _Full involuntary_ Muscle firmness _Tone decreased_
Skin: bony prominences _Intact_ Lesions _Facial lacerations_
Color changes _0_ Gait _―_ Posture _―_ Absent body part _0_
Intravenous, drainage, suction, etc. (specify) _I.V._
Actual Weight _―_ Reported weight _49_
Height _36"_
Temperature _99°_
During history and examination:
Orientation _no response to stimuli_ Pupils _Equal; react to light_
Convulsions _None_ Grasp ideas and questions (abstract, concrete)? _0_
Language spoken _Eng_ Voice-speech pattern _―_ Vocabulary _―_
Eye contact _―_ Attention span (distraction) _―_
1 |_____ 5
Nervous or relaxed _(Comatose)_

```
|_____5
|_____|
```
Assertive or passive   (Comatose)
Interaction with family member, guardian, other (if present)

Nursing Diagnoses (See Appendix I for answers.)

CASE 3

Nursing History and Examination, 10/27/81

Sixth admission for diabetic ketoacidosis of a 19-year-old white female with juvenile onset diabetes mellitus since age 5. Admitted with nausea and vomiting, abdominal pain, and blood glucose of 505 mgm. Medical evaluation states there is no obvious predisposing physical cause of ketoacidosis; admissions attributed to "noncompliance." Did not take insulin for 2 days prior to this admission.

Health-Perception–Health-Management Pattern: States that diet, exercise, and insulin are "all important" to her health, yet doesn't follow prescribed diet, does no exercise, and only takes insulin sporadically. Feels she understands the aspects of her disease well; has been able to understand instructions given to her by doctors and nurses. Does not follow recommendations sometimes "forgets" to take insulin or because it is "too much of a pain." She states that she probably would be healthier if she were "a good little diabetic" but that she knows she isn't. Believes she is susceptible to diabetic ketoacidosis since she has had five previous admissions; says this admission was due to a "virus"; doesn't believe that not taking insulin for last 2 days could cause current problem; states she overslept (11 A.M.) and it was too late to take insulin. Takes "night dose" at 5 P.M. States once went for a week without taking insulin. Doesn't consider herself to be very healthy, would give herself a "2 on a scale of 1 to 10."

Nutritional-Metabolic Pattern: Does not follow prescribed diet or count calories. *Breakfast*: eats cereal with tea or toast, butter, and tea. *Lunch*: eats peanut butter and butter sandwich with iced tea; usually has cereal or peanut butter again for dinner. States eats about 10 pieces of bread per day since this is what she eats whenever she gets hungry. She drinks six glasses sugar-free iced tea per day. Dislikes meat of any kind; doesn't care for poultry or fish. States that her family does not eat meals together; she gets her own meals. If her mother prepares a meat meal, she usually goes to her bedroom and feeds the meat to her cats. Usually eats alone; if does eat with parents, it's only when she makes the dessert, the only thing she knows how to cook. Has bought a vegetarian cookbook but says that she's too "lazy" to learn how to cook. Asked to see a dietician so that she can lose weight. Reports 5' 3", 135 lbs.

Elimination Pattern: No difficulty with bowels or urination, takes no laxatives. Does not complain of polyuria despite large fluid intake (approximately 2000 cc. per day reported).

Activity-Exercise Pattern: Reports no daily exercise pattern. Does not walk; feels she is weak and isn't able to do any activities. No activities outside her home. Has no physical disabilities but does not perform any activities other than watching T.V. or reading. Attended college for one semester but left and has no plans to return; unemployed.

Sleep-Rest Pattern: Usually retires 1 or 2 A.M., gets up at 7 A.M. to take insulin and eat. Usually naps in the afternoon for 2 hours when has nothing to do. Feels she is adequately rested. Takes no sleeping meds; no problems getting to sleep.

Cognitive-Perceptual Pattern: Reports no hearing difficulties. Wears glasses all the time for nearsightedness. No difficulty with recall. Considers herself to be "rather intelligent with I.Q. of 126" yet not "smart enough to be super like 140, the gifted." States has no difficulty learning and learns well with reading materials since things that she's told sometimes "slip right through", must be interesting and challenging in order for her to give any attention to them. Points out that English and literature are her favorite subjects; reports pleasure in getting a 750 score on her SAT.

REPORTED FUNCTIONAL LEVEL

Feeding	0	Dressing	0	Home Maintenance	0
Bathing	0 in bed	Grooming	0	Shopping	0
Toileting	0 in bed	General Mobility	(Bed Rest)		
		Bed Mobility	0	Cooking	0

FUNCTIONAL LEVELS CODE

Level O: Full self care

Level I: Requires use of equipment or device

Level II: Requires assistance or supervision from another person

Level III: Requires assistance or supervision from another person (s) and equipment or device

Level IV: Is dependent and does not participate

Self-Perception–Self-Concept Pattern: Considers herself to be physically weak and this prohibits her from doing things, such as joining the Army; doesn't think she could make it through basic training. She becomes annoyed at herself; considers herself to be "lazy." Believes parents are supportive enough when she needs them but states she usually doesn't tell them when things bother her and therefore remains "independent."

Role-Relationships Pattern: Lives with her parents; has a brother who is in the Air Force. Related that once she told her guidance instructor that she was living as a hermit after school and then the instructor picked "up the cue and had my whole family see the school psychologist." States that psychologist helped her mother to "change a lot and stop nagging" but that it did nothing for her. Reports no family problems but states that her family is "a bunch of strangers living under the same roof." Describes family as one which doesn't outwardly show emotions but feels that they give her what she wants (such as money). Feels her family gives her enough attention but "probably I could get used to receiving more from them." States diabetes is "no big thing" to her family since she's had it since age 5; "it is considered just the way it is." Family usually doesn't visit her in the hospital unless she asks them to, says she likes it this way. Has no friends, doesn't belong to any social groups, because she "has nothing in common with people her age." Likes to talk about herself; says enjoys talking about the "concepts" she is reading (Greek mythology), whereas girls her age like to talk "about boys or what clothes are *in* this fall." She sees her life as being "boring."

Sexuality-Reproductive Pattern: Reports normal menstrual cycle 28 days for 5 days duration. Presently on 2d day of menstrual cycle. Had no sexual relations. Dated in high school but no dating since graduation.

Coping-Stress Tolerance Pattern: States she has learned that "you can't do too much about things"; "you just wait and see what happens." Voice low during this discussion and sad facial expression. Regained composure quickly and changed subjects.

Value-Belief Pattern: States that she has not yet "gotten anything out of life that I have wanted"; says she would like "to do something useful and challenging with my life" but hasn't been able to identify these things. Might consider teaching. Won't be satisfied until able to "physically do something both useful and challenging." Doesn't want to waste time doing things aimlessly.

Examination

General appearance, grooming, hygiene: __Obese teenager in no acute distress; disheveled; hair dull and oily (unclean), uncombed__

Oral mucous membranes (color, moistness, lesions): __Pink, moist, no lesions__

Teeth: dentures __none__ cavities __multiple cavities__ missing __none__

Hears whisper? __Yes__

Reads newsprint? __Yes__ Glasses? __for reading and distance__

Pulse (rate): __100__ (rhythm): __Regular__

Respirations __20__ (depth): __Normal__ (rhythm): __Regular__

Breath sounds: __No wheezes, rales__

Blood pressure: __130/86__

Hand grip: __Strong__ Can pick up pencil? __Yes__

Range of motion (joints): __Within normal limits__ Muscle firmness: __Firm__

Skin: bony prominences; __Intact__ Lesions: __Knotty cutaneous deposits on arms and thighs from injections__

Gait: __not observed__ Posture: __Relaxed upright posture in bed__

Absent body part: __0__

Intravenous, drainage, suction, etc. (specify): __0__

Actual weight: __135__ Reported weight: __135__ Height: __5' 3"__

Temperature: __99°__

During history-taking and examination:

Orientation: __Yes__

Grasp ideas and questions (abstract, concrete)? __Both; good abstract ability__

Language spoken: __English__ Voice speech pattern: __Normal__

Vocabulary: __Extensive__

Eye contact: __Yes__ Attention span (distraction): __good attention span; very interested in sharing information about self__

<u>1   5</u>
Nervous or Relaxed: _____4_____
<u>1   5</u>
Assertive or Passive: _____3_____
Interaction with family member, guardian, other (if present)_ none present_

Nursing Diagnoses (See Appendix I for Answers.)

DIAGNOSTIC EXERCISES

A. DIAGNOSTIC RECOGNITION EXERCISE

Which of the following are useful descriptions of client problems (nursing diagnoses) on which to base nursing care:

1 Needs occupational therapy/boredom
2 Impaired verbal communication/uncompensated aphasia
3 Alteration in tissue perfusion (cerebral)/arteriosclerosis
4 Alteration in nutrition: less than body protein requirements/low financial resources
5 Potential fluid volume deficit
6 Chest pain/myocardial infarction
7 Stress

B. DIAGNOSTIC SELECTION EXERCISE, TYPE I

Select the best nursing diagnosis on which to base care:

Mr. G., aged 58, complains of increased, frequent urination and general malaise. He appears flushed and is having difficulty remembering events of the past 24 hrs. You note that he is exhibiting Kussmaul respirations. Blood sugar is 800 mg. percent. Mr. G.'s wife died one and one-half years ago. His son reports that "since then he's been low and drinking more heavily." There have been frequent crying episodes, eating and sleeping patterns are poor, and he has been neglecting personal hygiene. Mr. G. says he's "so lonely" without his wife.

1 Depression/loss of wife
2 Self-neglect syndrome/loss
3 Loneliness/loss of wife

4 Health management deficit/delayed grief resolution
5 Grief/loss of wife
6 Diabetes mellitus

C. DIAGNOSTIC SELECTION EXERCISE, TYPE II

Generate and evaluate diagnostic hypotheses after each set of data using list of diagnoses (Appendix A):

Mrs. A. is a 39 year old woman. It is 9 a.m. on her second day after a hysterectomy. When you walk in the room she is wearing her own nightgown and lying supine in the bed. The bed is in disarray. Her face is flushed, she's crying, and she turns away as you approach.

Diagnostic Hypotheses to Be Investigated?

You touch her arm in a gentle way, find the skin slightly warm to the touch. She says she is having pain at the operative site.

Diagnostic Hypotheses to Be Investigated?

She begins to tell you about her husband's visit last night. She says she felt so angry but "there was no reason"; refused to kiss her husband and even "told him to go and find another woman." You recall from the admission nursing history and assessment that she described her family and sexual relationships as good but that she had anticipatory anxiety, etiology undiagnosed.

Diagnostic Hypotheses to Be Investigated?

You say very gently, "When you think about it now, why do you think you were so angry?" She says, crying, "He reminds me how incomplete I am now; I'm finished as a female." You say, "Oh, no wonder you feel upset, I think we should talk about this. But first let me take your temperature and then let's sit and talk."

Diagnostic Hypotheses to Be Investigated?

T = 101°

Diagnostic Hypotheses to Be Investigated?

D. DIAGNOSTIC FORMULATION EXERCISES

See Appendix G for examples.

See Appendix I for answers.

ANSWERS TO DIAGNOSTIC EXERCISES

A. DIAGNOSTIC RECOGNITION EXERCISE

Item 1 *Needs occupational therapy/boredom* is not a nursing diagnosis. Need for care is described before describing the problem. If signs of boredom are present, further investigation is required.

Item 2 *Impaired verbal communication/uncompensated aphasia* represents a useful description on which to base care; it is a nursing diagnosis. The client would be helped to compensate for aphasia.

Item 3 *Alteration in tissue perfusion (cerebral)/arteriosclerosis* is a serious condition but usually not within the diagnostic competencies of a nurse. If this diagnostic judgment is made, the client should be referred for medical evaluation. Probably the client has nursing diagnoses but they are not described by this label. Alteration in tissue perfusion is accepted for clinical testing (see Appendix A), but it is difficult to justify that nursing care can resolve this problem.

Item 4 *Alteration in nutrition: less than body protein requirements* is a nursing diagnosis which employs accepted diagnostic labels. A more concise description would be, protein deficit/low financial resources.

Item 5 *Potential fluid volume deficit* is a well-formulated potential problem that provides a basis for care when risk factors are delineated.

Item 6 *Chest pain/myocardial infarction* is a concise expression of the accepted diagnostic category, alteration in comfort: pain. A modifier (chest) is employed to specify anatomical location. The stated etiology does not provide a basis for nursing intervention because nurses do not treat a myocardial infarction. If chest pain is a new symptom or current orders for pain medication or other drugs are inadequate to control pain, these observations should be referred to the physician. The pain may also signify decreased activity tolerance or a pain self-management deficit that requires health education. Further data is needed to determine if this is chronic pain (angina) or a sign of a complication. Chest pain/myocardial infarction represents inadequate formulation of a nursing diagnosis and inadequate assessment.

Item 7 *Stress* is not a useful description of a problem. The term represents an inference that requires further exploration to identify the problem and etiology before a plan of care can be designed.

B. DIAGNOSTIC SELECTION EXERCISE, TYPE I

Item 1 *Depression/loss of wife* represents inadequate problem formulation. Data suggest depression is a sign of another problem.

Item 2 *Self-neglect syndrome/loss* represents superficial problem formulation. Data suggests this is a sign of another problem.

Item 3 *Loneliness/loss of wife* represents superficial problem formulation. Does not provide a basis for clustering all the related data.

Item 4 *Health management deficit/delayed grief resolution* is the best nursing diagnosis within the set on which to base care. Permits clustering all data in one concise expression and focusing nursing care on grief resolution.

Item 5 *Grief/loss of wife* does not adequately represent the data available; grief is an expected reaction to loss of a wife, therefore no problem is communicated on which to base care.

Item 6 Diabetes Mellitus is a medical diagnosis, not a nursing diagnosis. Disease-related nursing care can be organized on the basis of this description.

C. DIAGNOSTIC SELECTION EXERCISE, TYPE II

Diagnostic hypotheses generated from the *first set* of data include: (1) *wound infection* (Is flush due to fever and a possible wound infection?), (2) *atelectasis* (Is flush due to fever and possible pulmonary complications? This complication is of low probability in lower abdominal surgery.), (3) *urinary retention* (Are the cues—bed in disarray, lower abdominal surgery, crying, and face flushed—signs of discomfort due to retention? This is a low probability on the second day unless there has been a post-operative history of retention.) (4) *incisional pain* (Are the signs of discomfort caused by pain? A likely pain site is the operative wound.), or (5) *fluid volume deficit* (Is flush and signs of discomfort on the second post-operative day caused by a history of low fluid intake?). The cues bed in disarray, face flushed, and crying at 9 a.m. suggest the possibility of sleep disturbance related to any of the above hypotheses. Adding the cues—turns away as you approach and hysterectomy—suggests unexpressed anger and situational depression over loss. A hypothesis to direct cue search could be formulated broadly as *ineffective coping related to loss* or more specifically as *perceived sexuality impairment.*

The test for skin warmth evident in the *second set* of data further supports the hypotheses—wound infection, pulmonary complications and fluid volume deficit. Pain at the operative site is a cue that also points to wound infection or to incisional pain without the presence of infection.

The *third set of cues* supports the hypothesis of *perceived sexuality impairment.* Information in the *fourth data set* suggests the nurse is testing the hypothesis of perceived sexuality (or reproductive) impairment. A likely etiological hypothesis is *loss (hysterectomy).* Note the priority for hypothesis investigation; the plan is to investigate previously generated hypotheses related to conditions manifesting fever—wound infection, atelectasis, and fluid volume deficit.

In the *fifth data set* information is obtained to support the hypotheses—wound infection, fluid volume deficit, and the low probability hypothesis of *pulmonary complications.* Amount and sufficiency of last voiding would decrease the risk of missing the problem of urinary retention. The nurse would quickly collect further data on these possibilities and call a physician.

Pain perception may be heightened by the psychological problem. A judgment has to be made whether to: (1) collect further data related to pain management, (2) offer the client the post-operative narcotic ordered, or (3) offer the opportunity to discuss perceptions and feelings about sexuality or reproductive loss, or (4) a combination of these actions.

Data support tentative nursing diagnoses formulated either as *perceived sexuality or reproductive impairment/loss (hysterectomy)* or as *ineffective coping/perceived loss of sexuality.* Further data would help formulate the diagnosis more specifically or data may support the possibility of a normal process of grieving. Pain management and any surgical-related care would be determined after medical evaluation of the client.

D. DIAGNOSTIC FORMULATION EXERCISES (APPENDIX G)

Case 1: Nursing Diagnoses

1 *Anticipatory Anxiety (Miscarriage)/Identification with Mother's Miscarriage; Knowledge Deficit (Activity Tolerance and Health Management During Pregnancy)*

States too much activity could cause miscarriage; activity (tennis, walking, sexual) self-restricted "so nothing happens to baby."
Client's mother had two miscarriages and client doesn't want this to happen.
Wants to be "careful and sure nothing happens to baby."
Resigned secretarial job because of pregnancy, time pressures in job; expected date of confinement—35 weeks.
Sleep onset delayed "since stopped work."
Increase of fatigue attributed to pregnancy.
Thinks she will be "good, careful mother."
Using maternity clothes before clothes get tight and press on baby.

"Every new mother is a little fearful and anxious in case something happens to baby."

Medical exam: no health problems; pregnancy progressing normally.

Will devote time to "getting things ready;" friends and neighbors work; few to talk to; days "seems long;" afternoon naps, 2 hrs.

3 *Health Management Deficit/Lack of Knowledge* (Breast Self-Exam)

a No pattern of breast self-exam.
b States doesn't know how to examine.

Case 2: Nursing Diagnoses

1 *Potential Airway Obstruction*

Comatose
Drooling at intervals
Unresponsive to stimuli
PO_2 78mm

2 *Total Self-Care Deficit (Level 4)/Comatose State*

Unresponsive to stimuli
No voluntary movement of extremities

3 *Parental Guilt/Perceived Responsibility (Accident); Fear of Child's Death*

Hasn't insisted son use seat belts.
States feels "guilty about accident, although not my fault."
"Why couldn't I be the one to die"; relates coma to approaching death.
Father pacing in room states will "feel better" when mother returns from out of town trip to visit sister.

Case 3: Nursing Diagnoses

These data describe a complex client-situation. Although a great deal of information was collected, more is needed for diagnosis. The case demonstrates that in complex situations, all the data needed cannot be collected in a busy hospital unit at admission. Secondly, time is needed to think about alternative interpretations and what diagnostic hypotheses would direct further cue-search.

Further data on family dynamics, support systems, and the client's insight and inclination to deal with problems are needed. Historically, focusing on noncompliance/knowledge deficit has not been effective (sixth admission for ketoacidosis). Underlying problems exist.

Ethically it is important to remember that this 19-year-old client's rights should not be violated in data collection. Calling the family to verify data or to gather further information without this client's knowledge could be viewed as a violation of rights. It may also jeopardize the nurse-client relationship. When encountering a client who volunteers the type and amount of information previously presented, the question of why should be raised. Does the behavior signify a plea for help, a testing of the nurse's reaction, or both? Mutual understanding needs to exist regarding the client's choice to deal with her life situation. If help is being requested then the problems interfering with her disease management, as well as general health management, can be further explored and identified. At some point the client and nurse may decide that one or both parents should be included.

Non-compliance (disease management) is a presenting problem but probably only a sign of more serious problems. Nurses perceiving themselves to have inadequate diagnostic or treatment skills in the possible developmental problems that this client and family exhibit may seek consultation. A mental health–clinical nursing specialist may be consulted.

Two possible hypotheses can serve as a basis for (1) clustering current data and (2) guiding further cue search.

Chronic Situational Depression

19 year old
Disheveled; hair dull and oily (unclean)
Sixth admission for diabetic ketoacidosis (blood glucose 505 mgm.)
Doesn't consider self healthy; would give herself "2 on a scale of 1 to 10"
Usually eats alone
States she has learned that "you can't do too much about things"; "You just wait and see what happens"
Voice low during this discussion and sad facial expression
Feels she is physically weak and not able to do any activities
Not yet "gotten anything out of life that I have wanted"
Would like to do something "useful and challenging with my life" but hasn't been able to identify these things
No friends; doesn't belong to any social groups because "has nothing in common with people her age"
Perceives her life as "boring"
No insulin taken 2 days prior to admission; doesn't believe this could cause her current problem
Overslept (11 A.M.) and too late to take insulin; night dose at 5 P.M.
States once went week without taking insulin
States diet, exercise, insulin important to health
States doesn't follow diet; forgets to take insulin; too much of a "pain"
No exercise; takes insulin sporadically
States understands her disease
Believes susceptible to ketoacidosis (five previous admissions)
Knotty, cutaneous deposits on arms and thighs from injecting
No daily exercise
Asked to see dietician so that she can lose weight
Weight (reported 135 lbs.); Height 5' 3"
Attended college for one semester; no plans to return
Unemployed 19 year old
Considers self "rather intelligent; IQ of 126; not smart enough to be super like 140, the gifted"
Pleased with 750 score on SAT

States things must be interesting and challenging in order to hold attention

English and literature are favorite subjects

Might consider teaching

Not satisfied until able to "physically do something both useful and challenging

Doesn't want to waste time doing things aimlessly

Likes to talk about self and "concepts" she is reading about (e.g. Greek mythology); girls her age talk "about boys, clothes"

Dated in high school; not dating since graduation

Dysfunctional Family Dynamics

Perceives family as "a bunch of strangers living under the same roof"; don't show emotions but give her what she wants (such as money)

States family gives enough attention but "probably I could get used to receiving more from them"

Usually eats alone

No activities outside home

Psychologist helped mother to "change a lot and stop nagging"

Lives with parents; brother in Air Force

Believes parents are supportive when needs them

Usually doesn't tell parents when things bother her and therefore remains "independent"

States family does not eat meals together; gets own meals

Bought vegetarian cookbook (doesn't eat meat); says too "lazy" to learn to cook

Diabetes "no big thing" to family as she has had it since age 5

Family doesn't visit hospital unless asked; likes it that way

ANNOTATED BIBLIOGRAPHY

DIAGNOSIS

I Concept of Nursing Diagnosis

Bonney, V., & Rothberg. J. *Nursing diagnosis and therapy: An instrument for evaluation and assessment.* New York: National League for Nursing, 1963. Contains early definition of nursing diagnosis and tool for assessment of functional problems. Assessment form was developed to facilitate planning for nurse staffing for chronically ill and disabled clients.

Chambers, W. Nursing diagnosis. *American Journal of Nursing,* 1962, *62*:102–104. Early article on diagnosis that emphasizes the elements of observation, interpretation, and identifying nursing problems.

Clark, J. Should nurses diagnose and prescribe? *Journal of Advanced Nursing,* 1978, *4*:485–488. Discusses the value of nursing diagnoses and concludes that nurses should diagnose and prescribe if competent.

Gebbie, K., & Lavin, M. A. Classifying nursing diagnosis. *Missouri Nurse,* 1973, *42*:10–14. Defines nursing diagnosis, reviews status, and makes recommendations for future development.

Gordon, M. Conceptual issues in nursing diagnosis. In N. Chaska (ed.). *The nursing profession: A time to speak.* New York: McGraw–Hill, 1982. Identifies current issues in the identification, standardization, and classification of nursing diagnoses. Views the first step in implementing nursing diagnosis as a perception of autonomy and accountability on the part of nurses.

Gordon, M., Sweeney, M. A., & McKeehan, K. Development of nursing diagnoses. *American Journal of Nursing,* 1980, *80*:699. Discusses historical development of nursing diagnosis from 1960 to 1980. Traces changes in form and focus.

Gordon, M. The concept of nursing diagnosis. In symposium on the implementation of nursing diagnosis. *Nursing Clinics of North America, 14*:487–496. Philadelphia: Saunders, 1979. Discusses the concept of nursing diagnosis and related issues. Progress in identification and classification are summarized; resources for implementation cited.

Gordon, M. Nursing diagnosis and the diagnostic process. *American Journal of Nursing,* August, 1976, *76*:1276:1300. Defines nursing diagnosis, concept, and structure (PES), and the diagnostic process.

Gordon, M. Classification of Nursing diagnosis. *Journal of New York State Nurses' Association*, March, 1978, *9*:5–9. Identifies four major areas of nursing practice which require clinical diagnosis and eight issues in practice which could be clarified by use of standard nomenclature.

Kim, M. J., & Moritz, D. A. (eds.). *Classification of nursing diagnoses: Proceedings of the third and fourth national conferences on classification of nursing diagnoses.* New York: McGraw-Hill, 1981. Contains currently accepted nursing diagnoses and defining characteristics. Papers included on various subjects related to nursing diagnosis.

King, L. S. What is a diagnosis? *J. American Medical Association,* 1967, *202*:714–717. Argues that the concept of diagnosis is not only used in medicine. Diagnosis means to distinguish and involves discrimination. Discussion of the need for precision in diagnosis, a framework of well-defined categories, and knowledge about the categories.

Lash, A. A. Re-examination of nursing diagnosis. *Nursing Forum,* 1978, *17*:332–343. Reviews differences between medical diagnosis and nursing diagnosis in the literature from 1953 to 1976. Views nursing diagnosis as offering the professional autonomy and independent decision making, two criteria of a professional.

Levine, M. Trophicognosis: An alternative to nursing diagnosis. In American Nurses' Association, *Exploring progress in medical-surgical nursing practice.* ANA Regional Clinical Conference, 1965, *2*:55–70. Early paper on nursing diagnosis advocating use of a different term.

Little, D., & Carnevali, D. The diagnostic statement: The problem defined. In J. Walter, G. Pardee, & D. Molbo. *Dynamics of problem-oriented approaches: Patient care and documentation.* Philadelphia: Lippincott, 1975. Describes what a nursing diagnosis is and is not and the need for accurate, concise, neutral, nursing diagnoses that communicate nursing management. Possible coping deficits arising from medical diagnoses are defined.

Mundinger, M., & Jauron, G. Developing a nursing diagnosis. *Nursing Outlook,* 1975, *23*(2):94–98. Discusses problems encountered in defining and instituting the use of nursing diagnosis. Describes two parts of a nursing diagnosis. Examples of mistakes made by beginning diagnosticians are given.

Myers, N. Nursing diagnosis. *Nursing Times,* 1973, *69*:1229–1230. Emphasizes the importance of diagnosis to nursing process. Defines nursing diagnosis.

Price, M. R. Nursing diagnosis: Making a concept come alive. *American Journal of Nursing,* 1980, *80*:668–674. Discussion of structural components of nursing diagnoses, common errors in diagnosis, steps in the diagnostic process and how to use a diagnosis.

Rothberg, J. S. Why nursing diagnosis? *American Journal of Nursing,* 1967, *67*:1040–1042. Argues that diagnosis is essential to professional practice. Diagnosis ensures focus on the individual. Presents an early definition of the concept.

Soares, C. A. Nursing and medical diagnoses: A comparison of variant and essential features. In N. Chaska (ed.). *The nursing profession: Views through the mist.* New York: McGraw-Hill, 1978. Outlines the diagnostic process in nursing and compares it to the process in medicine. States that a nursing diagnosis must include the statement of the problem (a conflict in needs) and the indirect or direct causes associated with the problem.

II Concept of Diagnosis: Other Professions

Brown, L. B., & Levitt, J. L. Methodology for problem-system identification. *Social Casework,* 1979, *60*:408–415. Outlines a possible system of problem identification based on psychodynamic, behavioral, and task-centered social work practice.

Engle, R. L., & Davis, B. J. Medical diagnosis: Present, past and future. I. Present concepts of the meaning and limitations of medical diagnosis. *Archives of Internal Medicine,* 1963, *112*:512–519. Discusses medical diagnosis, diagnostic process, and the absence of a unified concept or organizing principle for disease classification. Presents five "orders of certainty" in the use of diagnostic terms clinically.

Engle, R. L. Medical diagnosis: Present, past, and future, II. Philosophical foundations and historical development of our concepts of health, disease, and diagnosis. *Archives of Internal Medicine,* 1963, *112*:520–529. Traces the concepts of health, disease and diagnosis in medicine.

Engle, R. L. Medical diagnosis: Present, past, and future. III. Diagnosis in the future. *Archives of Internal Medicine,* 1963, *112*:530–543. Formulates a concept of disease (genetic) and views medical diagnosis of the future incorporating the complexities of genetics. Discusses use of computers in diagnosis.

Engle, G. L. Clinical application of the biopsychosocial model. *Journal of Medicine and Philosophy,* 1981, *6*:101–123. Suggestion for extension of the biomedical model in medicine to a biopsychosocial approach. Implication of the new model in the care of a client with acute myocardial infarct is presented and contrasted with the traditional approach.

Lazare, A. Hidden conceptual models in psychiatry. *New England Journal of Medicine,* 1973, *288*:345–351. Four conceptual models—medical, psychologic, behavioral, and social—used in clinical psychiatry are discussed. Argues that it would enhance communication among physicians if the use of these models were made explicit.

III Nursing Diagnosis in Specialties, Settings, or Services

Bruce, J. A. Implementation of nursing diagnosis: A nursing administrator's perspective. *Nursing Clinics of North America,* *14*:509–516. Philadelphia: Saunders, 1979. Discusses the need for planning and assessment of staff's interest and capabilities prior to implementation. Need for administrative support is stressed. Example is given of a format for a nursing care plan, using diagnosis in psychiatric nursing.

Dalton, J. M. Nursing diagnosis in a community health setting. *Nursing Clinics of North America,* *14*:525–532. Philadelphia: Saunders, 1979. Emphasizes that the primary service in home health care is nursing and that this needs to be communicated in clear diagnostic terms to third party payors. A teaching tool and excellent examples of diagnoses are included.

Demers, B. Beyond endocarditis: How nursing diagnosis helps focus your care. *RN,*

1979, *42*:51–54. Discussion of nursing diagnoses observed in a client with endocarditis. States how diagnoses influenced care planning and outcome evaluation.

Leslie, F. M. Nursing diagnosis: Use in longterm care. *American Journal of Nursing,* 1981. *81*:1012–1014. Report of an epidemiological study of nursing diagnoses in longterm care. Incidence of nursing and medical diagnoses are reported. Evaluates current diagnoses and use of diagnoses in care. No diagnostician reliability ratings reported.

Mahomet, A. D. Nursing diagnosis for the OR nurse. *AORN Journal,* 1975, *22*(5): 709–711. Defines nursing diagnosis. Places nursing diagnosis within the context of nursing process and suggests ways to enhance care of the surgical patient.

McKeehan, K. M. Nursing diagnosis in a discharge planning program. *Nursing Clinics of North America, 14*:517–524. Philadelphia: Saunders, 1979. Overview of factors influencing a process model of discharge planning. Discusses the need for nurses to articulate discharge diagnoses so that the level of care required can be determined.

Mundinger, M. Nursing diagnoses for cancer patients. *Cancer Nursing,* 1978, *1*:221–226. Identifies common nursing diagnoses occurring in clients with cancer based on clinician's experience and the nursing literature.

Rossi, L. P., & Haines, V. M. Nursing diagnoses related to acute myocardial infarction. *Cardiovascular Nursing,* 1979, *15*:11–15. Identification of nursing diagnoses in CCU and PCCU phases of care.

Weber, S. Nursing diagnosis in private practice. *Nursing Clinics of America, 14*:533–540. Philadelphia: Saunders, 1979. Illustrates the use of nursing diagnosis in direct, indirect, and consultation services in a psychiatric-mental health practice. Important points about the relevance of nursing diagnoses to third party reimbursement are discussed.

IV Specific Nursing Diagnoses

Avant, K. Nursing diagnosis: Maternal attachment. *Advances in Nursing Science,* 1979, *2*:45–56. Describes a seven-stage approach to diagnosis and a study to validate criteria for the assessment of maternal attachment.

Burgess, A. W., & Homstrom. L. L. Rape trauma syndrome. *American Journal of Psychiatry,* 1974, *131*:981–986. Report of a study of 109 rape victims. Identification of diagnostic categories: rape trauma syndrome, compounded reaction, silent rape reaction, and defining characteristics. Use of the clinical study method in identifying diagnostic categories.

Gordon, M., Sweeney, M. A., & McKeehan, K. Nursing diagnosis: Looking at its use in the clinical area. *American Journal of Nursing,* 1980, *80*:672–674. Describes the use of accepted and nonaccepted diagnoses by nurses in an OB-GYN setting. High incidence problems and problem areas at discharge are identified.

Guzzetta, C. E., & Forsythe, G. L. Nursing diagnostic pilot study: Psychophysiologic stress. *Advances in Nursing Science,* 1979, *2*:27–44. Framework for study of psychophysiologic stress presented. Description of methodology for identification of etiological stressors, parameters, defining characteristics and stress level. Data contributed to identification of the diagnostic category.

Holstrom, L. L., & Burgess, A. W. Assessing trauma in the rape victim. *American Journal of Nursing,* 1975. *75*:1288–1291. Report on three diagnostic categories of sexual trauma: rape trauma syndrome, accessory-to-sex reaction, sex-stress syndrome.

Describes the clinical study method of identifying nursing diagnoses and outlines steps in establishing new diagnostic category.

LeSage, J., Beck, C., & Johnson, M. Nursing diagnosis of drug incompatibility. *Advances in Nursing Science,* 1979, *1*:63–77. Argues that drug incompatabilities are nursing diagnoses when the etiology is linked to phenomena which nurses are educated and licensed to treat. Should be evaluated relative to definition of nursing diagnosis and diagnosis for purposes of referral.

Martin, K. S. Nursing diagnosis of impaired parenting relative to the preschool child: A pilot exploration. In Sigma Theta Tau. *Monograph Series 79, Clinical Nursing Research: Its Strategies and Findings II.* Proceedings of the Sixth Annual Nursing Research Conference, September 15–16, 1978, Tucson, Arizona. Sigma Theta Tau, 1100 W. Michigan St., Indianapolis, Indiana, 46223, 1979. Report of a pilot study to identify signs and symptoms of the nursing diagnosis, impaired parenting. Epidemiological study in community health setting.

McCourt, A. E. Measurement of functional deficit in quality assurance. *Quality Assurance Update,* 5:1–3, American Nurses' Association, Congress for Nursing Practice, 1981. Discussion of the definition, evaluation, and documentation of self care deficits. A numerical coding system and critical defining characteristics of this accepted nursing diagnosis are presented.

Nicoletti, A., Reitz, S., & Gordon, M. Descriptive research on parenting. In M. J. Kim, & D. A. Moritz. *Classification of nursing diagnoses: Proceedings of the fourth national conference on classification of nursing diagnoses,* New York: McGraw-Hill, 1981. Examination of the cues recorded to support actual and potential alterations in parenting.

Sweeney, M. A., & Gordon, M. Nursing diagnosis: Implementation and incidence in an obstetrical/gynecological population. In M. Chaska (ed.) *The nursing profession: A time to speak.* New York: McGraw-Hill, 1982. Report of a study of discharge nursing diagnoses of 163 obstetrical/gynecological clients. Describes methodology and findings in this epedemiological study. Concludes that accepted list of nursing diagnoses requires expansion.

V Identification and Classification of Nursing Diagnoses

Bircher, A. On the development and classification of diagnoses. *Nursing Forum,* 1975, *14*:10–29. Proposes a mastery-competency classification system based on the organizing principle of Maslow's hierarchy of human needs. Defines nursing diagnosis, discusses the potential problems and dangers inherent in making a diagnosis, and outlines the values of nursing diagnosis.

Brown, M. The epidemiologic approach to the study of clinical nursing diagnosis. *Nursing Forum,* 1974, *13*:346–359. Discusses epidemiological method for establishing the prevalence, distribution, and causality of a nursing diagnosis. Outlines five criteria for the development of a taxonomy of nursing diagnoses.

Diers, D. *Research in nursing practice.* New York: Lippincott, 1979. Excellent discussion of factor-searching methodology. Useful for studies concerned with identification of diagnoses (naming theory or concept identification studies).

Dodge, G. H. Current works to define, classify nursing diagnoses. *AORN Journal,* 1975, *22*:327–328. Reviews development of nursing diagnosis and advantages of standardization.

Gebbie, K. M., & Lavin, M. A. Classifying nursing diagnoses. *American Journal of Nursing,* 1974, *44*:250–253. Report on the first national conference on nursing diagnosis and diagnoses identified.

Gebbie, K. M. (ed.). *Summary of the second national conference: Classification of nursing diagnoses.* St. Louis: 1976. Report of the second national conference and diagnoses identified. Section included on the development of taxonomies in medicine and research project on identification of nursing diagnoses.

Gebbie, K. M. Development of a taxonomy of nursing diagnoses. In J. Walter, G. Pardee, & D. Molbo (eds.). *Dynamics of problem-oriented approaches: Patient care and documentation.* Philadelphia: Lippincott, 1976. Advocates development of nomenclature by utilizing inductive and deductive reasoning and a classification system for taxonomy preparation.

Gebbie, K. M., & Lavin, M. A. (eds.). *Classification of nursing diagnoses: Proceedings of the first national conference on classification of nursing diagnoses.* St. Louis: Mosby, 1975. Report of the first national conference and diagnoses identified. Introduces diagnostic classification, principles of classification, and use of a nursing taxonomy.

Gordon, M., & Sweeney, M. A. Methodological problems and issues in identifying and standardizing nursing diagnoses. *Advances in Nursing Science.* 1979, 2:1–16. Identifies conceptual issues in research on nursing diagnosis and presents three models for identifying and validating diagnostic nomenclature. Inter-rater reliability of diagnosticians is discussed.

Jones, P. E. A terminology for nursing diagnoses. *Advances in Nursing Science,* 1979, 2:65–72. Reviews methods of describing nursing practice and taxonomy development. Describes a study to identify and validate diagnostic categories.

Lewis, E. P. The stuff of which nursing is made. (editorial). *Nursing Outlook,* 1975, 23:89. Briefly discusses the growing interest in identifying and classifying nursing diagnoses and differences between medical and nursing diagnoses. Endorses nursing's efforts to establish a classification system for nursing diagnoses and provide a more scientific basis for practice.

McKay, R. P. Research Q & A: What is the relationship between the development and utilization of a taxonomy and nursing theory. *Nursing Research,* 1977, 26:222–224. Defines taxonomy and classification system. Discusses major tasks in development of a taxonomy of nursing diagnosis and its relevance to theory development.

Proder, B. What you should know about nursing diagnosis. *Medical Record News,* August 1975, 87–90. Supports the need for a classification system and presents an approach for manual collection of data on patients with nursing diagnoses.

Roy, Sr. C. A diagnostic classification system for nursing. *Nursing Outlook,* 1975, 23:90–94. Explores the rationale for a classification system in nursing. Lists principles of ordering a taxonomy and approaches to development: the inductive approach and the deductive approach. A discussion of the implications of a diagnostic classification system in nursing practice, education and research is included.

Sokal, R. R. Classification: Purposes, principles, progress, prospects. *Science,* 1974, 185:1115–1123. Often-quoted article on classification and classification systems. Defines terms, purposes, and principles of classification.

VI Classification Systems

Campbell, C. *Nursing diagnosis and intervention in nursing practice.* New York: Wiley, 1978. Compilation of nursing diagnoses and interventions. The book is extensively cross referenced and indexed for use as a reference manual.

An in-depth look at DSM-III: An interview with Robert Spitzer (editorial). *Hospital and Community Psychiatry,* 1982, 31:25–32. Discussion of the recently published revision of the classification of mental disorders. Major changes seen in the new emphasis on psychosocial factors and a multiaxial evaluation system.

Giovannetti, P. Understanding patient classification systems. *Journal of Nursing Administration,* February, 1979, 4-9. Reviews the development and characteristics of patient classification systems for nurse-staffing purposes.

Kim, M. J., & Moritz, D. A. (eds.). *Classification of nursing diagnoses: Proceedings of the third and fourth national conferences on classification of nursing diagnoses.* New York: McGraw-Hill, 1981. Contains currently accepted nursing diagnoses and defining characteristics. Papers included on various subjects related to nursing diagnosis.

Lynch, W. J., & Mauss, N. K. Brain injury rehabilitation: Standard problem lists. *Archives of Physical Medicine and Rehabilitation,* 1981, *62*:223-226. Identifies nomenclature for describing functional problems (many of which are similar to currently identified nursing diagnoses). Difficulties encountered in evaluation of the validity and reliability of criteria used to determine presence or absence of problems and to arrive at agreement on terminology are discussed.

McLemore, C. W., & Benjamin, L. S. Whatever happened to interpersonal diagnosis? A psychosocial alternative to DSM-III. *American Psychologist,* 1979, *34*:17-34. Review of social behavior coding models. Suggests that psychologists consolidate their knowledge in the form of an interpersonal taxonomy due to the shortcomings of the Diagnostic and Statistical Manual—III of the American Psychiatric Association.

Simmons, D. A. *Classification scheme for client problems in community health nursing.* Rockville, Md.: U. S. Government Printing Office, 1980. Classification scheme of client problems in community health nursing, a large portion of which are nursing diagnoses similar to those developed by the National Conference Group. Results of government contract research done by the Visiting Nurse Association of Omaha.

United States Department of Health and Human Services. *Nutritional problem classification for children and youth.* Rockville, Md.: U. S. Government Printing Office, 1980. Nomenclature and classification system developed and tested by a task force of nutritionists. Problems and potential problems are classified and coded for use in information processing systems.

United States Department of Health, Education, and Welfare. *Social work problem classification for children and youth.* Rockville, Md.: U. S. Government Printing Office, Publication No. (HSA) 77-5202, 1976. Nomenclature and classification system developed and tested by task force of social workers. Problems and potential problems are classified and coded under seven groupings for use in information processing systems.

VII Nursing Conceptual Frameworks

Leininger, M. Caring: A central focus of nursing and health care services. *Nursing and Health Care,* 1980, *1*(3):135-144. Discusses a central concept in nursing. Increases awareness about possible divergences in nurses' and clients' perceptions, as for example, regarding the concept of caring.

Nursing Development Conference Group. *Concept formalization in nursing: Process and product.* Boston: Little, Brown, 1973. Traces the development of concepts of nursing in education and practice. Provides guidelines for structuring nursing knowledge.

Peterson, C. J. Questions frequently asked about the development of a conceptual framework. *Journal of Nursing Education*, 1977, *16*:22–32. Sections useful in understanding what is a concept, proposition, hypothesis, theory, law, conceptual framework. Remaining discussion more applicable to curriculum.

Stevens, B. J. *Nursing theory: Analysis, application, and evaluation.* Boston: Little, Brown, 1979. Chapters on common themes in nursing theory and criteria for evaluating theories are of interest. Discussion of nursing theory and practice trends contains a discussion of work in diagnosis in the early 1970s.

PROCESS

I Nursing Process

Bailey, J. T., & Claus, K. E. *Decision making in nursing.* St. Louis: Mosby, 1975. A systems model for clinical decision making is presented. Emphasis is on skills and techniques basic to management of client care.

Bruner, J. S., Goodnow, J. J., and Austin, G. A. *A study of thinking.* Wiley, New York: 1956. Advanced; useful for understanding concepts, defining characteristics, and strategies for concept attainment.

Goodwin, J. O., & Edwards, B. S. Developing a computer program to assist the nursing process: Phase I from systems analysis to an expandable program. *Nursing Research*, 1975, *24*:299–305. Presents a systems model of the nursing process which includes nursing diagnosis. Operationally defines nursing from a cognitive perspective.

Grier, M. R. Decision making about patient care. *Nursing Research*, 1976, *25*:105–110. Report of a study to test the applicability of a decision theory to nursing treatment decisions. Findings indicated that nursing care decisions can be understood by the analytical model and nurses can order actions according to desirability and likelihood of outcomes. Recommends nurses learn procedures for making decisions.

McCarthy, M. M. The nursing process: Application of current thinking in clinical problem solving. *Journal of Advanced Nursing*, 1981, *6*:173–177. Explores the components of nursing process from a problem solving model. Relates current research in medical problem solving to nursing. No discussion of nursing diagnosis.

Sculco, C. D. Development of a taxonomy for the nursing process. *Journal of Nursing Education*, 1978, *17*:40–48. Useful discussion and examples of clinical inference and hypothesis generation. Focus is on examples of two levels of clinical inference, complex and highly complex. Codes components of the nursing process but does not develop a taxonomy of levels.

Walker, L., & Nicholson, R. Criteria for evaluating nursing process models. *Nurse Educator*, 1980, *5*:8–9. Five criteria are proposed to evaluate nursing process models: knowledge base, fluidity of steps, applicability, compatibility, and consistency.

Ware, A. Using nursing prognosis to set priorities. *American Journal of Nursing*, 1979, *79*:921–924. Discusses the concept of prognosis, how to determine prognosis, and how to set priorities.

II Diagnostic Process: Data Collection

Aspinall, M. J. Development of a patient–completed admission questionnaire and its comparison with the nursing interview. *Nursing Research*, 1975, *24*:377–381.

Study to compare effectiveness of assessment by questionnaire and by interview. More errors were made by unstructured interview and this method consumed more time. Important limitations of the study are cited.

Bates, B. *Guide to physical assessment*. J. B. Lippincott, Philadelphia: 1979. Presents content and method of physical assessment.

Block, B., & Hunter, M. L. Teaching physiological assessment of black persons. *Nurse Educator*, 1981, *6*:24–28. Increases awareness of variables such as race, that influence data collection.

Buckhout, R. Eyewitness testimony. *Scientific American*, 1974, *231*:23–31. Discussion of biases in observation which is applicable to data collection in nursing.

Ekman, P., & Friesen, W. V. *Unmasking the face: Guide to recognizing emotions from facial expressions*. Englewood Cliffs, N.J.: Prentice-Hall, 1975. Assessment guidelines for identifying facial expressions and underlying feelings. Also presents information about emotional states and skill training exercises.

Froelich, R. E., & Bishop, F. M. *Clinical interviewing skills* (3d edition). St. Louis: Mosby, 1977. Focuses on conducting a clinical interview of a client and influences that affect interviewing. Emphasis is on basic skills in history taking. Questions throughout that involve the reader in learning.

Jacoby, M. K., & Adams, D. J. Teaching assessment of client functioning. *Nursing Outlook*, 1981, *29*:248–250. Discusses systematic ordering of data in nursing diagnosis. Offers guidelines for students.

King, L. S. Signs and symptoms. *Journal of the American Medical Association*, 1968, *206*:1063–1065. Attempts to discriminate by definition the terms, signs and symptoms.

Moritz, D. A. Nursing histories: A guide, yes; a form, no! *Oncology Nursing Forum*, 1979, *6*:18–19. Use of checklist for nursing histories is viewed as a questionable practice. Argues that the way each area in an assessment is pursued and described varies with the concerns and patterns encountered in clients.

Pilette, P. C. Caution: Objectivity and specialization may be hazardous to your humanity. *American Journal of Nursing*, 1980, *80*:1588–1590. Explores the idea that dehumanized care providers may provide dehumanized care; cites the perils of total objectivity in assessment. Guidelines provided for recognizing and treating dehumanization.

Rosenhan, D. L. On being sane in insane places. *Science*, 1973, *179*:250–258. Relevant to assessment. Report of a study involving admission of pseudopatients to a psychiatric hospital and the influence of setting on diagnosis. Demonstrates how preconceptions can influence judgment and labeling of clients.

Shamansky, S. L., & Pesznecker, B. A community is. . . . *Nursing Outlook*, 1981, *81*:182–185. Useful in developing community assessment format. Defines the concept of a community in its "who, where, when, and why dimensions."

Spector, R. E. *Cultural diversity in health and illness*. New York: Appleton-Century-Crofts, 1979. Useful ideas about culture and symptoms, healing, folk remedies, and cultural expectations for assessment. Examines health and illness from the perspective of Asian-, black-, Hispanic- and native-American communities.

United States Department of Health, Education, and Welfare. *Basic concepts of environmental health*. Rockville, Md.: U.S. Government Printing Office, Publication No. (NIH) 77-1254, 1970. Provides information to gain an appreciation of environmental assessment. Summary of an environmental task force report on atmospheric pollutants, occupational safety, food and water supplies, and waste disposal. Methods and resources for estimating risk for disease are discussed.

Watson, A. B., & Mayers, M. G. *Assessment and documentation: Nursing theories in action.* Thorofare, N.J.: Slack, 1981. Describes assessment from data collection to diagnosis, assessment algorithms, and documentation using problem-oriented recording methods.

III Diagnostic Process: Information Processing

Archer, C. O., & Swearingen, D. Application of Benjamin Franklin's decision-making model to the clinical setting. *Nursing Forum*, 1977, *16*:319–328. Presents a simple diagram for treatment decisions based on Franklin's prudential algebra.

Aspinall, M. J. Use of a decision tree to improve accuracy of diagnosis. *Nursing Research*, 1979, *28*:182–185. Report of a study demonstrating that use of a decision tree increased accuracy in identifying explanations for decreased cognitive functioning following surgery in a client with a history of cirrhosis.

Aspinall, M. J., Jambruno, N., & Phoenix, B. S. The why and how of nursing diagnosis. *MCN: American Journal of Maternal-Child Nursing*, 1977, *2*:355–358. Good discussion of the diagnostic process. Demonstrates multiple hypotheses generation. Exercises provided in nursing diagnosis and diagnosis for purposes of referral.

Aspinall, M. J. Nursing diagnosis—the weak link. *Nursing Outlook*, 1976, *24*:433–437. A research project utilizing a case study approach revealed that most of the nurses included in the study lacked the theoretical knowledge of the problem that could be responsible for the medical dysfunction described, and also lacked an approach or strategy to enable them to evaluate the cues to arrive at an identification of the problem.

Aspinall, M. J., and C. A. Tanner. *Decision making for patient care: Applying the nursing process.* Appleton-Century-Crofts, New York: 1981. Chapter on clinical decision making provides overview. Remaining chapters are on specific clinical topics, some of which are nursing diagnoses.

Bieri, J., Atkins, A. L., Briar, S., Leaman, R. L., Miller, H., & Tripoldi, T. *Clinical and social judgment.* New York: Wiley, 1966. Advanced discussion of clinical judgment about human behavior. Presents theory and research on cognitive, situational, and structural factors influencing judgment using an information processing approach.

Boulding, K. E. Human knowledge as a special system. *Behavioral Science*, 1981, *26*:93–102. Broadly applicable to "knowing" in general. Discusses human knowledge and the human learning process. Processes in learning to "know about" and "know how" are described.

Card, W. I. Clinical decision making: I. An analysis. *Health Bulletin*, 1977, *35*:207–212. Advanced discussion of inference in medical decision making. Application of decision theory to cost and efficiency of diagnosis and treatment.

Crum, M. R., & Rowlands, E. E. Open-mindedness, rigidity, and the tendency to change inferences among psychiatric nursing staff: A pilot study. *Nursing Research*, January-February, 1978, *27*:42–47. Report of a pilot study to test the relationship between open-mindedness, between rigidity, and the tendency to alter inferences on the basis of new information. The variable, open-mindedness, but not rigidity, was found to be significant in the sample of nurses and aides.

Cutler, P. *Problem solving in clinical medicine: From data to diagnosis.* Williams and Wilkins, Baltimore: 1979. Basic references for beginning medical students on problem solving and data synthesis.

Dixon, N. Choice errors: Some hazards of decision making. *Nursing Mirror,* February 17, 1977, *25*:59–61. Discusses importance of decision making in nursing and biases that can enter into the process.

Doona, M. E. The judgment process in nursing. *Image,* 1976, *8*:27–28. Discusses the importance of clinical judgment in nursing. Analyzes phases and types of judgment.

Durand, M., & Prince, R. Nursing diagnosis: Process and decision. *Nursing Forum,* 1966, *5*:51–64. Defines nursing diagnosis and discusses steps in decision making.

Elstein, A. S., Shulman, L. S., & Sprafka, S. A. *Medical problem solving: An analysis of clinical reasoning.* Cambridge, Mass.: Harvard University Press, 1978. Advanced level discussion of literature on clinical reasoning, research studies, and summary of heuristics in diagnostic problem solving.

Field, M. Causal inferences in behavioral research. *Advances in Nursing Science,* 1979, *2*:81–92. Discusses current views on the concept of causality in behavioral sciences.

Fodor, J. A. The mind-body problem. *Scientific American,* 1981, *244*:114–123. Discusses traditional and current schools of thought regarding behavior and its causation.

Fredette, S., & O'Connor, K. Nursing diagnosis in teaching and curriculum planning. *Nursing Clinics of North America, 14*:541–552. Philadelphia: Saunders, 1979. Students will be interested in the examples given of increasing competency in diagnosis as a learner proceeds in the educational program. Discussion of nursing diagnosis can be the focus of theoretical and clinical study in educational programs.

Gordon, M. Nursing diagnosis and the diagnostic process. *American Journal of Nursing,* August, 1976, *76*:1276–1300. Defines nursing diagnosis, concept and structure (PES), and the diagnostic process.

Gordon, M. Predictive strategies in diagnostic tasks. *Nursing Research,* 1980, *29*:39–45. Report of a study describing how nurses narrow the universe of possibilities in identifying postoperative complications. Strategies are described and the lack of influence of inferential ability as measured by GRE and MAT scores. Does not deal with nursing diagnoses.

Green, P. E. Psychiatric nursing and the diagnostic process. *J. of the National Association of Private Psychiatric Hospitals,* 1974, *6*:19–26. Physician describes the unique contribution of data on behavior patterns by nurses to client's medical diagnosis. Notes that nurses avoid reporting judgments. (A reader obtains the impression from this article that nurses accumulate significant data for diagnosing dysfunctional health patterns.)

Hammond, K. R., Kelly, K. J., Castellan, N. J., Schneider, R. J., & Vancini, M. Clinical inference in nursing: Use of information-seeking strategies by nurses. *Nursing Research,* 1966, *15*:330–366. Advanced; has relevance to design of studies on diagnostic process. Discusses methodology and results of a small study on information-seeking strategies.

Hammond, K. R., Kelly, K. J., Schneider, R. J., and Vancini, M. Clinical inference in nursing: Information units used. *Nursing Research,* 1966, *15*:236–242. Advanced; has relevance to design of studies on diagnostic process. Study of cues used by nurses. Inconsistency found in information discrimination among nurses in this study conducted in the early 1960s.

Hammond, K. R. Clinical inference in nursing: A psychologist's view point. *Nursing Research,* 1966, *15*:27–38. Advanced; presents an analysis of cognitive tasks encountered by nurses. Author emphasizes the processing of physical cues to disease and sees increased complexity because nurse must think "as" the doctor thinks when making judgments.

Hammond, K. R., Kelly, K. J., Schneider, R. J. & Vancini, M. Clinical inference in nursing: Analyzing cognitive tasks. *Nursing Research*, 1966, *15*:134–138. Advanced; has relevance to design of studies on diagnostic process. Study in early 1960s of nurses' action-responses to cues. Subjects asked to report symptoms or signs not diagnoses. Suggests nurses' tasks involve complex, multicue inferences with multiresponse options.

Hammond, K. R., Kelly, K. J. Schneider, R. J., & Vancini, M. Clinical inference in nursing: Revising judgments. *Nursing Research*, 1967, *16*:38–45. Advanced; has relevance to design of studies on diagnostic process. Study in early 1960s of how nurses revise inferences about cues.

Henle, M. On the relationship between logic and thinking. *Psychological Review*, 1962, *69*:336–378. Advanced discussion of two views on the relation between logic and thinking. Suggests errors are not due to deviations from logical thinking but rather changes in the material from which reasoning proceeds. Role of logical processes in everyday life discussed.

Jacquez, J. A. (ed.). The diagnostic process. Proceedings of a conference, University of Michigan Medical School. Ann Arbor: Malloy Lithographing (photolithoprinted), 1964. Contains papers presented on taxonomy, diagnostic process, computerization, and evaluation of diagnostic skills. Discussion at an advanced level.

Kelly, K. Clinical inference in nursing. A nurse's viewpoint. *Nursing Research*, 1966, *15*:23–26. Describes nursing inferences (judgments) as probabilistic, complex, and having high social significance. Traces historically the expectations of nurses in the area of clinical inference.

Kelly, K. J. An approach to the study of clinical inference in nursing. *Nursing Research*, 1964, *13*:314–322. Advanced; has relevance to theory and design of studies on diagnostic process. Applies Brunswick's Lens Model to clinical inference and an empirical analysis of nurse-action. Argues that there is a critical need for quantitative description.

Klug, C. A. Judgment and creative thinking. *Image*, 1973, *5*:10–15. Relates judgment to creativity and suggests creativity in judgment can be learned. Applicable to therapeutic judgments about nursing care.

Knill-Jones, R. P. Clinical decision making. II. Diagnostic and prognostic inference. *Health Bulletin*, 1977, *35*:213–222. Advanced discussion of how the probability of a diagnosis or outcome is altered as data accumulates. Application of probability and decision theory to clinical inference.

Lazare, A. The psychiatric examination in the walk-in clinic: hypothesis generation and hypothesis testing. *Archives General Psychiatry*, 1976, *33*:96–102. Useful in regard to discussion of hypothesis generation and testing.

Marriner, A. The decision making process. *Supervisor Nurse*, 1977, *8*(2):58–67. Good discussion of decision making steps. Discussion in the context of the supervisory role but the principles discussed are applicable to nursing process.

Matthews, C. A., & Gaul, A. L. Nursing diagnosis from the perspective of concept attainment and critical thinking. *Advances in Nursing Science*, 1979, *2*:17–26. Report of a study to examine cognitive processes used in nursing diagnosis. Critical thinking, concept mastery, cue utilization, and attainment of diagnoses were studied.

McBride, A. B. How attribution theory can shape therapeutic goal setting. In American Nurses' Association. *New directions for nursing in the '80's*. Kansas City: American Nurses' Association, 1980, 73–82. Relevant to the concept of etiology. Describes attribution theory as dealing with the perceived cause of a situation. Behavior is affected by causal inferences. Attribution theory is useful in understanding clients' explanations and the meaning they ascribe to events. It is also applicable to the nurse's attribution of cause (etiology). This theory is applied to parenting, reactive depression, and wife abuse.

Nicksic, E. Problem patients or problem nurses. *American Journal of Nursing*, 1981, *81*:317–319. Discusses how care providers can produce problems, deny the credibility of clients, and label clients as problems.

Sarbin, T. R., Taft, R., and Bailey, D. E. *Clinical inference and cognitive theory*. Holt, Rinehart, and Winston, New York: 1960. Advanced; discusses the logic of clinical inference, cognitive organization, variations in inference, and validity of inference. Predates the concepts of diagnostic strategies.

Tversky, A., & Kahneman, D. Judgment under uncertainty: Heuristics and biases. *Science,* 1974, *185*:1124–1131. Advanced discussion of bias in human judgment.

Wadsworth, M. Health and sickness: The choice of treatment. *Nursing Digest*, September/October, 1975, *3*:50–51. Discusses ideas about causation of illness relevant to nursing. Concludes that the client's view is critical in diagnosis.

Ward, C. H., Beck, A. T., Mendelson, M., Mock, J. E., & Erbaugh, J. K. The psychiatric nomenclature: Reasons for diagnostic disagreement. *Archives of General Psychiatry*, 1962, *7*:198–205. Report of a study; contains excellent discussion of diagnostic disagreement applicable to nursing.

APPLICATION

I Nursing Diagnosis: Practice Issues

Chance, K. S. The Quest for Quality: An Exploration of Attempts to Define and Measure Quality Nursing Care. *Image*, 1980, *12*:41–45. Defines quality as applied to nursing care and reviews the major concepts in quality care assessment.

College of Nursing, Texas Woman's University. *Monograph, Fall 1979: Nursing Diagnoses*. Denton, Texas: College of Nursing, 1979. Overview of status of nursing diagnosis and three research studies (concept attainment, relation between logical reasoning and diagnosis, and a study of restlessness).

Connecticut Nurses' Association. Do nurses diagnose? *Connecticut Nursing News*, 1975, *48*:7. Discusses the confusion that has resulted in various court cases due to the absence of a uniform definition for "diagnosis."

Dodge, G. H. Forces influence move toward nursing diagnoses. *AORN Journal*, 1975, *22*:157–158. Identifies professionalism, accountability, quality assurance, emphasis on prevention, and justification of services as forces influencing a move toward nursing diagnoses.

Feild, L. Implementation of nursing diagnoses in clinical practice. *Nursing Clinics of North America*, 1979, *14*:497–508. Stresses the need to view nursing diagnosis in the context of nursing process. Guidelines, derived from change theory, that should be considered in implementation are discussed.

Fortin, J. D., & Rabinow, J. Legal implications of nursing diagnosis. *Nursing Clinics of North America*, 1979, *14*:553–562. Review of the legalities of nursing diagnosis. The argument is presented that if problems are not conceptualized and, therefore, not treated or not documented, the nurse may be held liable.

Ginzberg, E. The economics of health care and the future of nursing. *Nurse Educator*, 1981, *6*:29–32. An economist offers predictions about future economic influences on education, practice, and collegiality. Section on reimbursement.

Gordon, M. Determining study topics. *Nursing Research*, 1980, *29*:83–87. Various topics used to designate populations for quality assurance in nursing are reviewed. Argues why evaluation of nursing care should be based on nursing diagnoses and suggests ways this can be done. Examples given.

Henderson, V. On Nursing Care Plans and Their History. *Nursing Outlook*, June, 1973, *12*:378–379. Traces the history of nursing care plans and concludes that coordination of care requires a written plan.

Hershey, N. The influence of charting upon liability determinations. *Journal of Nursing Administration*, 1976, *6*:35–38. Discusses the importance of charting when a legal issue arises.

LaMontagne, M., & McKeehan, K. Profile of a continuing care program emphasizing discharge planning. *Journal of Nursing Administration*, 1975, *5*:22. Use of nursing diagnoses in discharge planning to prepare a nursing referral form that is comprehensive, concise, and problem-oriented. Quality of a plan depends on how referrals are written and communicated to the community agency.

McCloskey, J. C. The Problem-Oriented Record vs. the Nursing Care Plan: A Proposal. *Nursing Outlook*, August, 1975, *23*:492–495. Raises questions about the traditional care plan. Suggests eventually nurses will write orders in the order book or plans will be computerized.

McCourt, A. E. Measurement of functional deficit in quality assurance. In American Nurses' Association, Congress for Nursing Practice. *Quality Assurance Update*, 1981, *5*:1–3. Discussion of the definition, evaluation, and documentation of self care deficits. A numerical coding system and critical defining characteristics of this accepted nursing diagnosis are presented.

Moore, K. R. What nurses learn from nursing audit. *Nursing Outlook*, 1979, *27*:254–258. Discusses audit as an aspect of quality assurance, advocates use of nursing diagnosis.

Reider, K. A., & Wood, M. J. Problem-orientation: An experimental study to test its heuristic value. *Nursing Research*, 1978, *27*:25–29. Study demonstrating that the problem-oriented record system substantially increased nursing staff's ability to identify client problems.

Roy, Sr. C. The impact of nursing diagnosis. *AORN Journal*, May, 1975, *21*:1023–1030. Discusses the contribution of nursing diagnosis to implementing standards and the future impact of nursing diagnosis on nursing practice and education.

Schmadl, J. C. Quality assurance: Examination of the concept. *Nursing Outlook*, 1979, *27*:462–466. Defines quality assurance—what is assured, for whom, and how it is done.

Shoemaker, J. How nursing diagnosis helps focus your care. *RN*, *42*:56–61. Describes nursing diagnosis as a simple, practical way of improving care, steps in the diagnostic process, and required diagnostic skills are discussed.

Werley, H. H., & Grier, M. R. (eds.) *Nursing information systems*. New York: Springer, 1981. Report of a Research Conference on Nursing Information Systems, June, 1977. Sections on nursing diagnosis, clinical decision-making, standardization of nomenclature, use of diagnosis in client classification-nurse staffing, and other topics related to information processing.

Young, D. E., & Ventura, M. R. Application of nursing diagnosis in quality assessment research. In American Nurses' Association, Congress for Nursing Practice. *Quality*

Assurance Update, 1980, *4*:1–4. Discusses the application of nursing diagnosis in development of diagnostic, outcome, and process criteria for three accepted nursing diagnoses. Argues that combining medical and nursing diagnoses more clearly defines the population to be assessed than using medical diagnoses alone.

II Theory Development and Nursing Diagnosis

Henderson, B. Nursing diagnosis: Theory and practice. *Advances in Nursing Science*, 1978, *1*:75–83. Background and development of the concept of nursing diagnosis. Identifies nursing diagnosis as theory development in nursing.

Kritek, P. B. Commentary: Development of nursing diagnosis and theory. *Advances in Nursing Science*, 1979, *2*:73–79. Describes development of nursing diagnoses as a theoretical activity in nursing. Examines implicit values in diagnosis and the need to make values explicit.

Kritek, P. B. The generation and classification of nursing diagnoses: Toward a theory of nursing. *Image*, 1978, *10*:33–40. National effort to generate and classify nursing diagnoses described as first level theory building. Compares work in nursing diagnosis to characteristics of significant theories.

NAME AND TITLE INDEX

SUBJECT INDEX